BRIDGING THE GAP BETWEEN PRACTICE AND RESEARCH

Forging Partnerships with Community-Based Drug and Alcohol Treatment

Sara Lamb, Merwyn R. Greenlick, and Dennis McCarty, *Editors*

Committee on Community-Based Drug Treatment

Division of Neuroscience and Behavioral Health

INSTITUTE OF MEDICINE

NATIONAL ACADEMY PRESS
Washington, D.C. 1998

NATIONAL ACADEMY PRESS • 2101 Constitution Avenue, N.W. • Washington, DC 20418

NOTICE: The project that is the subject of this report was approved by the Governing Board of the National Research Council, whose members are drawn from the councils of the National Academy of Sciences, the National Academy of Engineering, and the Institute of Medicine. The members of the committee responsible for the report were chosen for their special competences and with regard for appropriate balance.

The Institute of Medicine was chartered in 1970 by the National Academy of Sciences to enlist distinguished members of the appropriate professions in the examination of policy matters pertaining to the health of the public. In this, the Institute acts under both the Academy's 1863 congressional charter responsibility to be an adviser to the federal government and its own initiative in identifying issues of medical care, research, and education. Dr. Kenneth I. Shine is president of the Institute of Medicine.

This study was supported under Contract No. 270-96-0008 from the Substance Abuse and Mental Health Service Administration's Center for Substance Abuse Treatment and the National Institute on Drug Abuse.

Library of Congress Cataloging-in-Publication Data

Bridging the gap between practice and research : forging
partnerships with community-based drug and alcohol treatment / Sara
Lamb, Merwyn R. Greenlick and Dennis McCarty, editors.
    p. cm.
Includes bibliographical references and index.
ISBN 0-309-06565-8 (cloth)
    1. Drug abuse—Treatment—Research—United States. 2.
Alcoholism—Treatment—Research—United States. 3. Drug
abuse—Research—United States. 4. Alcoholism—Research—United
States. I. Lamb, Sara. II. Greenlick, Merwyn R. III. McCarty,
Dennis, Ph. D.
    RC564.65 .B75 1998
    362.29'.0973—ddc21

                    98-25418

Printed in the United States of America

The serpent has been a symbol of long life, healing, and knowledge among almost all cultures and religions since the beginning of recorded history. The image adopted as a logotype by the Institute of Medicine is based on a relief carving from ancient Greece, now held by the Staatliche Museen in Berlin.

COMMITTEE ON COMMUNITY-BASED DRUG TREATMENT

MERWYN R. GREENLICK (*Chair*),* Professor and Chair, Department of Public Health and Preventive Medicine, Oregon Health Sciences University, Portland, Oregon

GAURDIA E. BANISTER (since July 1997), Director of Behavioral Health Services, Providence Hospital, Washington, District of Columbia

BENJAMIN P. BOWSER, Professor, Department of Sociology and Social Services, California State University at Hayward, Hayward, California

KATHLEEN T. BRADY, Associate Professor, Department of Psychiatry, Center for Drug and Alcohol Programs, Medical University of South Carolina, Charleston, South Carolina

VICTOR A. CAPOCCIA, President, CAB Health and Recovery Services, Inc., Salem, Massachusetts

THOMAS J. CROWLEY, Professor, Department of Psychiatry and Executive Director, Addiction Research and Treatment Service, University of Colorado School of Medicine, Denver, Colorado

EMILY JEAN HAUENSTEIN, Associate Professor of Nursing, University of Virginia School of Nursing, Charlottesville, Virginia

DENNIS McCARTY, Director, Substance Abuse Group, Institute for Health Policy, Heller Graduate School for Advanced Studies in Social Welfare, Brandeis University, Waltham, Massachusetts

A. THOMAS McLELLAN, Professor of Psychiatry, University of Pennsylvania, Philadelphia, Pennsylvania

STEVEN M. MIRIN, Medical Director, American Psychiatric Association, Washington, District of Columbia

LISA NAN MOJER-TORRES, Attorney, Lawrenceville, New Jersey

DAVID L. ROSENBLOOM, Project Director, Join Together and Associate Professor of Public Health, Boston University School of Public Health, Boston, Massachusetts

JAMES L. SORENSEN, Professor, Department of Psychiatry, University of California at San Francisco, San Francisco, California

JOSEPH WESTERMEYER, Professor, Department of Psychiatry, and Adjunct Professor, Department of Anthropology, University of Minnesota and Clinical Chief of Psychiatry, Minneapolis VA Medical Center, Minneapolis, Minnesota

---

*Institute of Medicine member

Preface

There are several aspects of this study that contribute to its specific character. The first is that the study was sponsored by both the Center for Substance Abuse Treatment (CSAT) and the National Institute on Drug Abuse (NIDA). The joint sponsorship was particularly apposite because the study's mission was predicated on the concept that there is value in enhancing collaborative relationships between the drug abuse research community and the world of community-based treatment programs. The symbolism of this collaboration between two, sometimes disparate, elements of the federal government responsible for supporting the respective communities facilitated the development of a collaborative perspective from the beginning of the study.

Consequently, this was not a search for villains. The process of the study was as collaborative as possible and the report is offered with the message that working together can help all of us in the field achieve individual objectives and serve the public good more effectively. The second feature that influenced this study is that it is one in a series of outstanding Institute of Medicine (IOM) studies of drug abuse issues conducted recently by study committees of the IOM's Division of Neuroscience and Behavioral Health. During the same period there have been a series of landmark reports and studies in the area by CSAT, NIDA, and other Substance Abuse and Mental Health Services Administration (SAMHSA) and National Institutes of Health (NIH) agencies. Chapter 1 reviews some of these studies and places this one in the context of the work of the last decade. The committee worked hard to keep focused on its charge and to avoid plowing ground that had been so well cultivated by the work of others. Many times this required an act of will, as the issues in this field are so compelling. The result of this discipline is that readers will need to look in one or another of the studies referenced in this report for more complete discussion of some topics.

An important study, funded by SAMHSA and carried out by the Mathematica organization, was released in March after the committee concluded its deliberations. The study assessed the costs and effects of requiring parity for mental health and substance abuse treatment within health insurance. This study is relevant to the report because of our recommendation that purchasers of care should take research findings into account in making purchasing decisions (see Recommendation 7). An identified barrier to the implementation of this recommendation was the different treatment of substance abuse services from other medical care services under health insurance, a difference that would be eliminated by achieving parity. This study was particularly timely because the Mental Health Parity Act was passed by Congress and became effective January 1, 1998. Parity bills were also introduced in 37 states last year, some of which included substance abuse services.

The Mathematica study indicates that full parity for mental health and substance abuse services would only increase health insurance premiums an average of 3.6 percent—in a group of health plans that reflect nationwide coverage. Most important for this study, it was estimated that substance abuse treatment contributes only .02 percent of the increase. The Mathematica study also reported that state parity laws on the books to date have had only small effects on premiums and that employers have not attempted to avoid parity laws by becoming self-insured.

The Mathematica findings are consistent with testimony before the committee that insufficient funding for treatment is a major obstacle to the integration of knowledge from treatment research into clinical practice. Because of the financial constraints of the field, many of those we talked with in the treatment community were extremely frustrated with research that provided evidence of effectiveness of treatments they would be unable to adopt because of limited treatment budgets.

The committee was also taken with the observation the drug abuse field included policy barriers deriving from an ideological or political perspective that prevented the free flow of some kinds of research knowledge into treatment programs. For example, the committee noted that treatment programs (and even treatment research) funded from or organized within the criminal justice system had a restricted set of options available. Consequently, in some instances it was not possible to integrate less expensive treatments that were of proven effectiveness.

The specific charge to the committee is discussed in Chapter 1 and is included in its entirety as Appendix A. As Chair, I proposed early in the process that we guide our task by testing three assumptions, beyond the basic assumption that the ultimate purpose of the study was to improve the effectiveness and efficiency of the treatment of addictive disorders in the United States:

1. drug abuse research will be improved and the knowledge creation process will be aided by the two-way communication and long-term collaboration between community-based treatment program staff and researchers;

2. community-based treatment programs will benefit, in a number of ways, from participating in drug abuse research; and

3. research findings exist that are not being universally used within treatment and the treatment programs (and their patients/clients) would benefit if these findings were appropriately implemented.

It is important to note that the committee and the treatment providers who participated in this study readily agreed that their definition of critical drug abuse research included the full research spectrum—from clinical research, through services research and sociobehavioral research, to program evaluation and quality improvement activities. Basic biological research was out of the scope of our charge and therefore isn't discussed in our report.

The report includes two distinctly different kinds of recommendations. The first kind of recommendations are formal policy and technical recommendations that could be (in our view) adopted directly by CSAT, NIDA, and other federal or state agencies. The second kind are normative recommendations to the two other audiences to which the report is being addressed—the treatment community and the research community. While the former are the recommendations most sought by the sponsors of the study, committee members recognized the many cultural barriers to the integration of research activities into community-based treatment programs, and these barriers exist in the subcultures of both the research and the treatment community. Because the strong subcultures have, at their heart, a critical set of beliefs and values we believe the cultures can only be changed by a change in some of their beliefs and values. The normative recommendations are focused on changing those elements of the cultures.*

There are so many acknowledgments that must be recorded. The first acknowledgment is to the wonderful committee members who were my

---

*These normative recommendations are put forward in the text under Recommendations 1 and 2, as well as the text of Chapters 1 and 5.

colleagues for this study. Drug abuse is not my substantive area, so I relied heavily on the committee members for their knowledge of the drug abuse field. All committee members had a hands-on role in the preparation of this report. That the committee's expertise is wide and deep is obvious to all in the field and that expertise guided the substance of this report. But of equal importance to the study was the spirit that emerged during the committee process. The interaction among the study director, the committee chair, and the committee members is as critical to the product as it is to the process. And this process was as fruitful and harmonious as any I have observed in serving on IOM committees over the past 25 years.

Of special note is the work of an executive writing group that was formed comprising myself, Victor Capoccia, Dennis McCarty, James Sorensen, from the committee membership, and Sara Lamb, the study director, and Constance Pechura, who was the Director of the IOM Division of Neuroscience and Behavioral Health during the life of the study. Drs. Sorensen, Capoccia, and McCarty were primarily responsible, with their own writing groups, for the first drafts of Chapters 2, 3, 4, and 5. They were wonderfully collaborative and constructive colleagues. Dr. McCarty, in addition to taking primary responsibility for Chapter 5, contributed creatively and substantially to the overall writing and is recognized as a co-editor of the report.

Dr. Pechura was extremely supportive throughout this process. She attended our meetings, piloted us through difficult technical, scientific, and political waters, and provided inspiration to us during difficult times. She was our friend and counselor.

The study was supported by a talented staff. Amelia Mathis was extremely professional as she staffed the committee. She always had the process under control with a firm, but friendly hand. She mothered us when we needed mothering and was unflappable in times of stress. She was always ready to go the extra step when that was needed. Research Associate Carrie Ingalls provided exceptional research and organizing skills, as well as support team management for the first half of the study. Thomas Wetterhan provided excellent administrative and technical support to the project and also assumed responsibility for providing research assistance in the last half of the study. His extensive knowledge of the systems, procedures, and resources of the IOM served the project well through the final challenging months of coordinating writing group activities, report preparation, and report review.

Finally, while the committee owns the findings and the recommendations, the ultimate responsibility for any IOM study always rests with the study director. This study was the first undertaken by study director Sara Lamb and she took over a study that was already behind schedule. She did an excellent job, learning both the substance of the field and the complexities of the process. My task as chair was made so much easier because she was such an able, competent, and staunch partner.

Merwyn R. Greenlick, Ph.D., *Chair*
Committee on Community-Based Drug Treatment

Acknowledgments

The Committee on Community-Based Drug Treatment and the study staff are grateful for the assistance received from many individuals and organizations over the course of the study. The names of those who participated in our workshop and roundtable discussions are listed in Appendix B. The opportunities for knowledge exchange provided by these interactive discussions were crucial to the deliberations of the committee and to the shaping of its subsequent recommendations. A number of individuals made special contributions to the committee's work and served as consultants in a variety of important ways: Joseph Brady, Deborah Haller, Constance Horgan, Arnold Kaluzny, Harold Perl, Everett Rogers, and H.R. (Rick) Sampson. The contributions of Constance Horgan, Arnold Kaluzny, and Everett Rogers are specifically referenced in the report.

The committee would like to recognize the individuals who helped identify and recruit a diverse and articulate group of participants for our public workshops: Douglas Anglin, UCLA Drug Abuse Research Center; Linda Kaplan, National Association of Alcoholism and Drug Abuse Counselors; Luceille Fleming, Ohio Department of Alcohol and Drug Addiction Services; Linda Grant, Washington Association of Alcoholism and Addiction Programs; Judge Richard Knolls, Second Judicial District, Bernalillo County, New Mexico; Phillip May, Center for Alcohol, Substance Abuse and Addictions (CASAA) at the University of New Mexico; Gwen Rubinstein, Legal Action Center; and Linda R.Wolfe-Jones, Therapeutic Communities of America.

The committee is greatly indebted to Phillip May and his staff at

CASAA, particularly Phyllis Trujillo, for making it possible for us to hold a workshop at the University of New Mexico; and to Dr. May and Lynn Brady, Executive Director of the Behavioral Health Services Division of the New Mexico Department of Health, for providing the committee with an overview of the community-based drug treatment system in New Mexico.

A number of persons contributed to this report by meeting with individual committee and staff members in their home states and sharing their information with the committee. The committee thanks the following state officials who gave us the benefit of their experience: Barbara Cimaglio, Office of Alcohol and Drug Abuse Programs, Oregon Department of Human Resources; and Cynthia Turnure and Patricia Harrison, Chemical Dependency Program Division, Minnesota Department of Human Resources; as well as the treatment providers who generously invited us to visit their programs: Dale Adams, Resada Alcohol and Drug Abuse Program, Las Animas, CO; Nancy Jo Archer, Hogares, Inc., Albuquerque, NM; Gaurdia Banister, Seton House of Providence Hospital, Washington, DC; Jane Spence and Bradley Anderson, Recovery Resources, Kaiser Permanente, Portland, OR; Ann Uhler, Comprehensive Options for Drug Abusers (CODA), Portland, OR; and Fredi Walker and Michel Lilly, Boston Detoxification Center, Boston, MA. The committee is especially grateful to those individuals who allowed their stories to be used in this report: Michael Kirby, Chilo Madrid, Selbert Wood, Carol Leonard, Richard Suchinsky, and those who chose to remain anonymous.

The perspective of the committee was broadened by many individuals, particularly by the contributions of two who were appointed to the committee, but were unable to continue because of conflicts in their teaching and research commitments. Spero Manson and Robert Fullilove both continued to be available to committee and staff. Robert Fullilove participated in both public workshops and served as the host for the provider panel for the first workshop. The committee and staff also appreciate the assistance and support provided by our project officers, Mady Chalk at the Center for Substance Abuse Treatment and Gerald Soucy at the National Institute on Drug Abuse.

Too numerous to mention are the many staff at the IOM who provided expert support at various stages of the project. The committee staff, however, wishes to particularly acknowledge Susan Fourt and Patricia Kaiser for library services throughout the study and Claudia Carl for piloting this report through review. The report was improved by the copy editing of Paul Phelps, as well as the assistance of two staff members from the Kaiser-Permanente Center for Health Research: senior editor Gary Miranda and library services coordinator Nancy Hunt.

This report has been reviewed by individuals chosen for their diverse perspectives and technical expertise, in accordance with the procedures approved by the National Research Council's Report Review Committee. The purpose of this independent review is to provide candid and critical comments that will assist the authors and the IOM in making the published report as sound as possible and to ensure that the report meets institutional standards for objectivity, evidence, and responsiveness to the study charge. The content of the review comments and draft manuscript remain confidential to protect the integrity of the deliberative process. We wish to thank the following individuals for their participation in the review of this report: James W. Curran, Emory University; Arthur J. Schut, Iowa Substance Abuse Directors' Association; Anderson Spickard, Vanderbilt University; Donald M. Steinwachs, Johns Hopkins University School of Hygiene and Public Health; Cynthia Turnure, Minnesota Department of Human Services; and Joan Ellen Zweben, 14th Street Clinic and East Bay Community Recovery Project.

While the individuals listed above have provided many constructive comments and suggestions, responsibility for the final content of this report rests solely with the authoring committee and the IOM.

Contents

EXECUTIVE SUMMARY   1

1 INTRODUCTION   16
The Study Process and Report Organization, 19
Historical Background, 21
Definitions and Current Context, 23
Summary, 25

**2 THE GAPS BETWEEN RESEARCH, TREATMENT,
AND POLICY**   27
Overview, 29
Evidence for the Gaps, 30
Barriers to Closing the Gaps, 40
Summary, 51

3 APPROACHES TO CLOSING THE GAPS   56
Overview, 56
Technology Transfer Models, 57
Organizational Change Models, 59
Practice Guidelines and Scorecards in Addictions Treatment, 61
Consensus Conferences and Evidence-Based Reviews, 63
Top-Down Incentives Models, 64
Models that Incorporate Trust-Building Experiences, 66
Summary, 69

4   BENEFITS AND CHALLENGES OF RESEARCH
    COLLABORATION FOR COMMUNITY-BASED
    TREATMENT PROVIDERS   73
    Overview, 75
    Benefits and Challenges of Research/Practice Collaborations, 75
    Factors Affecting Linkage Between Practice and Research, 78
    Summary, 86

5   BENEFITS AND CHALLENGES OF COMMUNITY-BASED
    COLLABORATION FOR RESEARCHERS   89
    Overview, 90
    Historical Approaches to Collaboration for Research, 90
    Models for Collaboration, 95
    Lessons from Demonstration Initiatives, 102
    Guidance for Grant Review, 106
    Summary, 107

6   FINDINGS AND RECOMMENDATIONS   111
    Strategies for Linking Research and Practice, 111
    Strategies for Linking Research Findings,
        Policy Development, and Treatment Implementation, 114
    Strategies for Knowledge Development, 116
    Strategies for Dissemination and Knowledge Transfer, 116
    Strategies for Consumer Participation, 118
    Training Strategies for Community-Based Research Collaboration, 119

APPENDIXES
A   Statement of Task   123
B   Workshops and Roundtable: Agendas and Participants   125
C   Commissioned Paper: Drug Treatment Programs and Research:
    The Challenge of Bidirectionality   135
        Benjamin P. Bowser
D   Commissioned Paper: The Treatment of Addiction:
    What Can Research Offer Practice?   147
        A. Thomas McLellan and James R. McKay
E   Commissioned Paper: The Substance Abuse Treatment System:
    What Does It Look Like and Whom Does It Serve?
    Preliminary Findings from the Alcohol and Drug Services Study   186
        Constance M. Horgan and Helen J. Levine
F   National Institutes of Health Consensus Development
    Statement on Effective Medical Treatment of Heroin Addiction   198
G   Useful Internet Resources—Examples   226

H List of Currently Available CSAT Treatment Improvement
  Protocols (TIPs)   233
I Opportunities for Collaboration   235
  Joseph Westermeyer
J Summary of Interviews with Minnesota State
  Alcoholism-Addiction Leaders   246
  Cindy Turnure and Patricia Harrison

INDEX   251

Acronyms

AA	Alcoholics Anonymous
ADSS	Alcohol and Drug Services Survey, sponsored by the Substance Abuse and Mental Health Services Administration
AHCPR	Agency for Health Care Policy Research
CASAA	Center on Alcohol, Substance Abuse, and Addictions at the University of New Mexico
CBO	community-based organization—in this report used to refer to community-based drug and alcohol treatment organizations
CCOP	Community Clinical Oncology Program of the National Cancer Institute
CME	continuing medical education
CSAT	Center for Substance Abuse Treatment
DATOS	Drug Abuse Treatment Outcome Study, sponsored by the Substance Abuse and Mental Health Services Administration
DSM-IV	*Diagnostic and Statistical Manual of Mental Disorders—* Fourth Edition
EAP	employee assistance program

HEDIS	Health Plan Employer Data and Information Set, developed by the National Committee on Quality Assurance
HIV	human immunodeficiency virus
HMO	health maintenance organization
IRB	Institutional Review Board, implements Title 45, Part 46 of the Code of Federal Regulations, Protection of Human Subjects, NIH Office of Protection from Research Risks
JCAHO	Joint Commission on Accreditation of Healthcare Organizations
LAAM	levo-alpha-acetylmethadol or levomethadyl acetate, trade name: Orlaam®
NASADAD	National Association of State Alcohol and Drug Abuse Directors
NIAAA	National Institute on Alcohol Abuse and Addiction
NIDA	National Institute on Drug Abuse
NIH	National Institutes of Health
ONDCP	Office of National Drug Control Policy
SAMHSA	Substance Abuse and Mental Health Services Administration
TIE	Treatment Improvement Exchange, sponsored by the Substance Abuse and Mental Health Services Administration
TIP	Treatment Improvement Protocols, maintained by the Substance Abuse and Mental Health Services Administration

BRIDGING THE GAP BETWEEN PRACTICE AND RESEARCH

In our scientific culture, knowledge is generally what can be known through science. But science understands some relationships by excluding others, including many that concern practice. Science rests on the power of abstraction. Wisdom may entail appreciation of contextuality.

Ann Lennarson Greer in "The shape of resistance . . . the shapers of change."

Executive Summary

As the United States approaches the twenty-first century, drug abuse remains one of our most intractable problems and only a small proportion of the approximately 9.4 million addicted and dependent individuals receive treatment in a given year. Further, despite the great strides made in research on the etiology, course, mechanisms, and treatment of addiction, serious gaps of communication exist between the research community and community-based drug treatment programs. Closing these gaps will not only be critical to improving drug and alcohol treatment, but will also be important to improving the nation's public health. Yet, to address the gaps, strategies are required to forge partnerships among diverse groups, such as researchers, treatment professionals, policymakers at all levels, consumers, as well as the public and private health sectors. These partnerships must be forged in a health care delivery and financing environment that is undergoing rapid change.

Community-based drug and alcohol treatment programs, the mainstay of our current addiction treatment system, developed during the 1970s and 1980s. Since then the financing of care has changed dramatically, and demands for accountability and efficiency are increasingly stressing the ability of these programs to survive. Within this context, this Institute of Medicine committee was charged with examining the community-based drug abuse treatment system with the goal of facilitating new strategies for partnership and increasing synergy among those working in a variety of settings to reduce the individual and societal costs of drug addiction (see Box 1).

BOX 1
The Committee's Task

The task of the committee was to:

1. Identify relevant treatment strategies and promising research approaches, including the development of a typology linking specific treatment strategies with amenable research approaches.
2. Identify mechanisms by which community-based treatment programs are participating in research, including subsequent use of that research.
3. Identify mechanisms for technology transfer.
4. Identify barriers that may hinder conduct of research or the application of research results in the treatment setting.
5. Identify barriers that hinder the communication of treatment practices back to the researchers.
6. Identify innovative yet practical strategies for overcoming these barriers.

The findings and recommendations of the committee are directed toward increasing communication, interaction, and activities, especially research activities, to enhance knowledge transfer between community-based drug treatment organizations (CBOs) and the research community. Committee members believe a bidirectional flow of information among treatment providers, researchers, and policymakers will enhance the quality of treatment-based research, increase treatment effectiveness, inform policy, and help CBOs to thrive in an increasingly challenging and complex environment (see Figure 1).

The audience for this report is quite broad and includes federal, state, and local policymakers, drug treatment researchers, community-based treatment providers (including their professional organizations), and consumers, as well as sponsors of research and treatment programs. Others with interest in this report will include managed care programs, professionals involved with employee assistance programs, behavioral health researchers, behavioral health providers, criminal justice and social welfare programs, as well as foundations interested in public health, education, and professional training.

An early challenge for the committee was agreeing on a definition of community-based treatment organizations in order to frame the study. Ultimately, the consensus achieved among committee members was that *program accountability may come the closest to capturing the essence of social identity in the definition of "community-based."* The extent to which a program is accountable to elements of a specific community defines the program's interests, mission, and the social setting it serves. In the inquiry

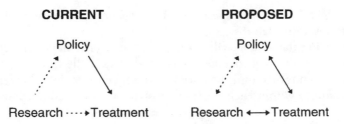

FIGURE 1   Need for bidirectional communication.

underlying its recommendations, this committee sought to include the widest range of drug treatment programs possible and was careful not to exclude from discussions and consideration those programs that defined themselves as community-based. Likewise, the committee was cautious not to exclude, a priori, any significant programs of interest by a determination that they were not "community-based." Thus, the public workshops included representatives from a diverse group, ranging from small local programs that would be considered community-based by the most restrictive definition, to large and complex programs sponsored by entities such as the Department of Veterans Affairs, academic medical centers, state court systems, and managed care organizations.

The committee obtained information from a rich variety of sources. For example, *roundtable and workshop discussions with providers, researchers, and policymakers* were held and *site visits* made by the committee and staff to solicit a broad base of input from representative stakeholders in 19 states. These meetings included individuals with expertise at all levels of government, drug courts, Native American health, school-based programs, drug abuse counseling, and research, among others.

New treatment, research, and policy questions flow out of changes in the policy environment as well as the new scientific understanding of brain biology and the mechanisms of addictions. It is important, therefore, to accelerate the exchange of information and knowledge among the research, treatment, and policy areas in order to bring the benefits of treatment research to the drug treatment consumer and to society. The evidence for the barriers between research, treatment, and policy is discussed in Chapter 2. Chapter 3 describes approaches to bridging the gap among stakeholders in this field, including technology transfer, organizational change, practice guidelines, use of consensus conferences and evidence-based reviews, top-down incentives and, most importantly, models that incorporate trust-building experiences. Chapters 4 and 5 address the challenges of the research/practice collaboration from the perspectives of the treatment providers and the researchers, respectively. The appendixes contain tools to assist those trying to bridge the gaps.

Changing the system will require treatment providers, reseachers, and policymakers working together to ask and answer the right questions and to jointly commit to implementation. Consequently, while this report proposes changes within each area, its most important recommendations are for the joint activities and investments which are necessary to produce systemic changes.

FINDINGS AND RECOMMENDATIONS

The committee's review of the challenges faced by community-based drug treatment providers, current research in this field, models for collaboration between research and practice, community-based organizations, and dissemination strategies led to findings and recommendations in six areas: (1) strategies for linking research and practice, (2) strategies for linking research findings with policy development and treatment implementation, (3) strategies for knowledge development, (4) strategies for dissemination and knowledge transfer, (5) strategies for consumer participation, and (6) training strategies for community-based research collaboration. The committee believes that attention to its recommendations will lead to improvements in clinical practices and will enhance the value of treatment research to clinicians, investigators, policymakers, consumers of treatment, and the public generally. The committee is also aware that many others (e.g., professional organizations, commissions, foundations, policy institutes, and prior IOM committees) have plowed this ground and sown seeds that have not always flourished. However, the value of the potential harvest is so great that it is essential we persevere in its cultivation.

Strategies for Linking Research and Practice

Despite some striking examples of strong collaborations between community-based drug and alcohol abuse treatment programs and research institutions, it was apparent that relatively few investigators work closely with community treatment programs, and even fewer programs participate actively in research.

Research participation becomes a possibility for treatment providers when community-based organizations are compensated for the costs of research participation and when program staff and investigators collaborate in construction of hypotheses, research design, and data collection, analysis, and interpretation.

The level of participation in research collaborations depends on the stage of organizational development of the treatment program, compatibility of the research with the organization's mission and culture, and its financial stability. Thus, research roles may vary from relatively passive participation (completing surveys and submitting data to state databases) to involvement as a partner in the development of research questions, data collection, and data interpretation. However, incentives for all parties must be strategically aligned if real progress is to be made.

The committee identified barriers to closing the gap between treatment, research, and policy. These barriers range from organizational factors, stigma, and social policy to cultural differences and funding problems, all of which can be strong disincentives for the collaboration needed to advance the field.

A pervasive theme heard in our workshops was the need for communication, mutual respect, and trust. Values of researchers and providers often differ and these differences must be recognized and resolved. The conduct of community-based research is an intensely interpersonal enterprise and trust relationships must be cultivated, at different levels of the organization, with community residents, and often with members of other agencies connected to the CBO. These relationships often take years to build.

The trust necessary for long-term collaboration is generally based on a history of increasing involvement. Successful collaborative programs from other health fields include support for a permanent infrastructure that facilitates long-term development. The National Cancer Institute's Community Clinical Oncology Program (CCOP) uses this strategy to bring state-of-the-art oncology research to community-based cancer treatment programs. CCOP facilitates research collaborations and enhances the ability of treatment programs to apply research findings to the general patient population. Development of a similar mechanism for use in community-based drug and alcohol abuse treatment could catalyze research/practice collaborations and stimulate improvements in practice. CCOPs are not inexpensive and they present a significant managerial challenge. The infrastructure alone at each clinical site can exceed $200,000. However, the infrastructure recommendation that follows does not necessarily require a model with that complexity. It could begin as a demonstration project involving the funding of one full-time-equivalent staff person and some computer support to a small set of diverse treatment sites. This level of support could be the target, whichever of the various network collaboration models was implemented.

Based on these findings, the committee offers two recommendations and identifies certain key characteristics that will facilitate their successful implementation.

RECOMMENDATION 1. The National Institute on Drug Abuse and the Center for Substance Abuse Treatment should support the development of an infrastructure to facilitate research within a network of community-based treatment programs, similar to the National Cancer Institute's Community Clinical Oncology Program (CCOP) networks.

To be successful, the infrastructure and network development will depend on commitment from the community-based treatment programs and researchers. Certain key areas will need to be addressed to foster partnership. For the community-based treatment programs, these include:

- encouraging, and, when appropriate, participating in biomedical, social-behavioral, treatment effectiveness, and services research;
- seeking collaboration with researchers to build information systems that enhance the delivery of clinical services, improve program management and operations, and contribute to research databases;
- enhancing quality improvement strategies and fostering the development of organizational learning; and
- promoting staff education on current research and creating strategies to encourage adoption of clinical protocols that hold promise to improve treatment services.

Likewise, for treatment researchers, the following approaches are suggested:

- encouraging, and, when appropriate, seeking collaborative opportunities with CBOs;
- recognizing the burdens of research on programs and consumers and providing fair compensation for the time and resources required to participate in studies;
- remaining sensitive to any potential their work has to harm consumers or treatment programs;
- guarding against the misuse of their research findings and the findings of other researchers in the development of funding and regulatory policies and the design of clinical protocols;
- supporting, through their work and their policy participation, consumer education on state-of-the-art clinical services; and
- recognizing the value of consumer participation by providing information accessible to consumers about the benefits of research, by including consumers on study advisory groups and by integrating informed consumer opinion in research proposals and study designs.

RECOMMENDATION 2. The National Institute on Drug Abuse and the National Institute on Alcohol Abuse and Alcoholism should develop research initiatives to foster studies that include community-based treatment programs as full partners.

Issues to be addressed by these initiatives include the following:

- including representatives from the treatment community in the development of the research initiative and in the review of proposals;
- showing sensitivity to the needs and constraints of community-based programs;
- requiring, in the proposal, an assessment of the study's burden and impact on the treatment program and its clients, as well as its potential relevance and practicality for CBO implementation;
- requiring active, early, and permanent participation of treatment staff in the development, implementation, and interpretation of the study;
- emphasizing the consideration of gender, gender identity, race, and urban/rural issues in research priorities; and
- providing a rapid funding mechanism to promote small research projects on emerging issues affecting treatment (e.g., managed care, welfare reform, performance measurement).

Strategies for Linking Research Findings, Policy Development, and Treatment Implementation

State and federal policies sometimes hinder the diffusion of knowledge flowing from research that is relevant to drug abuse treatment. Selective prohibitions on the use of state and federal funds can inhibit the application of proven research findings. Language in the Substance Abuse Prevention and Treatment Block Grant, for example, prohibits the use of federal funds for needle exchange, despite studies demonstrating this improves the effectiveness of outreach to a population at highest risk for HIV infection. A similar restriction on the use of funds for client payments inhibits the implementation of behavioral reinforcement strategies. Local laws and policies restrict the development and operation of methadone services. Moreover, state and federal officials have generally not used funding mechanisms to facilitate collaboration between treatment programs and researchers, to foster adoption of new and effective treatments, or to improve the design of clinical research.

The committee believes that the coordination of state and federal programs is important to facilitate active collaboration and improvement of drug and alcohol treatment. Two recommendations are offered emphasizing the role of states in this collaboration, accompanied by approaches to undergird needed support.

RECOMMENDATION 3. State authorities should provide financial incentives for collaborative investigations between CBOs and academically oriented research centers; and should support structures to foster broad participation among researchers, practitioners, consumers, and payers in the development of a treatment research agenda, including studies to measure outcomes and program operations.

RECOMMENDATION 4. CSAT and the states need to cooperate in the development of financial incentives that encourage the inclusion of proven treatment approaches into community-based treatment programs. This approach should include making additional funds available for implementing targeted treatment approaches.

To improve treatment, the following are considered critical areas to address:

• Creating mechanisms to ensure the adoption of treatments proven to be effective and development of requests for proposals that support implementations of specific treatments within local community-based settings.

• Providing support for the development of management information systems within community-based drug treatment programs, including consultation for system planning. These data systems should not be a one-way conduit to a state database but should also provide information to the treatment programs in a usable format and become the basis of public reports on outcomes.

• Encouraging state substance abuse authorities to expand researcher, provider, and consumer participation in the development of licensing standards, staff development requirements, and initiatives to enhance consumer participation. Licensing standards provide the basis for monitoring treatment outcomes and processes and for managing progress toward desired patient outcomes. The best staff development standards require ongoing staff training and education (e.g., through publications, seminars, enrollment in continuing education, and attendance at training sessions that disseminate information on emerging developments in clinical care). Consumer participation standards provide consumers with information on state-of-the-art treatment techniques; also, outcomes measurement systems are best developed with input from families and patients.

Strategies for Knowledge Development

Practitioners and policymakers requested more research on treatment effectiveness and studies that help programs operate more effectively and identify interventions that serve clients more effectively. The complexity of the contemporary economic and policy environment increases the importance of health services research and the dependence of policymakers on the data and results from research investigations.

The committee's findings suggest that expanding the range of studied treatment settings, treatment modalities, and treatment populations may result in more broadly applicable treatment research findings. These observations led the committee to make two specific recommendations in this area.

RECOMMENDATION 5. CSAT and NIDA should develop mechanisms to enable state policymakers to monitor service delivery in community-based treatment programs and to determine if consumers receive services empirically demonstrated as effective and to ascertain if the treatment dosage and intensity are sufficient to be effective.

RECOMMENDATION 6. NIDA and NIAAA should continue to support "real world" services research and cost-effectiveness studies and include the development of services research in their strategic plans.

Strategies for Dissemination and Knowledge Transfer

The committee found at least four factors that inhibit diffusion of drug abuse treatment knowledge: (1) the structure of treatment delivery systems; (2) the diversity of the clients, providers, and other stakeholders; (3) the stigmatization of people who are dependent on alcohol and other drugs; and (4) an inadequate base of knowledge about technology transfer specific to the field. Differences in perspective among consumers, clinicians, researchers, and policymakers also inhibit knowledge dissemination and use.

Because providers and payers are often unaware of the latest research, the committee found a pressing need to create consensus in the field about which treatments have been proven to be effective and which have been proven to be ineffective. Further, the research agendas of the federal agencies should continue to be fueled by agreement in the field on which models have not received adequate study. The fruits of this consensus process should be widely distributed.

Key to improving knowledge dissemination will be cooperation and collaboration across federal agencies, states, professional organizations, and consumer groups, among others. The committee recommends two general approaches to establish the needed collaboration.

RECOMMENDATION 7. CSAT, NIDA, NIAAA, and AHCPR are the federal agencies that should develop formal collaborations, where appropriate, to synthesize research, reduce the barriers to knowledge transfer, and provide updated information about drug and alcohol treatment strategies to purchasers of health care.

A variety of approaches could be utilized to accomplish these goals. For example, expert panels of investigators, practitioners, program administrators, policymakers, and consumers could be convened by NIDA, NIAAA, and CSAT to generate up-to-date consensus recommendations for community-based drug and alcohol treatment programs based on current research. NIDA-, NIAAA-, and AHCPR-sponsored research on drug treatment knowledge dissemination would help to reduce barriers to the transfer of treatment knowledge and encourage treatment programs and policymakers to adopt proven treatments. Research findings need to be prepared in a form and disseminated within channels that enhance availability and acceptability to community-based treatment programs—especially front-line treatment staff. Continued support for and improvement of electronic and print publications directed to treatment programs and consumers is necessary, and other media, such as public access television should be considered.

CSAT, NIDA, and NIAAA also have an important role in the development of information to enable purchasers of care to take research findings into account explicitly in making purchasing decisions. At the same time, purchasers should develop treatment criteria that ensure treatments of proven effectiveness are adequately funded and should consider withholding funding when the science base shows the treatment to be unequivocally ineffective.

RECOMMENDATION 8. CSAT, in collaboration with state substance abuse authorities, professional organizations, and consumer organizations in the addiction field, should continue the development of evidence-based treatment recommendations (including consideration of short- and long-term outcomes) for use by clinicians of all disciplines involved in the treatment of drug and alcohol use disorders.

To ensure that these treatment recommendations have a positive impact on health care, these agencies and groups should work to encourage their use. Measurement of the impact of guidelines on clinical care delivery will optimally include short-, intermediate-, and long-term treatment outcomes.

Strategies for Consumer Participation

Consumers are rarely involved in the issues of how drug abuse treatment research is supported and conducted. Although many community-based treatment programs were founded by men and women in recovery and counselors in recovery make up a significant portion of the workforce, there are few advocacy groups for patients and their families. In view of the stigma and legal hazards attached to illicit drug abuse, the reluctance to advocate is understandable but unfortunate. Consumer advocacy for state-of-the-art services has improved care for individuals with cancer, and with HIV/AIDS. Drug abuse treatment may enjoy similar benefits if drug treatment consumers become informed consumer advocates.

RECOMMENDATION 9. CSAT and NIDA, in collaboration with state substance abuse authorities, should develop public awareness programs to encourage consumers and their families to recognize high quality treatment programs so they will begin to demand that treatment programs include research-proven treatment approaches within their treatment models.

These groups should consider a variety of approaches to accomplish this goal. These include:

- Encouraging provider quality scorecard development to assure that consumer-oriented quality and satisfaction data, including short- and long-term outcomes data, are available to the public. Scorecard development is an early stage but growing movement in health care generally and could provide useful information about community-based treatment programs.
- Reviewing and updating the formats and content of communication vehicles to assure that treatment and research information is accessible to consumers and to the community-based treatment organizations.

It is also critically important that representatives of consumers and their families, with the support and assistance of the research, treatment, and policy communities, promote local as well as national advocacy groups to work with state funding agencies, insurers, managed care organizations, and self-insured employers to encourage the use of valid and reliable measures of treatment outcomes. Such measures serve as a basis for evaluating the efficacy of specific treatment modalities and the cost effectiveness of treatment programs, individual treatment providers and networks of care. State and federal governments, employers, and purchasing alliances could then be encouraged to use these data to inform their health care purchasing and contracting decisions. Consumer groups should also advocate for the development of standards of care in community-based clinics, treatment networks, integrated delivery systems, and managed care networks. Such standards could be used in accreditation of treatment programs and are best if based on findings from clinical research, as well as broadly accepted clinical consensus.

Training Strategies for Community-Based Research Collaboration

In order to foster collaborative research in this field, it is necessary to enhance special skills needed for the next generation of drug abuse researchers. Despite the many prior recommendations for addressing this problem, both clinical and research training programs need to be more attentive to the need for collaboration to improve treatment in this field. The committee made three recommendations specific to preparing trainees for active participation in clinical research studies.

RECOMMENDATION 10. NIDA and other research funding agencies should support predoctoral and postdoctoral research training programs that provide experience in drug abuse treatment research and health services research within community-based treatment programs. Programs funded should have the full and active participation of community-based treatment programs and should include resources to fund the costs of participation for the treatment programs.

RECOMMENDATION 11. University training programs in the health professions should:

- enhance exposure of students to didactic teaching about substance abuse and dependence;
- require didactic teaching as well as supervised clinical experiences in community-based treatment settings;
- teach students to interpret substance abuse treatment research and apply research findings in their clinical practices;
- work with professional organizations to enhance continuing education about the addictions within the residency training curriculum of the various health professions; and
- support researchers seeking to enhance collaborative relation-

ships with treatment programs by offering tuition credit for CBO staff involved in funded collaborative research.

RECOMMENDATION 12.   NIDA, CSAT, and other appropriate funding agencies should create research training programs for staff members of community-based treatment programs to strengthen the ability of the treatment programs to include research activities and to adopt the findings of research into their treatment approaches. Training programs should promote research training for clinical staff through fellowships and tuition remission, and incentives for attending professional meetings.

* * *

To enhance the likelihood that these recommendations are given serious consideration by the agencies to which they are addressed, the assistance of private foundations is also needed. Foundations could play an important role by developing grant programs to:

• Support training in clinical and services research in the addiction disorders. These grants should emphasize skills needed for participating in collaborative research and the translation and implementation of treatment research into local community settings.

• Support training for consumers and their families to become effective advocates and to develop advocacy organizations to promote state-of-the-art treatment and treatment research, as well as consumer participation in policy areas such as the development of standards of care.

TABLE 1 Summary of Recommendations

Strategies	Recommendations	Primary Responsibility
I. Linking research and practice	1. Develop research infrastructure and network of community-based drug treatment organizations (CBOs)	NIDA, CSAT
	2. Research initiative for collaborative studies within CBOs	NIDA, NIAAA
II. Linking research, policy development and treatment implementation	3. Promote university/CBO studies and develop treatment research agenda	States
	4. CBO incentives to implement targeted treatments	CSAT, states
III. Knowledge development	5. Assist states to develop treatment and outcomes monitoring system	CSAT, NIDA
	6. Support services research and cost-effectiveness studies	NIDA, NIAAA
IV. Dissemination and knowledge transfer	7. Coordinate activities to synthesize research and provide information to payers	CSAT, NIDA, NIAAA, AHCPR
	8. Develop evidence-based treatment recommendations—with broad constituency participation	CSAT
V. Consumer participation	9. Develop public awareness programs to increase demand for proven treatment	CSAT, NIDA

TABLE 1 Continued

Strategies	Recommendations	Primary Responsibility
VI. Training for community-based research collaboration	10. Support pre/post doctoral training for community-based research collaboration	NIDA, other NIH training programs
	11. Provide teaching, supervised clinical experience and CME in addiction treatment— for all health professions	University training programs
	12. Create research training programs for CBO staff through fellowships and other incentives	CSAT, NIDA, university programs

1

Introduction

Drug abuse remains one of our nation's most intractable problems. Only a small proportion of the approximately 9.4 million addicted and dependent individuals receive treatment in a given year. In fact, almost 80 percent go untreated, a figure that has changed little in the 1990s while the number needing treatment has increased (Epstein and Gfroerer, 1998). The stigma of drug abuse and the political and financial barriers encountered at all levels impede efforts to increase treatment. The care of patients with addictive disorders is characterized by a high degree of variability in the application of treatment methodologies and patient placement decisions. In addition, the field has been plagued by approaches to treatment that have not been based on evidence beyond anecdotal reports and belief systems. Dogmatic thinking about etiology and treatment of addictive disorders, as well as changes in the financing environment, has led to the application of treatment concepts without reference to their appropriateness or efficacy for particular classes of patients.

At the same time, however, there is a paucity of data on the efficacy of specific treatments and their short- and long-term outcome, as well as on the relationship between clinical and demographic characteristics of patients with addictive disorders and their responses to particular treatment modalities. These difficulties are greatly complicated by the fact that patients often have a limited ability to comply with treatment regimens, a high incidence of relapse, and high levels of other coincident psychiatric, psychosocial, and medical problems. Perhaps as many as half of those needing treatment for drug and alcohol abuse also need treatment for co-occurring mental illness.[1] Thus, the clinical complexities inherent in treating such patients has fostered a tendency to apply multiple treatment modalities without thinking through or knowing which treatments may be most effective for a specific patient, or considering the sequence in which such treatments should be applied.

This situation has major implications for the treatment of addictive disorders and, thus, for public health. The absence of an evidence-based approach to addiction treatment, coupled with a lack of valid and reliable measures of treatment outcome, has induced skepticism on the part of purchasers of care, policymakers, and consumers as to the value of treatment for drug and alcohol abuse and dependence. Skepticism and the stigma attached to these disorders, which are perceived by many as volitional and suggestive of moral weakness, has further led to discrimination in benefit design and reluctance by payers and managed care organizations to allocate resources to the care of such patients.

Community-based drug treatment organizations (CBOs) provide the backbone of drug and alcohol treatment today and their capabilities have not kept up with the rising problem of addiction, nor with the major scientific advances that have been made in understanding the biopsychosocial basis of addiction (IOM, 1996, 1997a). Such organizations receive the majority of their funding from public dollars, through state and local appropriations and federal block grants to states. In 1997 public funds accounted for two-thirds (65 percent) of the reported revenues in drug and alcohol treatment programs (Horgan and Levine—Appendix E). In the current environment of fiscal restraint and burgeoning need, there is great interest in strengthening the community-based drug treatment organizations and in helping these providers better utilize research findings on effective treatment strategies.

This report examines these issues and presents the findings and conclusions of an Institute of Medicine committee convened at the request of the Substance Abuse and Mental Health Services Administration's Center for

---

[1]There are perhaps 10 million individuals who have co-occurring mental illness and substance abuse problems, including alcohol abuse and dependence. NIAAA's Ninth Special Report to Congress indicates that 13.7 million meet DSM-IV criteria for either alcohol abuse or alcohol dependence (NIAAA, 1997). And the most recent SAMHSA estimate for individuals needing treatment for drug abuse and dependence is 9.4 million (Epstein and Gfroerer, 1998). Even adjusting generously for the overlap between the two groups, it appears that co-occurring mental illness is a very large problem in treating individuals for alcohol and drug abuse. Based on recent survey data cited in Horgan and Levine (see Table 7, Appendix E), it appears that the proportion of facilities providing both substance abuse and mental health services is increasing.

Substance Abuse Treatment (CSAT) and the National Institute on Drug Abuse (NIDA).[2]

This committee was asked to accomplish the following tasks (see Appendix A):

1. identify relevant treatment strategies and promising research approaches, including the development of a typology linking specific treatment strategies with amenable research approaches;
2. identify mechanisms by which community-based treatment programs are participating in research, including subsequent use of that research;
3. identify mechanisms for technology transfer;
4. identify barriers that may hinder conduct of research within or the application of research results in the treatment setting;
5. identify barriers that hinder the communication of treatment practices back to the researchers; and
6. identify innovative yet practical strategies for overcoming these barriers.

The committee hopes that its findings and recommendations will foster increased bidirectional communication, interaction, and activities aimed to enhance knowledge transfer between CBOs and the research community. Committee members believe a bidirectional flow of information will enhance the quality of treatment-based research, increase treatment effectiveness, and help CBOs to thrive in an increasingly challenging and complex environment. The participation of policymakers will be essential if this is to happen. Thus, the audience for this report is quite broad and includes federal, state, and local policymakers, drug treatment researchers, community-based treatment providers (including their professional organizations), and consumers, as well as sponsors of research and treatment programs. Others with interest in this report may include managed care programs, professionals involved with employee assistance programs (EAPs), behavioral health researchers, behavioral health providers, and those involved with criminal justice and social welfare programs. And finally, there is an important role for foundations, because, while many of the needs identified in this report are interstitial with regard to the missions of the agencies to

---

[2]CSAT is the federal agency mandated by Congress to expand the availability of effective treatment for alcohol and drug problems. As one of the National Institutes of Health, NIDA's mission is to provide the research and add to the knowledge of drug abuse and addiction and its effective treatment, including educating the public and broadening the dissemination of research findings to improve drug abuse treatment practice and policy.

whom these recommendations are addressed, they are areas of significant interest for a number of foundations.

THE STUDY PROCESS AND REPORT ORGANIZATION

To accomplish its task, the committee met four times between April and December 1997. Through these meetings and other activities summarized below, the committee obtained information from a rich variety of sources. For example, *roundtable and workshop discussions with providers, researchers, and policymakers* were held and *site visits* made by the committee and staff to solicit a broad base of input from representative stakeholders. The workshop and roundtable discussions, held in Washington, D.C., and Albuquerque, New Mexico, yielded data of critical interest to the committee. These workshops were designed to allow researchers, providers, and policymakers to discuss the issues with each other and with members of the committee. A list of participants and the topics discussed are included in Appendix B.

The first workshop was held in Washington, D.C., with participants from 14 states. Providers, researchers, and policymakers presented in separate panels, each hosted by a member of the committee. Providers spoke of the gap between research and practice, as well as the language and culture barriers that hinder collaboration. They expressed concern that research findings were sometimes misinterpreted and misused in the search for lowest-cost alternatives, but they also expressed their need for relevant and practical research, conducted and disseminated in ways that would help them improve treatment and demonstrate cost effectiveness. Other major concerns of this group were the changing policy and regulatory environment, shrinking treatment options and capacity, and growing need for infrastructure and training resources. Examples included, a state where providers were given only ten days to implement new legislation requiring screening and evaluation for all DUI (driving while under the influence) arrestees and another state where a facility was facing the requirement to work with multiple HMOs with one outdated computer and just one person who knew how to use it.

Policymakers, as well as providers, spoke of the long lag time for research findings to reach them and the need for better strategies for translating research information to meet their needs. It was suggested that policymakers and researchers take lessons from business: design audience-specific information and market it aggressively. Policy panelists stated that federal and state policymakers needed to know what worked, and that Congress wanted evidence to support community-based treatment organizations as the front line of prevention and treatment.

Researchers and providers spoke of financial and political barriers to the implementation of proven research findings. For example, behavioral incentive programs proven highly effective in treatment of cocaine addiction are not very practical for a midwest CBO receiving $340 per case per year, about a third of the cost of the incentive program. Researchers talked of the difficulty getting funded for community-based research, the special pitfalls of the NIH grant review process for applied research proposals, and the challenge of doing research in a nonacademic treatment setting. Providers and researchers agreed on the difficulties of getting funding to cover the true costs of participating in research. This workshop concluded with a discussion focused on the impact of stakeholder interactions and how these interactions—or their lack—affected treatment of drug abuse, the need for more and different collaborative research and better strategies to translate results into findings relevant to the intended audience.

The second workshop, held in Albuquerque, New Mexico, was co-hosted by the Center on Alcoholism, Substance Abuse and Addiction (CASAA) at the University of New Mexico and provided input from stakeholders in western states. Participants described successes and failures in research collaboration and dissemination of research findings, as well as the challenges of integrating clinical experience with research design. This meeting provided an opportunity to obtain an overview of community-based drug treatment in a richly multicultural and mostly rural state containing a very large Hispanic population and 26 Indian nations. In addition to researchers from CASAA, participants included representatives of the state substance abuse agency, the state legislature, the city of Albuquerque, Albuquerque public schools, New Mexico drug courts, the Navajo Nation, and the regional representative of the National Association of Alcohol and Drug Abuse Counselors. Participants from Arizona, California, Colorado, Texas, and Washington attended the Albuquerque workshop, representing providers, researchers, and counselor organizations and the Window Rock Navajo Reservation.

Additional input from drug treatment providers and policymakers in the District of Columbia was obtained through two meetings attended by committee staff. The first was a special meeting of the District of Columbia Health Policy Council to discuss drug abuse and mental health needs where it was reported that less than 10 percent of the estimated 76,000 substance abusing individuals in D.C. received any form of treatment. The second was a meeting for District providers of drug abuse treatment held at Seton House of Providence Hospital. The discussion focused on the dilemma faced by treatment providers in an area of shrinking social as well as treatment services. The lack of social services is a special concern to providers with clients who may never have held a job, perhaps do not speak English or have not learned to read, and do not have family or community support to "wraparound" their treatment. At the earlier D.C. committee workshop, this issue was also raised as an area where research could help funding and regulatory agencies understand the difference between habilitation needs and rehabilitation needs "and perhaps, thank us, instead of penalizing us, for taking these difficult patients."

Finally, to supplement these meetings, individual committee members made site visits to treatment programs and state agencies in their area to explore issues relevant to the study. Site visits were also made by members of the committee staff (see Acknowledgments for list of sites visited).

Another important source of information was *invited presentations to the committee on special topics*. These topics included: diffusion of innovation and dissemination; models of collaboration; research agenda building; drug services survey data; requirements of federal and state policy; and, finally, the implications of the current research grant review process for efforts to form and maintain research collaborations with community-based treatment organizations.

Four additional activities completed the major data gathering phase of the study:

1. preparation of commissioned papers (Appendices C, D, and E);
2. review of journals and other publications that disseminate drug abuse research findings;
3. review of research literature and relevant websites; and
4. review of survey and other data sources (e.g., State Alcohol and Drug Abuse Profile Data, CSAT's Uniform Facility Data Set, and NIDA's Drug Abuse Treatment Outcome Study).

This report is organized into six chapters including this introductory chapter, which provides an overview of the major issues and study process. The second chapter examines the gaps between research, treatment, and policy in detail. Chapter 3 describes approaches for closing these gaps. The potential benefits and challenges confronting community-based treatment providers are the subject of Chapter 4. Chapter 5 discusses these benefits and challenges from the researcher perspective and presents models of successful collaboration. The committee's findings and recommendations are presented in Chapter 6.

HISTORICAL BACKGROUND

To understand the current state of community-based drug treatment, it is useful to consider key aspects of the development of the drug treatment system in the United States. Prior to the 1960s, community-based, noninstitutional services for drug abuse were almost nonexistent. Drug dependent individuals who received treatment were most likely to receive limited and ineffective care in state mental hospitals, county jails, federal hospitals, and penal facilities. Alternatives developed during the 1960s and 1970s in response to state legislation that decriminalized public intoxication and federal legislation that permitted community services for the treatment of drug addiction. Stimulated by federal initiatives, such alternatives accompanied the trend to deinstitutionalize the mentally ill from state mental hospitals, develop community mental health centers, and fund alcoholism and drug abuse treatment programs (Besteman, 1992; IOM, 1990a,b).

Historically, access to treatment for drug abuse was more limited than for alcohol treatment. Prior to the 1960s, treatment for opiate, cocaine, and marijuana dependence was generally restricted to two federal public health hospitals located in Lexington, Kentucky, and Fort Worth, Texas (IOM, 1990b, 1997b; Jaffe, 1979). The first therapeutic community for drug addiction, Synanon, opened in 1958 and demonstrated that a program using group confrontation and staff in recovery could promote stable recovery from heroin addiction. Second generation therapeutic communities developed during the early 1960s and incorporated public funding and professional staff into the model. Methadone and methadone maintenance treatment, first implemented in New York City, also developed during the early 1960s (Courtwright et al., 1989; IOM, 1990a, 1997b).

In 1966 a system of community-based treatment centers was authorized by the Narcotic Addict Rehabilitation Act of 1966 (P.L. 89-793) (Besteman, 1992). Two years later, a 1968 census of drug treatment programs identified 183 agencies located primarily in states with major metropolitan areas (New York, California, Illinois, Massachusetts, Connecticut, and New Jersey) (Jaffe, 1979). Most of the facilities had opened recently; over 75 percent were less than five years old and only two (the federal hospitals) had been operational for more than 20 years (Jaffe, 1979). In 1971, President Nixon created the Special Action Office for Drug Abuse Prevention (SAODAP), predecessor to the Office of National Drug Control Policy, to coordinate his "war on drugs." The first director of SAODAP, Dr. Jerome Jaffe, was determined to improve access to treatment by shifting services from prisons and hospitals to community-based services, primarily because institutional services were too expensive and it was impossible to meet the demand for care (Jaffe, 1979).

These initiatives, and the funding authorized to implement their requirements, resulted in two critical shifts in the delivery system of care for addiction. First, groups of men and women in recovery were encouraged to incorporate as private not-for-profit entities and to open detoxification centers, halfway houses, therapeutic communities, and outpatient treatment centers. Thus, the recovering community was empowered to participate fully in the development of the continuum of care and to draw upon their personal experiences with recovery in the design and implementation of services. Second, by 1995, more than 8,000 facilities were providing drug or combined alcohol and drug treatment in the 50 states and the District of Columbia. All of these facilities receive some funding from their state alcohol and drug abuse agencies, and in most cases fully 80 percent of their revenue came from public sources (Gustafson et al., 1997).

DEFINITIONS AND CURRENT CONTEXT

This committee was funded by CSAT and NIDA to study community-based drug treatment. While the committee focused its data collection primarily on drug abuse treatment and research, it recognized that alcohol is also a drug and one that plays a large part in community-based drug treatment. Hence recommendations are included for the National Institute on Alcohol Abuse and Addiction (NIAAA), and the term drug abuse as used in this report should be interpreted to include alcohol abuse when that is appropriate in the context.

The first challenge for the committee was the need to define community-based organization in order to frame the study. The committee reviewed several approaches for doing this, including the approach taken by a previous IOM committee that emphasized the multifaceted nature of community-based care and need to pay special attention to the needs of community groups that are vulnerable and underserved (IOM, 1994). An earlier monograph from NIDA, defined a community-based organization as, "a noninstitutional provider located in the community where its user population resides" (Cartwright and Kaple, 1991). This latter definition seemed overly restrictive to the committee in light of the current environment in which increasing numbers of providers of community drug treatment are associated with medical and other institutions. Ultimately, there was a consensus among committee members that *program accountability may come the closest to capturing the essence of social identity in the definition of "community based."* The extent to which a program is accountable to major elements of a specific community defines the program's interests, mission, and the social setting it serves. So, in an important sense, the community itself may define community-based.[3]

An important aim of this study is to increase bidirectional interaction and knowledge exchange between the research community and the drug treatment community. In considering definitional issues, then, the committee believed that this aim would not be well served by a highly restrictive definition of community-based treatment programs. Consequently, in the

---

[3]A paper by committee member Benjamin P. Bowser, reflecting the work of a subcommittee formed to address this problem is included as Appendix C. This paper discusses the importance of community, the many ways of defining community, and the meaning of "community-based" in the context of drug abuse treatment programs.

inquiry underlying its recommendations, this committee sought to include the widest range of drug and alcohol treatment programs possible and was careful not to exclude from discussions and consideration those programs that defined themselves as community-based. Likewise, the committee was cautious not to exclude, a priori, any significant programs of interest by a determination that they were not "community-based." Thus, the public workshops included representatives from a diverse group of treatment programs, ranging from small programs who would be considered community-based by the most restrictive definition, to large and complex programs sponsored by larger entities, such as the Department of Veterans Affairs, academic medical centers, state court systems, and managed care organizations.

One of the important cultural elements that differentiates among community-based treatment programs is the set of beliefs that each uses to define the knowledge base about how to deliver effective drug treatment. There are at least two main types of programs in this regard. First, there are programs in which treatment models are based largely on the experiential knowledge of staff, especially those in recovery from drug abuse problems. This is the tradition of the "twelve-step" programs, following the model of Alcoholics Anonymous (AA). Such treatment providers have confidence in their knowledge because it has been tested in a most important test—their own recovery. Also in this category are programs that are identified with religious organizations and bring an element of faith to their treatment approach. Since faith is built into the foundation of their treatment approach, their religious beliefs fuel their organizational culture, including, to some extent, their fundamental "knowledge" about the nature of appropriate treatment for drug abuse problems. On the other hand, there is a set of organizations more closely related to the general health care system or to the traditions of the behavioral sciences. Because these treatment programs share much of the culture of medicine and the behavioral sciences, their organizational cultures include more of their scientific beliefs and values about the nature of treatment. Such a perspective suggests that, in programs in this second category, the therapist's knowledge about what is appropriate in treatment is defined by the fruits of scientific medical or behavioral research.[4]

---

[4]Some of this argument follows a perspective put forth by Edward Suchman. In discussing different world views among consumers of health care, Suchman argued that some people had, what he called, a "cosmopolitan" view of the world, while others had a "local" view. And he proposed ways to differentiate those approaches to and explanations of life. He proposed that those views also led to unique and different orientations toward health and illness. He suggested that people with a "cosmopolitan" view of the world were more likely to have, what he referred to as, a "scientific" orientation to health and disease. Those with a "local" life view would be more likely to have a "parochial" orientation to health and illness (Suchman, 1966).

It was not, however, the a priori assumption of this committee that one or the other kind of program is "better" in some fundamental way, although many might agree that a close link to medical sciences—especially in the current environment—is most desirable. In fact, there is very little scientific data available on relative treatment effectiveness by categories of treatment programs. Yet, this categorization does provide the opportunity to consider different models of relationship between researchers and the treatment programs, depending on the specific orientation and organizational culture of the different types of programs.

In the environment today, all community-based drug treatment programs have seen an increase in drug use, an exploding epidemic of HIV and AIDS, an increase in tuberculosis, hepatitis, and other infectious diseases, an increase in comorbid psychological and psychiatric problems, and high levels of unemployment. However, treatment length, intensity, and service mix have decreased due to payor restrictions, despite increases in the acuity and complexity of multiple problems drug abuse patients experience. Community-based organizations are challenged to meet demand in this environment of rapid changes, with dwindling resources and uncertainty about the future. Most community-based organizations will survive, but some will not, and indeed some have already closed their doors. To remain viable, community-based organizations must learn to adapt and navigate in this new and uncertain environment. To do this they must have new tools, new skills, new incentives, and new partnerships.

SUMMARY

Community-based services for drug and alcohol addiction developed in response to many factors: poor care in state mental hospitals, discrimination and prejudice in general hospitals and private facilities, inhumane conditions in "drunk tanks," the expense of providing institutional services, and the need to rapidly expand the nation's capacity to provide treatment for drug abuse and alcoholism. The services that developed and served the nation during the 1970s and 1980s have shrunk during the early 1990s, and the organizations that provide them are challenged to survive as the nation approaches the twenty-first century. Competition for funding has increased, the financing of care has changed, and demands for accountability and efficiency are forcing free-standing community-based agencies to seek mergers with hospitals and health plans or to integrate with mental health and community health programs. Over 60 percent now report they are part of another organization (Appendix E, Table 1).

One of the major threats to the survival of this system is the widening gap between knowledge gained from basic scientific and treatment research and knowledge gained from clinical experience. This is accompanied by growing isolation of the clinical-provider communities from the research communities. Within this context, it is clearly critical to examine closely all elements of the community-based drug abuse treatment system with the goal of facilitating new strategies for partnership and increasing synergy among those working in a variety of settings to reduce the individual and societal costs of drug addiction.

REFERENCES

Besteman KJ. 1992. Federal leadership in building the national drug treatment system. In: Institute of Medicine *Treating Drug Problems*. Vol. 2. Washington, DC: National Academy Press.

Cartwright WS, Kaple JM, eds. 1991. *NIDA Research Monograph 113: Economic Costs, Cost-Effectiveness, Financing, and Community-Based Drug Treatment*. Rockville, MD: National Institute on Drug Abuse.

Courtwright D, Joseph H, Des Jarlais D. 1989. *Addicts Who Survived: An Oral History of Narcotic Use in America, 1923–1965*. Knoxville, TN: The University of Tennessee Press.

Epstein J, Gfroerer J. 1998. *Changes Affecting NHSDA Estimates of Treatment Need for 1994–1996: OAS Working Paper*. Rockville, MD: Office of Applied Studies, Substance Abuse and Mental Health Services Administration.

Gustafson JS, Reda JL, McMullen H, Sheehan K, McGencey S, Rugaber C, Anderson R, DiCarlo M. 1997. *State Resources and Services Related to Alcohol and Other Drug Problems: Fiscal Year 1995*. Washington, DC: National Association of State Alcohol and Drug Abuse Directors, Inc.

IOM (Institute of Medicine). 1990a. *Broadening the Base of Treatment for Alcohol Problems*. Washington, DC: National Academy Press.

IOM. 1990b. *Treating Drug Problems*. Washington, DC: National Academy Press.

IOM. 1994. *Reducing Risks for Mental Disorders: Frontiers for Preventive Intervention Research*. Washington, DC: National Academy Press.

IOM. 1996. *Pathways of Addiction: Opportunities in Drug Abuse Research*. Washington, DC: National Academy Press.

IOM. 1997a. *Dispelling the Myths About Addiction: Strategies to Increase Understanding and Strengthen Research*. Washington, DC: National Academy Press.

IOM. 1997b. *Managing Managed Care: Quality Improvement in Behavioral Health*. Washington, DC: National Academy Press.

Jaffe JH. 1979. The swinging pendulum: The treatment of drug abusers in America. In: Dupont RI, Goldstein A, O'Donnell J eds. *Handbook on Drug Abuse*. Washington, DC: U.S. Government Printing Office. Pp. 3–16.

NIAAA (National Institute on Alcohol Abuse and Alcoholism). 1997. *Ninth Special Report to the U.S. Congress on Alcohol and Health*. Rockville, MD: National Institute on Alcohol Abuse and Alcoholism.

Suchman E. 1966. Health Orientation and Medical Care. *American Journal of Public Health* 56:97–105.

2

The Gaps Between Research, Treatment, and Policy

A committee member interviewed the director of a substance treatment program in a western state serving 37 male and 15 female substance-dependent patients who live on site for 90 days. They may stay another 30 days in less heavily supervised housing. When it started in 1972 the program aimed at "traditional" alcoholics, but most patients now have alcohol and other substance problems in combination. The staff is small and includes several recovering persons. Because of managed care reimbursement changes in recent months, the program faces a budget deficit this year. Over the years the program has come to rely heavily on block grant funding. Taking public funds, rather than relying on self-pay and other private sources, forces the program to accept more criminal justice referrals.

The program's board of directors primarily comprises older, conservative AA members. They are somewhat suspicious of changes, but they are willing to fund the program's deficit over the next year. Thereafter, if the financial problems are not solved, they probably will direct the program to revert to its former practice of

This chapter was edited by James L. Sorensen with contributions by Lisa Mojer-Torres, Kathleen T. Brady, Thomas Crowley, Emily Jean Hauenstein, A. Thomas McLellan, and Steven M. Mirin.

only housing alcoholic people as they attend AA. All counseling would be discontinued.

Relationship with Research

The program has never been involved in research. The director has no scientific training and has never applied for research funds. His board has encouraged him to apply for such funds, under the belief that if they receive research funds, they could use it for other purposes.

The director reports some interest in research based on his informal observation that perhaps one patient in five "makes it" to a consistently abstinent life. He would like to be able to predict which one out of five would be the successful one, and he would like to see more effective treatments for the other four out of five.

The director feels that involving his program in research might be good for staff morale because the staff is curious and wants to improve. He also worries that doing research probably would mean more work, and he expresses some concern that researchers might find his treatment to be ineffective. However, overall he feels the benefits would outweigh the risks. The director says that the program would be more likely to get into research if there were direct financial benefits. He feels that his Board would oppose introducing any more non-AA treatment as part of a research project.

Information Sharing on Treatment Advances

Regarding information dissemination, this director mentions "NIDA Notes" and says that a similar, brief publication focusing on treatment research would help him. The director receives most of his information about new treatments through peers in the state provider's association. He evaluates new treatment information based on a kind of "gut" feeling and his own extensive experience in the field. He is, for example, aware of naltrexone treatment for alcoholism, and he even attended a meeting sponsored by the drug's manufacturer. However, his program is not using naltrexone because he concluded that for his program, which has no medical or nursing staff, potential benefits from naltrexone would not offset the cost and effort needed to introduce it.

Summary

This man has worked for 25 years to help drug- and alcohol-dependent patients. This was the first time that a researcher had asked his opinion about the research-clinical interface. He provides shelter, support, strong encouragement of AA participation, and a small but caring treatment staff. Changes in his funding and requirements under the state block grant program and from managed care now force him to offer treatment to criminal justice patients with whom he feels less comfortable. Moreover, after 25 years in the field he is not sure that his program can survive financially for the next year. The board of directors is not very supportive of non-AA treatments. His work is consumed with making administrative changes to keep his program alive. He has no ill will toward research, and in fact supports the concept, but his program is struggling so much that it seems to him an unlikely site for conducting treatment research.

OVERVIEW

There are important gaps between the knowledge gained from research, everyday practice in community-based drug abuse treatment programs, and governmental policies about drug abuse treatment at the local, state, and national levels. Much has been learned about drug abuse treatment at each of these levels—research, treatment, and policy. Yet these groups make too little use of one another's knowledge base.

As the site visit report at the beginning of this chapter illustrates so well, there is often a wide cultural and experiential separation between the professionals who conduct empirical investigations and the men and women who apply research findings in treatment and policy settings. Researchers, moreover, study some treatments and leave other treatment modalities, settings, and populations underexamined. Sometimes it takes years for research results to affect treatment delivery. This lag in the diffusion of innovation has been well documented in other areas of health care (Eisenberg, 1986; Ferguson, 1995), but many components of drug treatment seem particularly resistant to incorporating research findings into treatment. Furthermore, relevant studies are slow to reach the desks of policymakers (Millman et al., 1990), and officials do not appear to rely heavily on policy analysis from research organizations (Lester, 1993). At the federal level the commitment to knowledge dissemination has waxed and waned over the years (Backer, 1991), but there are signs of a new upswing of interest in dissemination of information about research-proven drug abuse treatments.

The interactive communications thrust of the NIDA Drug Abuse Treatment Initiative is an example of this new interest.

EVIDENCE FOR THE GAPS

The evidence for the gaps begins with the different perspectives and priorities among researchers, treatment providers, and policymakers. The often overlooked consumer perspective is included as well. Examples of areas where there are clear gaps between research, treatment, and policy include pharmacotherapy, psychosocial interventions, and broader service delivery approaches (i.e., integrating drug and alcohol treatment with other medical treatment and social services, to address the multiple problems of many if not most addicted individuals).

Different Perspectives

Researchers perceive that many research-developed innovations have improved the treatment of drug abuse. For example, methadone maintenance treatment began as a research effort, and relapse-prevention techniques were honed by research investigations. Significant advances have been made in behavioral treatment of drug abusers (Stitzer and Higgins, 1995). The beneficial effect of including contingency-based counseling in methadone maintenance has been reported, as has the finding that contingency management is an effective way to promote abstinence during treatment for both heroin-dependent and cocaine-dependent patients. Studies have found that treatment intensity and systematic follow-up improve treatment results (Fiorentine and Anglin, 1997; Hoffman et al., 1994; Price, 1997; Simpson et al., 1997). Researchers believe that patient outcomes would be significantly improved if these, and other research-tested modalities, were fully utilized in treatment.

Treatment providers have a different perspective. Faced with the challenges of providing services on a daily basis, providers are often frustrated by what they see as the failure of research to provide them with relevant answers to their important questions. Many of their most important questions are in policy- and reimbursement-related areas that, at least until recently, have been under researched. They perceive that current policy provides little incentive for treatment programs to implement new research findings. For example, some states (currently, Idaho, Mississippi, Montana, New Hampshire, North Dakota, South Dakota, Vermont, and West Virginia) prohibit methadone treatment except for detoxification. One representative of a state provider association reported that reimbursement in that state was too low to allow the implementation of effective contingency models, even if direct payment to consumers were permitted by federal policy controlling the use of block grant money.

Those who define and implement policies have a third perspective and report yet another set of problems. They do not find the research literature easily accessible. They point to the oversupply of information at all levels, too little of which supports the cost-effectiveness of the programs they fund and administer. For information to be effective, they argue, it must respond directly and easily to the needs of increasingly time-pressed individuals and organizations. Providing information on complex and difficult technical issues poses special challenges for all involved (IOM, 1997b). Frustrated by the time lag and the flood of printed material, policymakers tend to rely on familiar sources to select and summarize the information relevant to them as the issues emerge (Young, 1997).

Policymakers and treatment providers both faulted researchers for having no concept of real time. One provider who participated in a multisite study comparing treatment modalities said that some programs were dead when the positive findings were reported five years after the study ended. However, the value of having the right information at the right time was illustrated by the workshop participant who reported that a timely cost-effectiveness study resulted in the 600 substance abuse treatment programs in Ohio receiving a 30 percent funding increase for the biennium (Ohio Department of Alcohol and Drug Addiction Services, 1996). A state agency director expressed the need for faster research turnaround this way:

> Much research now being published was conceived several years or a decade ago, when a much different system was in place—when today's problems were just beginning. Research funding should support more exploratory, quasi-experimental, clinically relevant studies. Secondary analyses and meta analyses of state agency data might reveal useful information. (Appendix J)

The consumer perspective is often overlooked. There is no popular literature pushing new research findings to consumers, as there is for other chronic disease conditions. Consumers generally have fewer options in selecting drug treatment programs than in other areas of medical care. When choice is available it is difficult to obtain information to make an informed decision and the individual may also find that the treatment of choice is not provided or not covered by their insurance. Few treatment consumers are effective advocates, and former consumers are busy building lives. Individuals needing treatment may want more treatment capacity to reduce waiting lists, more convenient locations and hours for treatment, better integration of drug abuse treatments with other needed medical and social services, counselors with more training, better detoxification facilities, more research into the causes and treatments of drug abuse disorders, and help in reducing the increased risk of drug problems among children of drug abusers. But, there is little structure for consumer input. The stigma and denial attached to addiction inhibit consumer action and social support.

Despite these handicaps, there is support for treatment and research for problems of drug dependence. Often it is built on the need to defend society from drug abusers, rather than on a need to help "victims" of addiction. Mayors and county officials may lobby their state and federal representatives for help in controlling drug problems with treatment. Judges and district attorneys can also be effective voices for change as they seek treatment resources for the growing drug court movement (Drug Strategies, 1997); but drug abusers rarely lobby for more treatment. Addicted persons are not in a strong position to ask society for help.

Research Findings That Are Underutilized in Treatment

The committee identified several examples of research findings that are not generally utilized or are underutilized in various components of the treatment system. They include pharmacotherapy and psychosocial treatments as well as service delivery approaches. The issues are introduced in this chapter to illustrate the consequences of the gaps between research, treatment and policy. They are discussed in greater detail in a paper by McLellan and McKay included as Appendix D.

Medications in the treatment of drug abuse disorders are underutilized in many community-based treatment settings. Methadone maintenance for treatment of opiate addiction provides an example of the difficulty implementing established findings and knowledge in this field. Adequately designed clinical trials have consistently shown that methadone maintenance treatment is effective only when methadone is given in adequate doses (Ball and Ross, 1991; Caplehorn and Bell, 1991). Despite this research finding, past surveys have found many treatment programs that prescribe inadequate methadone doses (Calsyn et al., 1991; D'Aunno and Vaughn, 1992), although this situation may be improving according to recent reports (Leshner, 1997).

The reasons for this low dosage of methadone may still include lack of adequate information concerning the effectiveness of higher doses, despite public statements of support by such authorities as the National Institutes of Health and Office of National Drug Control Policy. Ambivalent attitudes concerning the use of medications in the treatment of drug abuse disorders may also be a contributing factor. However, while this study was under way, an important and historic event took place which may be a hopeful indicator for change. In 1997 the National Institutes of Health convened a Consensus Development Conference on Effective Medical Treatment of Heroin Addiction, the first NIH conference on this topic. After hearing from many experts the consensus panel concluded that opiate addiction met the criteria of having effective medical treatment and established diagnostic criteria, and it made recommendations for improving treatment access and identified future research areas and training needs. The consensus statement from this conference is included as Appendix F.

Another example of this gap between research and practice is the underuse of naltrexone, a pharmacologic treatment (opiate-antagonist) which has long been shown to be effective in preventing relapse to opiate addiction in highly motivated patients (Brahen et al., 1978). Several well-controlled studies have also shown naltrexone to be effective as an adjunct to a variety of psychosocial rehabilitation interventions in the treatment of alcohol dependence (Volpicelli et al., 1992). In 1994, naltrexone received Food and Drug Administration (FDA) approval for use in the treatment of alcohol dependence.

However, naltrexone is not widely used in alcohol treatment outside of medical centers and some specialized treatment settings. The manufacturer of naltrexone estimates that approximately 80,000 individuals were treated with naltrexone in 1996 for all indications. Even allowing for a large margin of error, these figures indicate that naltrexone is prescribed for less than one percent of the persons who might benefit. The reasons for this low utilization are unclear, but they likely relate to some of the organizational constraints described above, including lack of available medical expertise, lack of cost reimbursement coverage, and lack of information concerning the cost-effectiveness of adding this medication to current treatment strategies.

A final example of an established research finding that has not been adopted widely in clinical practice is the integration of contingency management strategies in community-based treatment settings. The knowledge that positive reinforcement can increase desired behaviors has been empirically demonstrated in both laboratory and clinical settings. Over the years, these principles have been applied to drug abuse treatment in several ways. In a study of cocaine users, Higgins and colleagues used a system of vouchers which could be traded for material goods which individuals received when the routine urine testing proved negative (Higgins et al., 1994). This research, when compared to noncontingent vouchers, demonstrated a very beneficial effect of the voucher system in increasing drug-free urines. This study has since been replicated (Silverman et al., 1996) in a number of different treatment settings. Despite this, the use of positive reinforcement or a voucher-based system has not been widely implemented in treatment settings. Again, the barriers are multiple, including lack of information concerning the efficacy of these strategies as well as implementation difficulties due to payer policies. Several workshop participants expressed concern about these barriers and one provider reported that the average total treatment reimbursement in his state was less than the value of one set of vouchers. And certainly there is the public perception that people should not be paid for staying drug free.

Service Delivery Approaches

Drug abuse providers treat persons who are physically, emotionally, socially, and economically unstable. Standard treatments may target only one facet of their need. Service delivery methods, which involve bundling drug abuse treatment with other services that address the multiple disabilities of addicted individuals, have been shown to promote recovery and prevent relapse. Service delivery approaches include, for example, case management, rapid admission, programs geared to the special requirements of treating women with children, as well as so-called "wraparound services" such as medical care, job training, and social services. Providers who spoke with the committee saw the decline of such services in their communities as a significant barrier to successful treatment. Research based on data from NIDA's Drug Abuse Treatment Outcome Study (DATOS) reports a widening gap over the last decade between the need for services that go beyond basic drug abuse treatment and the supply of such services (Etheridge et al., 1995). An exception to this disheartening decline of supportive services is the DATOS finding that methadone programs are treating more medical problems than in the past. This report also mentions that methadone dosage levels have improved from earlier years (Leshner, 1997). Others have reported the need for and the contribution of supportive services to treatment outcomes (Ball and Ross, 1991; McLellan et al., 1994; Widman et al., 1997).

Adolescents with a drug abuse problem are another special needs population and one that is still growing overall despite the decline at younger ages (Johnston et al., 1997). When there is co-occurring mental illness or physical handicaps in this population the need for integrated services becomes even more important. Yet few are able to receive treatment from a single source. And if they do find treatment they may be subject to conflicting directions of mental health and substance abuse clinicians. Left to the mercies of these disparate systems, many such young people fall through the cracks (National Health Policy Forum, 1998).

Other special needs in consumers of drug abuse services also have motivated a services delivery approach to treatment. For example, drug abusers are at high risk of contracting the human immunodeficiency virus (HIV), and those with HIV have significant medical needs that cannot be managed in many treatment programs (e.g., HIV treatment, tuberculosis monitoring and diagnosis, and treatment of sexually transmitted diseases) (Selwyn, 1996). Many community-based treatment organizations (CBOs) that treat drug abuse are not equipped to manage on-going primary care for these complex needs. This has motivated some programs to integrate primary care services with drug abuse services for these special populations, typically in university-based settings, but the effectiveness of integrated services requires systematic evaluation. Similarly, drug abusing women and their children require a composite of services to effect positive outcomes (Rahdert, 1996) (see Box 2.1). In the California comprehensive model of care for drug-addicted women, the relationship between services offered and outcome is currently being evaluated (Brindis et al., 1997).

Evaluations of the effectiveness of service delivery methods have identified important variables in determining outcome, including patient factors at treatment, duration and intensity of treatment, and service delivery methods and their determinants (McLellan et al., 1996). Outcome studies of a wide variety of programs and service delivery methods demonstrate, when keeping patient characteristics, treatment intensity, and duration constant, some programs have much more success than others. In another study of subjects receiving methadone only, standard methadone treatment, and enhanced methadone services, the enhanced treatment group demonstrated the greatest improvement in the areas of personal adjustment and public health and safety risk (McLellan et al., 1993).

However, reviews of multimodal service delivery across a variety of settings indicate that many modalities had not been sufficiently evaluated (Floyd et al., 1996). Properly designed research is needed to assess the extent to which improvement in outcome can be expected using various increments of treatment intensity. This requires systematic variation in treatment dose as a key element in determining outcomes. In order to determine the most cost-effective mix of treatment and service delivery methods, much more well-designed health services research must be conducted in this area.

According to a state agency chief and research director who were interviewed by a committee member, state planners would like research in community programs to address such issues as:

- How brief can brief contacts be and still be effective?
- How much do interventions cost (including assessment, training, consultation, and administrative costs, cost efficacy and cost offsets)?
- Where should treatment be provided? Examples: medical center, home, workplace, telephone contacts? (See Appendix J)

Treatment Approaches That Are Understudied in Research

Just as research findings have been underutilized in the treatment community, there are treatment approaches that have been understudied by the research community. In committee roundtables providers said they needed

BOX 2.1
Pregnant and Parenting Women

She has been hiding her drinking, but doesn't know how much longer she can fool the people around her. She is ignoring the kids and feels guilty, seems like all of the time now. She is terrified that her ex-husband will find out that she's drinking so much and get the judge to take the children away from her. Maybe he should—"I'm a lousy mother anyway." Someone told her about a clinic where she could get sober. "Would it work for me? Can I afford it? Who will take care of my kids?"

The first place women go to get help is their primary care provider. Here, screening for substance abuse is uncommon, so substance abusing women go unrecognized. When these practitioners do discover their client's substance abuse they often are judgmental. This especially is true if the woman seeking help is pregnant or has young children. The provider has to decide whose rights to consider, the mother's or her children's. Most commonly the rights of the women are secondary. This can lead to loss of custody of her children, her unborn baby, and to prosecution for her. A woman will avoid this punitive environment often putting herself, her baby, and her other children at further risk.

Substance abuse is rising among young women and this has brought new challenges to the treatment community. Most treatment models are based on experience with men, and do not work well for women. Research has shown that women have better treatment outcomes if their treatment is based on a family model of care that includes gender-specific treatment. Therapeutic modalities shown to be effective for women include group therapy, treatment separated from males, and the use of female therapists. Comprehensive services that include the needs of children like day hospitalization for their mother, residential treatment, and prevention services for them also seem promising.

Federal legislation in recent years has spawned the growth of women's services within existing treatment venues and the development of a significant number of new programs. The treatment community in California for example, has used these legislative initiatives to develop a continuum of programs that extend from prevention to residential treatment. The rapid development of women's programs has not permitted systematic evaluation of treatment effectiveness. *This is a unique opportunity for the research and treatment communities.* Researchers have the chance to study treatment through all stages of its development and implementation. CBOs that treat women may be more receptive to research since their organizations are relatively new, often based on scientific theory, and less entrenched than those providers with a longer treatment tradition. The development of evidence-based treatment for women is an opportunity to set a research agenda that is bidirectional, collaborative, and creates partnerships between researchers and providers.

SOURCES: Abcott (1994); Brindis et al. (1997); Brindis and Theidon (1997); Garcia (1993); Grella (1996); Kaufman (1996); Light et al. (1996); Mallouh (1996); Naegle (1988); Pokorni and Stanga (1996); Ripple and Luthar (1996); Samsioe and Abreg (1996); Streissguth (1993).

practical, relevant research results that they could implement with the resources available to them. Some representatives of community-based drug treatment programs expressed the belief that researchers were not knowledgeable about community-based treatments. They suggested providers should be involved in research from the beginning to help formulate research questions that were important to them, rather than just serving as a research site for investigating researchers' ideas. As the paper by McLellan and McKay points out there is a strong need to identify clinical and policy issues that should be the focus of future research to fill the gaps between what is known and what needs to be known (see Appendix D). The committee found little evidence of research that systematically examines the distribution of treatment research across different kinds of modalities of drug abuse treatment.

The National Institute on Drug Abuse recognizes that very few researchers are studying therapeutic communities, and the research that has been done tends to focus on assessing their overall effectiveness rather than investigating how they work, why, or for whom (Chasnoff et al., 1996). Consequently, NIDA has given a prominent role in its new treatment initiative to increasing research with therapeutic communities (Leshner, 1997).

The treatment modality most commonly available is the outpatient modality. Outpatient programs offer counseling to drug abusers or their families. The term "outpatient" encompasses a variety of treatment programs that may have little in common, except that they do not offer a place to live (Sorensen and Bernal, 1987). The 1990 NIDA sponsored Alcohol and Drug Research Study found that outpatient "drug-free" treatment accounted for approximately half of the total treatment, and were offered in 71 percent of all facilities (Batten et al., 1993). Preliminary data from a SAMHSA study carried out by the same researchers in 1997 showed that outpatient nonmethadone treatment accounted for more than 60 percent of total treatment in a national sample of drug and alcohol treatment facilities (see Appendix E).

Other nontraditional treatment programs may be more widespread than research evidence would indicate. For example, acupuncture treatment of addiction is commonplace in the growing drug court movement. The National Acupuncture Detoxification Association points out that acupuncture is used in over 200 programs across the United States. There have been many studies of its potential usefulness but until now these studies have generally provided equivocal results because of design, sample size, and other factors. A review of 22 controlled clinical trials of acupuncture for addiction treatment concluded that the strength of positive findings varied inversely with the methodological rigor of the study (Ter Riet et al., 1990). Widespread support for acupuncture has persisted despite these review findings. An NIH consensus development panel reviewed this issue in November 1997 and concluded there are promising results in some areas (e.g., dental and postoperative pain and chemotherapy nausea and vomiting); in other situations (e.g., addiction, stroke rehabilitation, and asthma), acupuncture may be useful as an adjunct treatment or included in a comprehensive management program. They cited the emergence of plausible mechanisms for the therapeutic effects of acupuncture as encouraging and concluded that "there is sufficient evidence of its potential value to conventional medicine to encourage further studies. There is [also] sufficient evidence of acupuncture's value to expand its use into correctional medicine and encourage further studies of its physiology and clinical value" (NIH, 1997).

Studies of patient factors, treatment factors, and community factors in treatment outcome research are all needed, as are studies of the effect of payment level and political environment on treatment outcome. Treatment provider professionals have a variety of questions that could be addressed in research but are not receiving sufficient attention. Patient factors have been much more widely studied than have treatment setting or modality, perhaps because there are few measures of treatment setting or treatment services. Treatment providers speaking to the committee recommended directing research attention to such challenging problems as community resistance to the placement of drug treatment facilities, the so-called "NIMBY" (not in my back yard) problem. This is a problem that requires measurement of neighborhood and organizational systems, as well as individuals. Several workshop participants commented on the role that the different perspectives of researchers and treatment programs played in determining what research was done. One participant reported that in her state the treatment and research communities held differing views of addiction, one favoring the disease model and the other a behavioral model, which presented a barrier to research collaboration. There are substantially different views about the desired "outcome" of an addiction treatment. For example, studies using an outcome of "percentage improvement" in needle use will have little credibility with a clinician who believes that abstinence is necessary for recovery to occur.

Many clinical trials exclude the classes of patients that are most prevalent in community-based agencies, and consequently findings from such research do not seem relevant when viewed by treatment providers. To illustrate, studies of treatment techniques for cocaine abusers commonly screen out potential participants who are also abusing alcohol. This not only limits the generalizability of the research, it also reduces the study's credibility to the provider community, because cocaine abusers normally present for treatment with alcohol abuse and a variety of other problems that would have led to their exclusion from much research. Another difficult but important population needing study is the large and seemingly growing number of individuals with co-occurring mental illness and substance abuse problems.

Stated in the vocabulary of health services research, the treatment community perceives there is a surfeit of "efficacy" research (studies conducted under controlled experimental conditions) and a shortage of "effectiveness" studies (where treatment modalities are studied under real-world conditions). Many of the treatments that receive research attention are resource-intensive interventions studied under rarefied conditions for fixed periods of time.

A comprehensive review of the treatment outcomes literature prepared for the committee is included as Appendix D. This review of what treatment has been studied offers some starting points for filling in the gaps between what is known and what needs to be studied. While the authors acknowledge that the existing literature is disappointing with regard to informing practice at the level of the community treatment program, they identify findings from controlled clinical research that have been significantly and repeatedly related to favorable outcomes and do suggest important directions for treatment practice in the real world. Their findings also suggest that a reader will get substantially different views about the outcome of treatment, depending upon the perspective taken regarding what "outcome" is and when, how, and by whom it is measured. The paragraph below illustrates the significance of this point.

> A quality assurance or service delivery evaluation of [an adduction] treatment [program] might conclude that the program "had very good outcomes" since there was no waiting for treatment entry and at discharge, more than 80 percent of the patients were "highly satisfied" with their counselor and clinician. A clinical researcher, having interviewed a sample of patients at admission to the program, and again six months following discharge, might conclude that the program "had mixed outcomes" since at the follow-up point, only 50% of the patients were abstinent (the intended goal of the program), but there was a 70 percent reduction in frequency of drinking and a 50 percent reduction in medical and psychiatric symptoms. Meanwhile, an economist or health policy analyst might have used Medicaid data tapes to compare the health services utilization rates of a sample of discharged patients, two years prior to their treatment admission and two years following their discharge. The conclusion here might be that "treatment had very poor outcome" since there had been no decrease in medical care utilization from the pre- to the post-treatment period, hence no "cost-offset" to the public. (McLellan and McKay, Appendix D).

Overall, there is a need to distinguish between what has been understudied and what has been studied substantially but found to be ineffective. In this field, as in other areas of health care, therapeutic practices remain prevalent in the field even though they have not been tested or shown to be effective. There is a pressing need to catalogue the treatments that have been proven to be effective and to develop a research agenda that will stimulate systematic review of the others.

Policies That Impede Treatment

Further, there is a need to review the policies that may put barriers in the way of the utilization of proven treatments and the development of new ones. For example, state regulations can be a barrier to the integration of methadone treatment into comprehensive treatment facilities and laws in some states prohibit methadone maintenance entirely. State regulation is an even greater barrier for treatment providers desiring to use newly developed medications. Each state is responsible for amending its narcotics regulations to permit treatment with new medications. This slow, cumbersome process can take several years and is a barrier to the development and implementation of new treatments (IOM, 1995). And finally, financing policies that bar the use of effective treatment strategies or that contribute to the decline of needed support services (e.g., medical, employment, and social services) should be examined within the context of closing the gaps and making the treatment system work.[1]

BARRIERS TO CLOSING THE GAPS

There are several sets of barriers to be overcome in order to reduce the gaps in understanding and communication across the research, treatment, and policy communities. Some of these barriers are held in common across the three communities. These barriers became readily apparent in the workshops and other data-collection activities carried out by the committee. Some of the principal barriers are described in the remainder of this chapter, and the following chapter identifies some potential solutions. However, as the British Navy story below illustrates (Box 2.2), innovations, even successful ones, do not sell themselves.

Structural Barriers

Community-based drug treatment organizations must comply with the directives and regulations of their funders. Like other publicly funded orga-

---

[1]See Chapter 5, Treatment Financing and Trends in Health Insurance, in *The Development of Medications for the Treatment of Opiate and Cocaine Addictions: Issues for the Government and Private Sector* for a concise review of the complexities of the financing disincentives in this field (IOM, 1995).

BOX 2.2
Controlling Scurvy in the British Navy:
Innovations Do Not Sell Themselves

In 1601, an English sea captain, James Lancaster, conducted an experiment to evaluate the effectiveness of lemon juice in preventing scurvy. The beneficial effect of lemon juice was so clear that one would have expected the British Navy to adopt citrus juice for scurvy prevention on all its ships. But it was not until 1747, about 150 years later, that James Lind, a British Navy physician who knew of Lancaster's results, carried out another scurvy experiment on the *HMS Salisbury*. The scurvy patients who got the citrus fruits were cured in a few days.

Certainly, with this further solid evidence of the ability of citrus fruits to combat scurvy, one would have expected the British Navy to adopt this technological innovation for all ship's crew on long sea voyages. And in fact, it did so. But not until 1795, 48 years later. Scurvy on Navy ships was immediately wiped out. And after only 75 more years, in 1865, the British Board of Trade adopted a similar policy, and eradicated scurvy in the merchant marine.

SOURCE: Condensed from a case illustration in Rogers (1995), originally based on a 1981 article by Frederick Mosteller.

---

nizations, they must justify their existence to their community, payers, and constituency. Concern with survival naturally diverts attention from the development and expansion of the treatment program. Under these circumstances, involvement in research or adoption of new treatments cannot compete with more immediate concerns.

The typical treatment organization is small, employing less than 30 workers. Resource constraints limit the type and range of services the organization can provide, and it often lacks the financial and human resources to participate in research. Even the introduction of new treatment modalities may be impossible for many CBOs without significant external financial support

The core staff will likely include a mix of counselors in recovery and those who were introduced to the field through graduate training. The number and mix of practitioners are sufficient to support a specific treatment program and achieve a sufficient revenue base. However, implementing new psychopharmacological therapies generally requires adding medical staff, and new behavioral interventions may require trained psychologists who are not a part of current staff (Stitzer and Higgins, 1995). CBOs are frequently unable to afford the additional professional time to implement new treatments (Naranjo and Bremmer, 1996). Even those with enough resources may be reluctant to spend the amounts required.

Managers play an important role in implementing organizational change. But many forces may impede them in the dissemination and application of research findings. Changes in Medicaid, for example, may mean changes in billing, documentation of patient care, and services provided. Changes in patient mix create new demands on managers. This is especially true in drug abuse, where treatment needs are specifically linked to the drug used. Since drug user choices are influenced by supply forces, there are often rapid shifts as new types of drugs become more readily available. Managers must be cognizant of drug trends in their constituency and adjust treatment services accordingly. Introduction of new treatment is, understandably, less compelling to managers than dealing with immediate challenges in the external environment.

Factors internal to the organization also occupy managers' attention. When managers are therapists, they may have difficulty providing leadership to implement new treatments. Treatment providers may be reluctant to change methods of treatment. Changes in treatment approaches take time and effort, and many front-line treatment providers do not feel they have the time for such retooling. To the extent that manager-providers share these same attitudes, the likelihood of implementing new treatments is decreased. The manager who is not a provider may be less reluctant to introduce change, but may also be less likely to understand the relevance of new treatment findings to the treatment program's constituency. If the manager is receptive to new findings, he or she may lack the technical or leadership skills to ensure their adoption into treatment.

Financial Barriers

Community-based drug treatment organizations are supported primarily by public funds through block grants, Medicaid, other local funding, and private health insurance. An increasing percentage of their clients come from criminal justice sources. Each of these payors has regulations that affect services provided by CBOs. To receive funding, organizations must comply with a multitude of payor-specific criteria—accurate diagnosis, justification of the medical necessity for the provision of services, documentation of care, and reports about client progress. Payers may limit the intensity and length of care provided. Patient care reporting and billing requirements vary widely across payors, but the CBO must meet all requirements in order to be paid for services.

By accepting block grant funding states accept provisions which affect how drug abuse treatment is delivered. Block grants require the states to ensure the provision of prevention services, outreach for injection drug users, and early intervention for those at risk for HIV. Currently, injection drug users and pregnant women receive priority. Treatment providers must provide mandated services to maintain their financial viability. Block grants also regulate what services can or cannot be provided, for example, generally restricting inpatient care, cash payments to patients, and needle exchange programs. The states pass on these requirements to the treatment provider.

Over-emphasis on drug courts and prison treatment programs can result in treatment funds being carved out or diverted disproportionately into the criminal justice system, with the ironic result that some people needing treatment, especially among the poor, have nowhere else to turn. Communities, in other words, should not require someone to throw a brick through a window in order to get treatment.

Treatment for Addiction:
Advancing the Common Good
Join Together (1998), p. 17.

Since most drug abuse treatment facilities derive a portion of their funding locally, they must also be responsive to community priorities and community opinions. In most communities, public opinion favors criminal justice intervention rather than treatment intervention. This is evidenced in drug interdiction policies at the federal level and community preferences for jailing those who have committed nonviolent offenses while abusing drugs or alcohol.

In order to maintain funding and community support, community providers must often avoid the use of treatments viewed as controversial. This, for example, could restrict the applicability of contingency management techniques. This apparently effective treatment modality is also controversial because it is viewed as rewarding drug abusers for their actions. Likewise, discharge of patients followed by their involvement in a very public crime has direct implications for local funding of drug abuse. In this environment CBOs proceed cautiously when considering the adoption of new treatments. In summary, many CBOs do not have sufficient organizational resources to implement new treatment findings while also dealing with the complexities of their real world political and financial environment.

Education and Training

A sequence of steps must occur for a provider organization to be successful in adopting new treatments. These steps include becoming aware of the new treatment, evaluating its utility in the local setting, trying out the new treatment, adopting the new treatment, and confirming that the new treatment works with local clients. These steps to provider adoption of new treatments require that education and training in the new treatment be provided by the organization. A number of factors contribute to making this a very challenging objective.

There are at least three categories of providers within the drug abuse treatment community: (1) licensed practitioners, educated, at a minimum, at the master's degree level and who have received specific education in drug abuse treatment; (2) nonlicensed practitioners (many with college training in another field) who receive on-the-job training in the provision of drug abuse treatment; and (3) the recovering drug abuser who also has received on-the-job training. (Recovering providers can also be in the other two categories.) One survey of 1,328 drug and alcohol counselors found that about 45 percent of respondents had graduate degrees. Nearly one out of two respondents (46 percent) identified themselves as in recovery. Counselors without degrees (81 percent) and those with associate degrees (72 percent) were more likely to report that they were in recovery. Of those with doctoral degrees 18 percent also reported that they were in recovery (Mulligan et al., 1989).

Professionals with graduate training also receive on-the-job training, but experience is not their only reference point for practice. These providers are more likely to be exposed to a model of life-long learning and to be familiar with the processes of acquiring new formal knowledge to improve their treatment.

Drug abuse treatment providers who gain knowledge primarily through experience and on-the-job training may not be as open or as able to participate in the adoption of new treatments that are outside their experience base. The apprenticeship model of training is more viable where a relatively narrow range of duties are performed and when the work environment is relatively predictable. Predictability is decreasing in jobs in most fields, and this is true in the drug abuse field as well. The introduction of new treatments affecting significant numbers of consumers can be destabilizing to an organization and the providers. Staff may not readily adapt to such a change, especially one that requires a change in their behavioral repertoire that takes them out of their "comfort zone."

Efforts to improve the standards of behavioral health care can also tend to undermine the worker trained in an apprenticeship model. State standards are harder to meet for providers trained in the apprenticeship model. Introduction of state provider-qualification requirements has fueled a debate within the drug abuse treatment community about what constitutes appropriate treatment. This debate may work against the adoption of new treatment modalities in CBOs.

Recovering people fear being taken over by people with letters after their name.

Beny Primm, M.D., Committee Workshop,
July 29, 1997, Washington, D.C.

Even when studies document that a treatment can be successfully implemented in a clinical setting, the challenge of the final stage of transfer to treatment programs is often daunting. It requires training staff in delivering the new treatment, changing attitudes of the providers so they embrace the new treatment, and providing evidence that the new treatment is effective in the local clinic situation. Each of these components of training poses problems for the treatment program. Training must be planned, systematic, and protective of the fidelity of the treatment. Researchers who establish treatment effectiveness are sometimes best able to translate the intervention. With the right skills, these researchers can provide the requisite training, anticipate the difficulties, assist in the process of changing provider attitudes, and encourage providers to "own" the research. If this transfer of ownership does not happen the prospects are poor for sustaining the intervention after the researchers are gone (Altman, 1995).

However, few incentives currently exist for researchers to participate in the final processes necessary for a successful adoption. Researchers may not have the skills or may be unwilling to engage in on-site training and mentoring of providers as they implement new treatments. When a CBO is ready to implement the new treatment findings, their research partners have often gone on to other studies. Researchers are generally interested in testing new treatment paradigms, and they are more likely to be funded when they design experimental research. These disincentives have impeded research translation. Neither research translation nor dissemination plans are explicitly weighted in the evaluation criteria for research grants. Dissemination activities count far less than scientific publications for academic promotion. Consequently, there is little organized effort to disseminate research to practice and those who do conduct such activities often do not have the organizational status to successfully carry out this difficult task. This is by no means a problem unique to community-based drug treatment. All too little effort goes into ensuring the use of evidence-based practices in any health care field.

Research is like insurance, it is often sold but seldom bought.

Robert O. Phillips, NAADAC Southwest Regional Vice President, Committee Workshop, September 8, 1997, Albuquerque, NM

Effects of Stigma

Stigma is a special problem for the drug abuse treatment field in many ways. As with other chronic, relapsing medical conditions, there is no cure for addiction, but the existing treatments allow for successful management of addiction and prevent the development of more expensive medical disorders. The major difference is the public's perception of chronic diseases, such as hypertension, diabetes, and asthma as clearly medical conditions, where addiction is more often viewed as a social problem or character deficit. There is no serious argument against supporting health care systems for hypertension, diabetes, or asthma, but there is still much debate regarding support for treatments of addiction (O'Brien and McLellan, 1996).

People who work in drug abuse treatment programs may face a very personal problem of stigma. In many places working in this field is considered a mark of failure. The existence of the programs is often in doubt. Public drug treatment programs often are inadequately funded and staffed and have long waiting lists. The NIMBY syndrome defeats many efforts to site new drug treatment facilities (see Chasnoff et al., 1996, and Box 2.3).

There are few advocates for drug abuse treatment. Persons who have other chronic disorders, or who have family members with those disorders, benefit from disease specific advocacy efforts like the American Heart Association, the American Cancer Society, or the American Lung Association. These organizations educate the public about these disorders, and they provide some (although usually limited) direct services to their "victims." They raise money to support research and educate policymakers to help obtain additional funds for research and treatment. Because people see those with heart disease, cancer, or birth defects as "victims," they are willing to contribute through private channels and with tax moneys to fight those disorders. Unlike these fields in which patient groups provide a strong voice for treatment and research, generally little is heard from people who suffer from addictive disorders.

Some advocacy groups have been successful however. The Gay Men's Health Crisis and other AIDS advocacy groups have been very successful

---

BOX 2.3
A Closed Door

At the request of his state drug abuse authority, one member of this committee opened a methadone clinic in a rural community. At a get-acquainted meeting with the city fathers, he was told bluntly that the community leaders did not want methadone treatment in their area. They were not interested in research data showing methadone's reduction of crime and health-care costs; they preferred that those who needed methadone treatment move to a city with a methadone clinic.

---

despite the double societal stigmas of their disease. The National Alliance for the Mentally Ill (NAMI) is an excellent example of effective advocacy efforts lead by family, friends, and supporters of those who suffer from mental illness. The National Alliance of Methodone Advocates (NAMA) also provides a working example of how those most affected by addiction can advocate for themselves.

Another stigmatizing factor is job status. To a greater degree than in other chronic disorders, the field of addiction has in the past had large numbers of workers who have themselves experienced the problem. This included physicians and nurses as well. Of all the health care treatment programs, drug abuse treatment may be the most frequent employer of its own graduates. Historically, and to some extent yet today, the ranks of counseling have been filled with significant numbers of former drug abusers, while the ranks of administrators have been less so (Brown, 1997). This disparity in status is often complicated by co-occurring ethnic differences.

Recovering workers have been increasingly accepted as effective counselors (Christensen and Jacobson, 1994), and there has been a growth in the development of certification programs for drug abuse counselors. Nonetheless, credentialing requirements tend to discriminate against experientially trained staff, and counselors in recovery are challenged to develop a more theoretical perspective and apply research in their clinical work.

The stigma of the field may also contribute to the lack of mainstreaming of substance abuse in the curricula of undergraduate and graduate programs in health-related fields. The recommendations of the 1995 conference on training sponsored by the Macy Foundation represent a step in the right direction as does the inclusion of this training objective, for the first time, in the National Drug Control Strategy (ONDCP, 1998).

The Macy report recommended training about drug and alcohol abuse for all primary care physicians (i.e., family-practice, internal medicine, pediatrics, and obstetrics-gynocology). Internal Medicine residency programs are now required to have this training (Josiah Macy, Jr. Foundation, 1995).

Subsequently an IOM committee also made training recommendations in this area. Their investigation led them to conclude that the lack of courses in addiction starts a cycle of shortages at every stage of the professional pipeline, and that as a result fewer undergraduates are exposed to scientific information about addiction, fewer graduate students and medical students express interest in the field, causing fewer administrators to seek faculty with addiction expertise, resulting in fewer young professionals on the faculty, and ultimately, fewer senior faculty to mentor those who might be interested in practicing addiction medicine or doing research in this field (IOM, 1997a).

Objective 4: Support and promote the education, training, and credentialing of professionals who work with substance abusers.

From Goal 3 of Strategic Goals and Objectives of the 1998 National Drug Control Strategy; ONDCP (1998), p. 27.

There appear to be few opportunities for training in a community setting, for either physicians or other health professionals. One such program, Physicians in Residence, provides a hands-on, five day program for residents which includes training and practice in interviewing, assessment and treatment planning, as well as participation in AA meetings. Residents left the program reporting confidence in their new skills, however, a follow-up evaluation suggested they needed continuing support to integrate and maintain these skills in a work environment where substance abusers were less interested in treatment (Levin et al., 1996). Addiction treatment training, as well as research training in community-based treatment facilities requires more opportunities for hands-on experience and continuing education.

Inadequate Knowledge Base About Technology Transfer

There is little information about spread of innovations in drug treatment and how treatment programs use research findings in their work. A qualitative approach to studying technology transfer occurs more frequently than quantitative procedures, and sophisticated research techniques are the exception rather than the rule. Typically, surveys in this field do not include questions about the adoption of new treatment techniques.

NIDA's main extramurally funded research study on technology transfer, according to Backer (1991), was conducted over a six-year period in the

1980s and concerned a method for providing employment-related training for ex-drug abusers (Hall et al., 1988; Sorensen et al., 1988). This random assignment study found that dissemination methods employing personal contacts (site visits and conferences) produced significantly more adoptions than did printed materials alone. There were also adopter site differences: residential programs were more likely to adopt the employment workshop than were outpatient programs.

Published case studies include a description of the implementation of NIDA's cocaine prevention program (Forman and Lachter, 1989). NIDA also sponsored a project to educate injection drug users about HIV risk reduction outside of drug abuse treatment clinics (Brown, 1995). Their dissemination model included extensive training and technical assistance with a newsletter publicizing the positive outcomes, and annual meetings of program administrators and practitioners. Another case study examined the difficulties of disseminating an alcohol withdrawal protocol and a phar-macotherapy technique (Naranjo and Bremmer, 1996). A case study of an international project called Effective Care in Pregnancy and Childbirth reviews and illustrates the principles involved in "retailing research" to bridge the barriers across the cultures of researchers and practitioners (Lomas, 1993). Technology transfer in drug abuse treatment appears to be a fruitful field for further work.

Policy Barriers

In the environment described above, it is easy for society to ration drug treatment, or reject certain forms of treatment. The usual argument advanced for funding drug abuse treatment is not that addiction is a treatable chronic disease, but that drug abuse treatment is cheaper than prison and cheaper than treating AIDS. Drug-dependence treatment is relatively cheap, although not readily available. Residential treatment programs provide intake evaluations, group and individual counseling, recreational therapies, urine monitoring, transportation to supervised work, regular reports to licensing and referring agencies, housing, and all meals at a daily cost less than the bill for sleeping overnight at a mid-price hotel and considerably less than the costs of staying in jail (Kaskutas, 1998). As shown in Figure 2.1, all federal spending on drug treatment has increased less than inflation in recent years.

Prejudice against addicts can also lead to policies that prevent the use of improved treatment approaches. Research has shown that prolonged maintenance treatment with methadone and other opioid agonists like LAAM (levo-alpha-acetylmethadol) and buprenorphine reduces mortality and morbidity among drug abusers and reduces crime in the community (see Appendix F). However, methadone maintenance treatment is banned in many

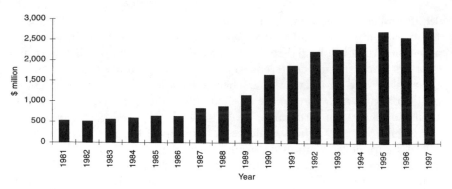

FIGURE 2.1   Federal drug abuse treatment spending, 1981–1997 (millions of dollars). SOURCE: ONDCP (1996, 1997)

communities because of moral disapproval and fear that it will encourage those needing treatment to stay and may attract additional addicts to their community. Similarly, some clinicians still encourage patients to reject methadone maintenance in favor of the less-effective methadone detoxification treatments. Others provide methadone doses that are too low to be fully effective and encourage patients to end maintenance treatment prematurely. Some criminal-justice agencies referring probationers for treatment refuse permission for them to receive methadone maintenance.

> The stereotype that drug abusers could change their behavior if they were sufficiently motivated is inconsistent with understanding the complex, multiple factors involved in addiction. When policymakers view drug abusers as untreatable or undeserving of public support, treatment programs, insurance coverage and training programs may be underfunded or abolished.
>
> *Dispelling the Myths About Addiction* (IOM, 1997a), p. 140.

So, consider the director of the treatment program described at the beginning of this chapter who learns of new research showing that naltrexone improves outcome in alcoholic patients and in heroin addicts on probation. His program is funded for interpersonal treatments by relatively inexpensive counseling staff. He cannot buy the expensive new medication, nor hire a physician to prescribe it, nor a nurse (or pharmacist) to dispense it. The director of such a program may well view the research that determined the effectiveness of naltrexone as impractical.

In one sense that director would be right, since society clearly rations health care in the field of drug dependence on a different basis than rationing occurs in other health care areas. Payment is available only for inexpensive treatments, while the research evidence for efficacy of other treatments is disregarded. Such rationing leads to waiting lists as the agency must cut treatment slots and serve fewer people. Decreasing the length of treatment and increasing counselor caseloads also blocks the utilization of new treatments of proven efficacy.

SUMMARY

Considerable resources flow into drug abuse research but it often takes years before research findings change drug abuse treatment. In a review of outcome studies addiction treatment was shown to be about as successful as treatment of other chronic disorders such as hypertension, diabetes, and asthma. Indeed, less than 50 percent of patients with insulin-dependent diabetes, and less than 30 percent of patients with hypertension or asthma, comply with their medication regimens, with consequently sizable rates of reoccurrence or worsening of condition. These rates are comparable to success rates for treatment of persons with addictive disorders, (O'Brien and McLellan, 1996). Treatment is the most effective way to cut drug use and drug abuse treatment is clearly cost-effective from a societal perspective (Caulkins et al., 1997; Gerstein et al., 1994; SAMHSA, 1997). Despite this evidence, less than 20 percent of those who need treatment are receiving it and there are many barriers to implementing better treatment and providing better access.

With the knowledge explosion taking place in understanding the biology of the brain and the mechanisms of addiction, it is difficult for the best informed and best intentioned treatment provider, researcher, or state substance abuse director to keep abreast of the science. As new treatment questions and new research answers flow out of the new scientific understanding, new policy questions arise. It is important to enhance the exchange of information and knowledge among the research, treatment, and policy areas in order to bring the benefits of treatment research to the drug treatment consumer and to society.

In summary, there are many gaps in communication among treatment, research, and policy, the three key segments of the drug abuse treatment community. These gaps are caused (or exacerbated) by a set of critical barriers to better communication and coordination. Other barriers include lack of advocacy efforts, and lack of training opportunities (and requirements) in substance abuse treatment and research for all health-related professions. In addition, many CBOs lack organizational resources to implement new treatment findings while they are struggling with the complexities of a shifting political and financial environment. The committee concluded that there are ways to overcome the barriers and narrow the gaps and the following chapter describes a variety of models to aid this effort.

REFERENCES

Abcott AA. 1994. A feminist approach to substance abuse treatment and service delivery. *Social Work in Health Care* 19(3–4):67–83.

Altman DG. 1995. Sustaining interventions in community systems: On the relationship between researchers and communities. *Health Psychology* 14:526–536.

Backer TE. 1991. *Drug Abuse Technology Transfer*. Rockville, MD: National Institute on Drug Abuse.

Ball JC, Ross A. 1991. *The Effectiveness of Methadone Maintenance Treatment*. New York: Springer-Verlag.

Batten JL, Horgan CM, Prottas JM, Simon LJ, Larson MJ, Elliott EA, Bowden ML, Lee M. 1993. *Drug services research survey phase I final report: Non-correctional facilities (revised)*. Institute for Health Policy, Brandeis University.

Brahen LS, Capone T, Bloom S et al. 1978. An alternative to methadone for probationer addicts: Narcotic antagonist treatment. *Contemporary Drug Issues* 13:117–132.

Brindis CD, Theidon KS. 1997. The role of case management in substance abuse treatment services for women and their children. *Journal of Psychoactive Drugs* 29(1):79–88.

Brindis CD, Berkowitz G, Clayson Z, Lamb B. 1997. California's approach to perinatal substance abuse: Toward a model of comprehensive care. *Journal of Psychoactive Drugs* 29(1):113–122.

Brown BS. 1995. Reducing impediments to technology transfer in drug abuse. In: Backer TE, David SL, Soucy G eds. *Reviewing the behavioral science knowledge base on technology transfer*. NIDA Research Monograph 155. Rockville, MD: National Institute on Drug Abuse. Pp. 169–185.

Brown BS. 1997. Staffing patterns and services for the war on drugs. In: Fox DM, Egertson J, Leshner AI eds. *Treating Drug Abusers Effectively*. Malden, MA: Blackwell Publishers. Pp. 99–124.

Calsyn DA, Saxon AJ, Barndt DC. 1991. Urine screening practice in methadone maintenance clinics: A survey of how the results are used. *Journal of Nervous and Mental Disorders* 179:222–227.

Caplehorn JRM, Bell J. 1991. Methadone dosage and retention of patients in maintenance treatment. *Medical Journal of Australia* 154:195–199.

Caulkins JP, Rydell CP, Schwabe WJ, Chisea J. 1997. *Mandatory Minimum Sentences: Throwing Away the Key or the Taxpayers' Money?* Santa Monica, CA: RAND Drug Policy Research Center.

Chasnoff IJ, Marques PR, Strantz IH, Farrow J, Davis S. 1996. Building bridges: Treatment research partnerships in the community. *NIDA Research Monographs* 166:6–21.

Christensen A, Jacobson NS. 1994. Who (or what) can do psychotherapy: The status and challenge of nonprofessional therapies. *Psychological Science* 5:8–14.

D'Aunno T, Vaughn TE. 1992. Variations in methadone treatment practices. Results from a national study. *Journal of the American Medical Association* 267:253–258.

Drug Strategies. 1997. *Cutting Crime: Drug Courts in Action*. Washington, DC: Drug Strategies.

Eisenberg JE. 1986. *Doctors' Decisions and the Cost of Medical Care*. Ann Arbor, MI: Health Administration.

Etheridge RM, Craddock SG, Dunteman GH, Hubbard RL. 1995. Treatmetnt services in two national studies of community-based drug abuse treatment programs. *Journal of Substance Abuse* 7:9–26.

Ferguson JH. 1995. Technology transfer: Consensus and participation. The NIH Consensus Development Program. *Joint Commission Journal on Quality Improvement* 21(7):332–336.

Fiorentine R, Anglin MD. 1997. Does increasing the opportunity for counseling increase the effectiveness of outpatient drug treatment? *American Journal of Drug and Alcohol Abuse* 23(3):369–382.

Floyd AS, Monahan SC, Finney JW, Morley JA. 1996. Alcoholism treatment outcome studies, 1980–1992: The nature of the research. *Addictive Behavior* 21(4):413–428.

Forman A, Lachter SB. 1989. The National Institute on Drug Abuse cocaine prevention campaign. In: Shoemaker P ed. *Communication Campaigns About Drugs: Government, Media, and the Public.* Hillsdale, NJ: Lawrence Erlbaum Associates.

Garcia SA. 1993. Maternal drug abuse: Laws and ethics as agents of just balances and therapeutic interventions. *International Journal of the Addictions* 28(13):1311–1339.

Gerstein DR, Harwood H, Fountain D, Suter N, Malloy K. 1994. *Evaluating Recovery Services: The California Drug and Alcohol Treatment Assessment (CALDATA).* Contract No. 92-00110. Sacramento, CA: State of California Department of Alcohol and Drug Programs.

Grella CE. 1996. Background and overview of mental health and substance abuse treatment systems: Meeting the needs of women who are pregnant or parenting. *Journal of Psychoactive Drugs* 28(4):319–343.

Hall SM, Sorensen JL, Loeb P. 1988. Development and diffusion of a skill training intervention. In: Baker TB, Cannon DS eds. *Addictive Disorders: Psychological Research on Assessment and Treatment.* New York: Praeger Scientific Press. Pp. 180–204.

Higgins ST, Budney AJ, Bickel WK, Foerg FE, Donham R, Badger GJ. 1994. Incentives improve outcome in patient behavioral treatment of cocaine dependence. *Archives of General Psychiatry* 51(7):568–576.

Hoffman JA, Caudill BD, Koman JJ, Luckey JW, Flynn PM, Hubbard RL. 1994. Comparative cocaine abuse treatment strategies: Enhancing client retention and treatment exposure. In: Magura S, Rosenblum A eds. *Experimental Therapeutics in Addiction Medicine.* Binghamton, NY: The Hayworth Medical Press. Pp. 115–128.

IOM (Institute of Medicine). 1995. *The Development of Medications for the Treatment of Opiate and Cocaine Addictions: Issues for the Government and Private Sector.* Washington, DC: National Academy Press.

IOM. 1997a. *Dispelling the Myths About Addiction: Strategies to Increase Understanding and Strengthen Research.* Washington, DC: National Academy Press.

IOM. 1997b. *Information Trading: How Information Influences the Health Policy Process.* Washington, DC: National Academy Press.

Johnston LD, O'Malley PM, Bachman JG. 1997. *Monitoring the Future Study.* Rockville, MD: National Institute on Drug Abuse.

Join Together. 1998. *Treatment for Addiction: Advancing the Common Good.* Boston, MA: Join Together.

Josiah Macy, Jr. Foundation. 1995. *Training About Alcohol and Substance Abuse for All Primary Care Physicians. Proceedings of a Conference.* Phoenix, AZ, October 2–5, 1994. New York: Josiah Macy, Jr. Foundation.

Kaskutas LA. 1998. Methodology and characteristics of programs and clients in the social model process evaluation. *Journal of Substance Abuse Treatment* 15(1):19–25.

Kaufman E. 1996. Diagnosis and treatment of drug and alcohol abuse in women. *American Journal of Obstetrics and Gynecology* 174(1):21–27.

Leshner AI. 1997. Introduction to the special issue: The National Institute on Drug Abuse's (NIDA's) Drug Abuse Treatment Outcome Study (DATOS). *Psychology of Addictive Behaviors* 11(4):211–215.

Lester JP. 1993. The utilization of policy analysis by state agency officials. *Knowledge: Creation, Diffusion, Utilization* 14:267–290.

Levin FR, Owen P, Rabinowitz E, Pace N. 1996. Physicians in Residence Program: An evaluation of a novel substance abuse training approach for residents in primary care specialties. *Substance Abuse* 17(1):5–18.

Light JM, Irvine KM, Kjerulf L. 1996. Estimating genetic and environmental effects of alcohol use and dependence from a national survey: A "quasi-adoption" study. *Journal of Studies on Alcohol* 57(5):507–520.

Lomas J. 1993. Retailing research: Increasing the role of evidence in clinical service for childbirth. *Milbank Quarterly* 71(3):439–475.

Mallouh C. 1996. The effects of dual diagnosis on pregnancy and parenting. *Journal of Psychoactive Drugs* 28(4):367–380.

McLellan AT, Arndt IO, Metzger DS, Woody GE, O'Brien CP. 1993. The effects of psychosocial services in substance abuse treatment. *Journal of the American Medical Association* 269(15):1953–1959.

McLellan AT, Alterman AI, Metzger DS, Grissom GR, Woody GE, Luborsky L, O'Brien CP. 1994. Similarity of outcome predictors across opiate, cocaine, and alcohol treatments: Role of treatment services. *Journal of Consulting and Clinical Psychology* 62(6):1141–1158.

McLellan AT, Woody GE, Metzger D, McKay J, Durrelll J, Alterman AI, O'Brien CP. 1996. Evaluating the effectiveness of addiction treatments: Reasonable expectations, appropriate comparisons. *Milbank Quarterly* 74(1):51–85.

Millman J, Samet S, Shaw J, Braden M. 1990. The dissemination of psychological research. *American Psychologist* 45:668–669.

Mulligan DH, McCarty D, Potter D, Krakow M. 1989. Counselors in public and private alcoholism and drug abuse treatment programs. *Alcoholism Treatment Quarterly* 6(3/4):75–89.

Naegle MA. 1988. Substance abuse among women: Prevalence, patterns, and treatment issues. *Issues in Mental Health Nursing* 9:127–137.

Naranjo CA, Bremmer KE. 1996. Dissemination of research results regarding the pharmacotherapy of substance abuse: Case examples and a critical review. *Substance Abuse* 17:39–50.

National Health Policy Forum. 1998. *Dual Diagnoses: The Challenge of Serving People with Concurrent Mental Illness and Substance Abuse Problems. Issue Brief No. 718.* Washington, DC: National Health Policy Forum.

NIH (National Institutes of Health). 1997. *NIH Consensus Development Conference Statement on Acupuncture: November 3–5, 1997.* Rockville, MD: National Institutes of Health.

O'Brien CP, McLellan AT. 1996. Myths about the treatment of addiction. *Lancet* 347:237–240.

ONDCP (Office of National Drug Control Policy). 1996. *The National Drug Control Strategy, 1996: Program, Resources, and Evaluation.* Washington, DC: Office of National Drug Control Policy.

ONDCP. 1997. *The National Drug Control Strategy, 1997: Budget Summary.* Washington, DC: Office of National Drug Control Policy.

ONDCP. 1998. *The National Drug Control Strategy, 1998: A Ten Year Plan.* Washington, DC: Office of National Drug Control Policy.

Ohio Department of Alcohol and Drug Addiction Services. 1996. *Cost Effectiveness Study 1992–1996: Final Report.* Columbus, OH: Ohio Department of Alcohol and Drug Addiction Services.

Pokorni JL, Stanga J. 1996. Caregiving strategies for young infants born to women with a history of substance abuse and other risk factors. *Pediatric Nursing* 22(6):540–544.

Price RH. 1997. What we know and what we actually do: Best practices and their prevalence. In: Egertson JA, Fox DM, Leshner A eds. *Treating Drug Abusers Effectively.* Malden, MA: Blackwell Publishers. Pp. 125–155.

Rahdert ER, ed. 1996. *Treatment for Drug-Exposed Women and Their Children: Advances in Research Methodology. NIDA Research Monograph 165.* Rockville, MD: National Institute on Drug Abuse.

Ripple CH, Luthar SS. 1996. Familial factors in illicit drug abuse: An interdisciplinary perspective. *American Journal of Drug and Alcohol Abuse* 22(2):147–172.

Rogers EM. 1995. *Diffusion of Innovations.* 4th Edition. New York: Free Press.

Samsioe G, Abreg A. 1996. Ethical issues in obstetrics. *International Journal of Fertility* 41(3):284–287.

Selwyn PA. 1996. The impact of HIV infection on medical services in drug abuse treatment programs. *Journal of Substance Abuse Treatment* 13(5):397–410.

Silverman K, Higgins ST, Brooner RK, Montoya ID, Cone EJ, Schuster CR, Preston KL. 1996. Sustained cocaine abstinence in methadone maintenance patients through voucher-based reinforcement therapy. *Archives of General Psychiatry* 53(5):409–415.

Simpson DW, Joe GW, Brown BS. 1997. Treatment retention and follow-up outcomes in the Drug Abuse Treatment Outcome Study (DATOS). *Psychology of Addictive Behaviors* 11(4):294–307.

Sorensen JL, Bernal B. 1987. *A family like yours: Breaking the patterns of drug abuse.* San Francisco, CA: Harper and Row.

Sorensen JL, Hall SM, Loeb P, Allen T, Glaser EM, Greenberg PD. 1988. Dissemination of a job seekers' workshop to drug treatment programs. *Behavior Therapy* 19:143–155.

Stitzer ML, Higgins ST. 1995. Behavioral treatment of drug and alcohol abuse. In: Bloom FE, Kupfer DJ eds. *Psychopharmacology: The Fourth Generation of Progress.* New York: Raven. Pp. 1807–1819.

Streissguth PA. 1993. Fetal alcohol syndrome in older patients. *Alcohol and Alcoholism* Suppl. 2:209–212.

SAMHSA (Substance Abuse and Mental Health Services Administration). 1997. *National Treatment Improvement Evaluation Study.* Rockville, MD: Substance Abuse and Mental Health Services Administration.

Ter Riet G, Kleijnen J, Knipschild P. 1990. A meta-analysis of studies into the effect of acupuncture on addiction. *British Journal of General Practice* 40(338):379–382.

Volpicelli JR, Alterman AI, Hagashida M, O'Brien CP. 1992. Naltrexone in the treatment of alcohol dependence. *Archives of General Psychiatry* 49:876–880.

Widman M, Platt JJ, Lidz V, Mathis DA, Metzger DS. 1997. Patterns of service use and treatment involvement of methadone maintenance patients. *Journal of Substance Abuse Treatment* 14(1):29–35.

Young WB. 1997. The market for information in health policy: Using the "Just-in-Time" strategy. In: Institute of Medicine. *Information Trading: How Information Influences the Health Policy Process.* Washington, DC: National Academy Press. Pp. 11–26.

3

Approaches to Closing the Gaps

OVERVIEW

Efforts to close the gaps among research, treatment, and policy traditionally focus on education, training, and/or dissemination of information within each separate arena. Even when such activities are effective, they have the potential to change only one group. Thus they generally fall far short of producing systemic change. Changing the system (as Figure 3.1 is meant to illustrate) will require the three groups working together to ask and answer the right questions and to jointly commit to implementation. Consequently, while this report proposes changes within each area, it also proposes joint activities that are needed to produce systemic changes.

Other areas of medical care have developed strategies to facilitate an integration of treatment, research, and policy. These include models for technology transfer, financial and other incentives to encourage organizational change, as well as methods to develop consensus on evidence-based practices and promote their use. The committee also found examples of collaboration that included the development of infrastructures and promoted trust-building between researchers and providers. Based on findings from the committee's workshops, site visits, briefings, and review of the

This chapter was edited by James L. Sorensen with contributions by Kathleen T. Brady, Thomas Crowley, Emily Jean Hauenstein, A. Thomas McLellan, and Steven M. Mirin.

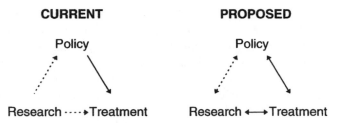

FIGURE 3.1 Need for bidirectional communication.

literature, several models are described here and in the following chapters that could help to bridge the gaps among stakeholders in this field:

- technology transfer models;
- organizational change models;
- practice guidelines;
- consensus conferences and evidence-based reviews;
- top-down incentives models;
- models that incorporate trust-building experiences;
- practice-based research networks (see Box 4.3); and
- collaboration case studies (see Chapter 5).

TECHNOLOGY TRANSFER MODELS

The knowledge base on technology transfer has grown rapidly in the last fifteen years. By one estimate the citations in this field exceeded 10,000 by 1995.[1] Experts make several distinctions that are useful in considering how to close the gaps between research, treatment, and policy in the drug-abuse area. They distinguish between technology transfer that is "hard" (e.g., equipment) and "soft" (e.g., counseling methods), and between technologies that are "high" (requiring substantial capital) and "low" (requiring relatively little investment). They differentiate between "embodied" technologies (involving a physical entity like a new drug) and "disembodied" technologies (e.g., a new counseling procedure) (Backer, 1991). Technology experts also distinguish between "information dissemination" activities (e.g., information clearinghouses) and "knowledge utilization" activities that provide assistance in adoption efforts after information is available.

A recent Institute of Medicine report (IOM, 1994) makes another use-

---

[1]For overviews of this area see the following works: (Backer, 1991; Backer et al., 1986; Glaser et al., 1983; Rogers, 1995a).

ful distinction when the goal is bidirectional communication, as it is in this study. In *Reducing the Risks for Mental Disorders*, the IOM committee used the term "knowledge exchange" because it emphasizes the need for two-way communication, including feedback. This report will do the same. By contrast, the term "dissemination" has a connotation of directionality, and is used when only a one-way flow of information is implied. Studies in the 1960s and 1970s established that information dissemination alone is usually insufficient to stimulate change in individuals or in organizations. Studies in the 1970s and 1980s explored more active methods of promoting information utilization and developed strategies to aid that end. Recent work has been concerned with consolidating these principles into programmatic strategies (Backer et al., 1995).

The National Institute on Drug Abuse and the Center for Substance Abuse Treatment both have technology transfer programs which include knowledge exchange as well as dissemination activities. NIDA dissemination tools include videotapes, program assessment packages, and clinical reports (see for example NIDA [1993]). Treatment topics (e.g., relapse prevention, methadone, and special population treatment issues) are addressed in videotapes. The NIDA web site (http://www.nida.nih.gov) includes "NIDA capsules," which describe the effect of individual drugs, extent of current use by age groups, and new research findings (see Appendix G). NIDA Infofax (1-888-NIH-NIDA) provides quick access to science-based facts on drug abuse and addiction. NIDA is placing increasing emphasis on knowledge exchange activities. The goal of the NIDA Treatment Initiative is to improve the quality of drug addiction treatment through reciprocal exchanges of ideas and information among the research, treatment and policy communities, and the public; and to stimulate research in areas of treatment most relevant to the public health. Treatment Initiative activities include national conferences on research and practice, and online town meetings to bring the latest drug abuse research findings to communities and to receive feedback about community needs (Leshner, 1997; NIDA, 1996).

CSAT produces a technical Treatment Assistance Publication Series (TAPS) that includes detailed clinical guidelines for such clinical activities as relapse prevention. CSAT by FAX is a one-page newsletter featuring recent developments in treatment (see Appendix G). It is faxed to all treatment programs that receive any CSAT funding and was regularly mentioned by providers participating in the committee workshops and site visits as something they valued. The CSAT dissemination program includes a Treatment Improvement Protocol (TIPS) series that covers a wide variety of treatment topics ranging from infectious disease screening to drug specific treatment recommendations (see Appendix H). Providers attending the workshops were familiar with the TIPS publications but considered their length and lack of a standard format to be a barrier in clinic use. An evaluation of this program is currently under way. A CSAT knowledge exchange activity is the Treatment Improvement Exchange (TIE) program to promote information exchange between CSAT staff and state and local alcohol and drug abuse agencies. TIPS and CSAT by Fax are both available on the Treatment Improvement Exchange. TIE is accessible via the CSAT web site (http://www.samhsa.gov/csat/csat.htm) or directly (http://www.treatment.org). While workshop participants who use the Internet appreciated this availability, it was evident that a significant number of providers still do not have effective access to this resource.

ORGANIZATIONAL CHANGE MODELS

An obvious goal of any organization is to maintain its viability. Organizational survival depends on the ability to provide a service or product that someone will buy or support. Increasingly, organizations must anticipate market forces and be able to accommodate rapid changes in their environment. Health care organizations, particularly those that are not-for-profit, traditionally have been somewhat sheltered from severe environmental and market forces. However, recent rapid changes in the financing of health care, including behavioral health care, are affecting community-based drug treatment providers.

As organization size increases, jobs within the organization become more differentiated. The workforce tends to be more stable because larger organizations are more likely to offer full-time employment, benefits, and other employee incentives. Organizational operations become formalized and may include specific procedures for innovation and implementation of new programs. Larger organizations are more likely to have adequate technology and other resources to sustain the extra work efforts that go into the adoption and implementation of new programs.

Many health care organizations have been unable to accommodate to a rapidly changing health care environment and have failed. This is particularly true of small to medium-sized mental health and drug abuse services that are poorly financed compared with organizations that provide mainstream health services. As a consequence, managers of CBOs, especially those that are small in size, focus primarily on maintaining organizational viability. This focus calls for a conservative organizational culture, a trim work force, and the ability to deliver a competitive product. The focus also stimulates attention to health care financing and other environmental changes that affect the resource base of the organization. In this climate, investing in innovation makes organizational sense only if it promotes organizational survival.

Not all organizations can support the kind of innovation necessary to implement the evidenced-based practice guidelines discussed below, for instance. For organizations with appropriate resources, however, being an early adopter of research findings may facilitate recruiting and maintaining a satisfied, high-quality workforce. Even when the innovation supports important organizational goals, innovative programming requires managerial support, adequate financial and human resources, and an organizational culture that values scientifically based practice, problem solving, and creativity (Crump et al., 1996). It is not only small CBOs that are finding it hard to meet these tests.[2] A description of the attributes associated with successful innovation is shown in Box 3.1.

The explicit goals of the organization may support innovation in treatment, but the organizational culture affects its outcome. Organizational culture has been described as the pattern of behaviors developed by groups to solve work-related problems and survive in their jobs (Coeling and Simms, 1993). It is manifested in the organization's beliefs and values, in its normative structure, and through artifacts or symbols (Seago, 1996). It is within this culture that the implicit goals of the organization take root. The culture's strength is determined by the degree of consensus among all levels of workers about which norms dominate and prevail in the actions of the organization. A strong organizational culture among the staff workers which is incongruent with management can defeat management efforts to introduce change (Nystrom, 1993).

Successful adoption of research findings in CBOs depends on careful matching of organizational characteristics, culture, and stages of development. This is discussed further in Chapter 4. Several authors have described an orderly process for adopting new treatments into CBOs when the implementation requires significant change within the organization (Altman, 1995; Nutbeam, 1996; Orlandi, 1996).

---

[2]Innovation is expensive. To support rapid innovation CBOs must be able to manage the up-front costs that are associated with implementation of new technology. This may include acquisition of the tools necessary to implement the programs (new medications, behavioral protocols, assessment measures), training of staff who will implement the new technology, renovation of existing facilities to accommodate the innovation, and acquisition of computer hard and software. CBOs capable of supporting the up-front costs also have to be able to project that the innovation will either pay for itself or generate a profit prior to investing in the new technology. Changing practice invariably means training of existing staff and may involve acquisition of new staff knowledgeable in the technology being adopted. The CBOs must be able to afford a core staff of varying levels of educational and professional expertise who are capable of applying research findings to practice.

BOX 3.1
**Attributes Associated With Innovations
Likely to Be Implemented**

• *Relative Advantage*—the degree to which a new idea is perceived as superior to the existing practice that it replaces.

• *Compatibility*—the degree to which an innovation is perceived by an individual as similar to previous experience or to beliefs and values.

• *Complexity*—the degree to which a new idea is perceived as relatively easy to understand.

• *Trialability*—the degree to which an innovation can be divided for experimental use by an individual.

• *Observability*—the degree to which a new idea can easily be seen by others.

SOURCE: Rogers EM. 1995b. Lessons for Guidelines from the Diffusion of Innovations. *Joint Commission Journal on Quality Improvement* 21(7):324–328.

PRACTICE GUIDELINES AND SCORECARDS IN ADDICTIONS TREATMENT

The development of practice guidelines might help close the gap among the three segments of the drug abuse field, as well as improve clinical outcomes and enhance the credibility of caregivers. Both payers and policymakers have voiced skepticism about the efficacy of treatment for substance use disorders. In part, this skepticism is based on anecdotal experience, along with biases rooted in stigma and a history of perceived abuses of the reimbursement system by some providers. To some extent these same barriers operate at the interface between the substance treatment community and the rest of health care system.

Guidelines are relatively new in this field. The American Society of Addiction Medicine (ASAM) has published placement criteria, and the American Psychiatric Association (APA) has published comprehensive practice guidelines for this patient population (APA, 1996). The psychiatric practice guidelines are based on review and synthesis of the currently available treatment literature, complimented where appropriate by the experience of a group of skilled clinician reviewers. Sequential drafts of the guidelines were reviewed by a national sample of individual clinicians and researchers, as well as numerous professional organizations and governmental agencies in the addictions field.

The psychiatric practice guidelines include principles of treatment applicable to all forms of substance use disorder, as well as sections on the assessment and management of patients with alcohol, cocaine, and opioid-related disorders. They provide a framework for choosing among treatment options and make specific recommendations wherever possible, based on the strength of available research findings as well as the perceived degree of clinical consensus among practicing clinicians. Treatments that have not been adequately tested in well-controlled trials, or treatments where there are conflicting reports about efficacy but which are consistent with expert opinion and generally accepted treatment principles, are recommended with a lower level of clinical confidence or alternatively, recommended to be applied only in specific clinical circumstances. These guidelines leave the ultimate judgment to the clinician, based on data presented by the patient and on the diagnostic and treatment options available. It is anticipated that the guidelines will be revised every three to five years to incorporate emerging research and clinical experience.

Despite the potential benefits of incorporating advances in clinical research into clinical care delivery, many barriers exist to the successful dissemination and adoption of evidence-based practice guidelines within the drug abuse treatment community. A number of factors may contribute to this situation. Chief among them is the heterogeneity in the background, training, and clinical perspectives of clinicians practicing within the addiction treatment community. With the notable exception of methadone maintenance, the relative paucity of clinically effective, medically based treatments for this patient population has helped foster a treatment culture in which many treatment approaches, including self-help and therapeutic communities, have flourished. Heavily influenced by both the experience and world views of recovering drug abusers, this segment of the treatment system has embraced a treatment philosophy and approaches to care that depend more on the motivational power of group support and on spiritual beliefs, than on methodologically sound studies of treatment effectiveness. In this context, guidelines based on data from clinical research, particularly research carried out in medical settings, may be seen as undermining treatment approaches less amenable to study by scientific methods.

Both the American Medical Association (Office of Quality Assurance, 1996) and the Institute of Medicine (IOM, 1992) have developed principles for practice guideline development and implementation. Not surprisingly, AMA recommends that guidelines be developed by, or in conjunction with, physician organizations. In addition, AMA recommends that guideline dissemination be coupled with a plan for measuring their impact on short- and long-term treatment outcome. Testing is important for guidelines in any field because of the potential for obtaining useful new information as well as avoiding unintended bad effects (Weingarten, 1997).

The IOM report on Clinical Guidelines for Practice (1992) recommended that guidelines should evolve as a result of a multidisciplinary process "that includes participation by representatives of key affected groups" who can identify, critically evaluate, and incorporate all important clinical and scientific evidence into the guidelines. The latter seems particularly relevant in developing clinical guidelines in the drug abuse field, if the target audience (i.e., community-based treatment programs) is to view the guidelines as credible. Multidisciplinary participation maximizes the chances for addressing practical problems in their use. A recent report recommended that guidelines be accompanied by a timetable for scheduled review and revision (IOM, 1997).

A number of studies have demonstrated that merely publishing guidelines does not change the practice patterns of targeted clinicians, but that there are strategies which enhance the likelihood of this occurring (Greco and Eisenberg, 1993; Rogers, 1995b). Strategies that work include direct endorsement by respected professional associations and clinical "opinion leaders," coupled with teaching sessions under their aegis, and the incorporation of guidelines into training and continuing education programs, as well as self-assessment, certification, and recertification examinations. The use of practice guidelines by third party payers and managed care organizations to inform decision making on benefit utilization also enhances their dissemination and ultimate acceptance. Incorporating measures of dissemination and incorporating guideline use in HEDIS surveys and JCAHO standards would facilitate this goal. It will be necessary to devise strategies by which the acceptability and ultimate utility of practice guidelines in drug and alcohol abuse treatment can be measured.

Compared to practice guidelines that have been developing for more than a decade, the science of consumer scorecards in health care is in an early state (Hanes and Greenlick, 1998). However, the movement is growing and a useful purpose could be served in the development of scorecards providing information about community-based treatment programs. Included in such scorecards would be information from consumer satisfaction and quality of life surveys, as well as other data on short- and long-term treatment outcomes assessing the effectiveness of the treatment program.

CONSENSUS CONFERENCES AND EVIDENCE-BASED REVIEWS

Closely linked to practice guidelines are consensus conferences and the development of evidence-based reviews, two other mechanisms that are being widely tested in other areas of the health care delivery to reduce the communication gaps among research, practice, and policy segments. The experience of the Agency for Health Care Policy Research (AHCPR) can provide some guidance in this area. As the question of practice variation and inefficiency in the health care system became a major focus at AHCPR, their first approach was the creation of a set of Patient Outcome Research Teams (PORT) and the implementation of a guidelines development process within the Agency. Several PORTs were funded, each with a focus on practice methods within a particular disease entity (Goldberg et al., 1994). The PORTs, studying practice in such areas as stroke, acute myocardial infarction, low-back pain, and knee replacement did some extraordinary work studying care in the various areas, and an extensive literature is emerging. The output from the PORTs was to fuel AHCPR's guideline development process.

The guideline development process did emerge and AHCPR became the official government agency creating guidelines in many important areas of clinical practice. But there were a variety of problems with the federal approach to guideline creation, including the evidence cited above that governmentally created guidelines was not the most effective way to influence clinical practice. Moreover, there was significant political fall-out from this process, including a move by one group of medical specialists to abolish AHCPR as a result of their unhappiness with the contents of a guideline. Cooler heads prevailed and the threat to the agency dissipated.

With experience came a rethinking of the guidelines/PORT model and AHCPR created a new model. The current thinking follows from the approaches discussed above, that guidelines are best created by sponsors closer to the actual clinical care, including managed care programs, medical specialty groups and the like. But the major impediment to guidelines creating is still the paucity of evidence reviews in many clinical areas. So AHCPR has now named twelve Evidence-Based Practice Centers to produce the evidence-based reviews intended to facilitate improvement in clinical practice. For the current status of this effort, see the AHCPR web site (http://www.ahcpr.gov). Further, AHCPR has created a national nomination process for assisting in determining priorities for the particular evidence-based reviews to be created. It is likely that a similar process would be extremely helpful in the area of substance abuse treatment.

Numerous impediments make it difficult for counselors, program managers, and state agency staff to sift through the research literature, critique it effectively, and select findings to implement in treatment. Techniques such as the consensus conference mechanism and the evidence-based reviews approach might begin to close the gap and to improve treatment, as well as to enhance the potential for broader use of treatment guidelines in drug abuse treatment. The first NIH Consensus Development Statement on drug abuse treatment is included as Appendix F and may also be found on the NIH Consensus Development Statement web site (http://consensus.nih.gov).

TOP-DOWN INCENTIVES MODELS

Workshop participants described a variety of "top-down" models, most of which could be fairly described as "money with strings" that would require recipients to do something that the proposer viewed as salutary. It was clear, however, that many treatment providers believe that money with strings can make it harder for them to successfully compete in an increasingly difficult world, and when that was the case they rejected the concept.

The discussion and deferral of plans to link federal funding for substance abuse treatment to performance objectives under the Performance Partnership Grants (PPG) Program illustrates the problem. In the opinion of the National Association of State Alcohol and Drug Abuse Directors and a National Academy of Sciences panel, performance measures for public health, substance abuse, and mental health are not ready for prime time. Both concluded that the science of performance measurement and the data available to support such a link are major stumbling blocks (Gustafson and Sheehan, 1997).

> Recognizing that data resources and measurement methods need improvement, the panel recommends that DHHS continue to work with states toward several infrastructure goals: developing common definitions and measurement methods; encouraging efficient development of data resources that support multiple public health, mental health, and substance abuse needs; incorporating state data priorities in national infrastructure development efforts; and promoting states' data collection and analytic capabilities.
>
> *Assessment of Performance Measures for*
> *Public Health, Substance Abuse, and*
> *Mental Health, Phase 1 Report;*
> NRC (1997)

One top-down model that was discussed would have suggested changes in the incentives that currently are attached to the state block grant money used to support treatment programs in most communities. The block grant program has requirements that states pass on to service providers. For example, states are required to assure expenditures for services to pregnant and parenting women, to injection drug users, and to provide access to HIV and TB services for testing and medication (GAO, 1995). In order to meet the requirements, states may offer treatment programs additional funds to deliver new services and to serve consumers with specified characteristics (e.g., using injection drugs, caring for children). States could also use funding strings to promote collaborations among community-based organizations and research groups. The Department of Veterans Affairs approach includes a money-with-strings strategy (see Box 3.2).

The introduction of managed care into the drug abuse treatment field has produced a new, and particularly difficult, set of requirements. Most treatment providers already are quite concerned with the "strings" that come with managed care money, but the quick response by treatment pro-

---

BOX 3.2
The VA Model—Top-Down Incentives Model

For the past seven years, the VA has used an in-service program of education and training to integrate research-based treatments into its approach to substance-dependent patients. This program has included national meetings for program leaders, interactive video teleconferencing for presentation of curriculum materials, the development of Centers of Excellence in Substance Abuse Treatment and Education as national education resource centers, quarterly conference calls with program leaders across the country, and small meetings to introduce technical treatments such as LAAM.

VA officials have learned that certain things do work in this process of change:

- "money with strings attached" that is, funds made available on a competitive basis for improvement and innovation in care delivery;
- strong medical and affiliated-health professional presence; Having well-educated leaders "makes a big difference" in the ability of programs to adopt technological advances, but may not affect administrative change within the system;
- good in-service education helps, but there is also a need for personal consultation, advice, "and hand-holding";
- media reports of changes in the VA system generate public interest and can push professionals to participate in the change process; and
- publications in the professional literature have little impact, but abstracting such literature to "separate the wheat from the chaff" would be helpful.

Richard Suchinsky
Associate Chief for Addictive Disorders,
Department of Veterans Affairs
Committee Workshop, July 27, 1997, Washington, DC

---

grams to the requirements of managed care programs, albeit against their wishes and desires, is an example of the power of this approach.

Top-down incentives were viewed by the committee as a powerful approach, but also a dangerous one. Money with dumb strings can lead to inappropriate actions and services, of which the committee heard several examples. The committee did agree that when top-down models are proposed, it must be with careful consideration of the potential negative consequences.

MODELS THAT INCORPORATE TRUST-BUILDING EXPERIENCES

Knowledge exchange and the development of two-way communication between treatment personnel and researchers requires the development of trust. Trust takes time to develop. Trust between researchers and practitioners builds over several years of shared experience in designing and carrying out service delivery research and is the key ingredient in establishing successful linkage between research and practice. Researchers who develop and implement interventions in the community need to design interventions that are useful to community systems after the formal phase of research ends. Thus in technology transfer it is essential to collaborate with the people who will need to live with the results of change and to foster effective long-term relationships between researchers and the community programs in which the research takes place (Altman, 1995).

Most drug abuse innovations involve procedural knowledge, such as treatment doses or behavioral change requirements, not hard technology such as a new medical device (Tenkasi and Mohrman, 1995). As a result, most innovations are not adopted literally. They are put into use through a process of "contextual adaptation" that matches the innovation to the environment. This is a human process involving creative synthesis by workers, a process of "reinventing innovations" by modifying them to fit varying local circumstances (Rogers, 1995a). Personal contact can also be a key to the adoption of new technology. For example, approaches that involve personal contact were found to result in greater adoption of a job seekers' workshop in drug treatment programs than dissemination approaches that provided only written materials (Sorensen et al., 1988). Personal consultation was similarly important in the VA successes described to the committee.

Once an innovation has been targeted for program adoption it may be necessary to have a period of transition in which the program adapts the innovation to its own culture (Diamond, 1995). The rituals of bureaucracy, such as organizational missions, policy statements, staff meetings, and in-service training—which exist in part to provide a way of reducing anxiety—can also be used to stimulate the transfer of the targeted innovation.

> It is probably impossible for those removed from the work to appreciate subtle differences in the work task. And so technology, defined broadly as the procedures and equipment we use, is always local.
>
> *Ann Lennarson Greer* in Greer (1995), p. 329

However, the "pull" for making local adaptations to a treatment model must be balanced with a concern for maintaining the efficacy of the treatment. For example, there has been considerable research over 20 years on the replication of the Program of Assertive Community Treatment (PACT).

A review of the research on this comprehensive community-based service delivery model for the seriously mentally ill has shown that positive client outcomes are achieved when the original model is followed with regard to organization, staffing, and practice patterns. The reviewer concludes that not implementing the program fully and not providing the necessary staff training will jeopardize the ability of the program to assist clients in becoming fully functioning members of their communities (Allness, 1997).

Several experts have recommended that researchers gain a deeper understanding of the treatment programs they hope to influence (Kavanaugh, 1995). Sobell adapts business techniques and encourages behavioral scientists to get "close to the customer" in developing and fostering close working relationships (Sobell, 1996). Brown suggests that, at a minimum, to develop effective technology transfer, the innovator must obtain input from potential adopters about the relevance, clarity, credibility, and adaptability of an intervention (Brown, 1995). Trust-building experiences can include site visits, jointly sponsored seminars and staff development activities, and short-term exchanges of staff.

The building of successful research-treatment partnerships, which recognize the contribution of both the research and treatment communities, is one way to build trust. Partnerships can be successfully organized with the community group as senior partner, the academic group as senior partner, or in a balanced partnership (Mittelmark, 1990). The committee heard from several administrators of community-based drug treatment programs who emphasized the need to work for a collaborative relationship. One pointed out that who takes the lead in a proposal depends on the funding agency: if it is SAMHSA, the CBO leads, if the funder is NIH, the leader is the university-based researcher.

These issues are not unique to drug abuse. In the area of cancer treatment, 80 percent of care is provided in the community and the quality of care can be quite variable. In an attempt to improve the quality of care provided in the local communities, various organizations have issued guidelines for effective treatment procedures, but like the Treatment Improvement Protocols in the drug abuse area, writing a guideline does not guarantee that providers will comply (Czaja et al., 1997; Ford et al., 1987; Klabunde et al., 1997).

The National Cancer Institute's Community Clinical Oncology Program (CCOP) provides a model for researchers and clinicians seeking to collaborate (Cobau, 1994; Kaluzny et al., 1993, 1996). To better integrate policy, research, and treatment and thereby assure access to improved care within local communities, CCOP involves primary care physicians and oncologists in the conduct and management of clinical trials, in cooperation with NCI-funded centers and clinical cooperative groups. CCOP has become a valuable resource to NCI for performance of a wide variety of investigational treatment, prevention, and control activities. The potential for adaptation of this model to the drug abuse treatment field is discussed in Chapter 5, with a recommendation following in Chapter 6. Chapter 5 includes other collaboration models as well. The practice-based research networks described in the next chapter (see Box 4.3) provides an alternative model developed in several medical specialties to involve clinicians in the development of knowledge to guide their practice.

Another trust-building model, the Agricultural Extension Service, has had a far-reaching impact on U.S. farm productivity in the past 50 years. As described to the committee by Everett Rogers of the University of New Mexico School of Communication, the agriculture extension model consists of a set of assumptions, principles, and organizational structures for diffusing the results of agricultural research to farmers. The success of the model is based on farmer participation in identifying local needs, serving on county-level committees to develop the research agenda, providing test plots for the agricultural research, and providing feedback to the state university researchers on the applicability of the results. It has built-in reward systems for farmers and researchers to encourage utilization of the new information. Agriculture extension specialists are in close social, political, and spatial contact with these county research committees and with agricultural researchers, which allows them to facilitate linking research-based knowledge to farmer problems. This model, funded by the U.S. Department of Agriculture, worked particularly well in diffusing agricultural production technology to family farmers in the early development of scientific farming (Rogers, 1995a; Rogers et al., 1976).

SUMMARY

Many of the approaches to closing the gap rely on infrastructure changes within both treatment and research organizations. The next chapter focuses on the issue from the perspective of the treatment programs, the following one focuses on changes needed within the research enterprise. Even when effectiveness studies document that a treatment can be successfully implemented in a clinical setting, technology transfer to local drug abuse treatment centers is difficult. New treatments typically are adopted and implemented by trained staff, who may be in short supply in many CBOs. Challenges in the final stage of treatment transfer include training staff in delivering the new treatment, changing attitudes of the providers so they embrace the new treatment, and providing evidence that the new treatment is effective in improving the health status of drug abusers.

Each of these components of training must be planned, systematically delivered, and protective of the fidelity of the treatment. Many have suggested that the transfer of new treatment knowledge occurs best in the context of a long-term relationship between a researcher and the sponsoring CBO (Nurco and Hanlon, 1996). In some places well trained and respected clinicians who have established trust with community treatment colleagues may be the best to transfer new knowledge. In either case, a collaborative model of community-based research appears to be the most appropriate model to facilitate the design of treatment research that is relevant to the CBO's values and mission, sensitive to its fiscal and human resources, and respectful of its culture and that of the population it serves. The conduct of community-based research is an intensely interpersonal enterprise, and these relationships must be cultivated at different levels of the organization, with community residents, and often with members of other agencies related to the CBO.

In developing a typology linking specific treatment strategies with amenable research approaches, it becomes clear that community-based research will be most likely to happen within the context of a structured collaboration between CBOs and researchers. This analysis favors approaches designed to develop such long-term collaborations, within which both investigators and providers become stakeholders and, consequently, become committed to the appropriate implementation of successful innovations created and tested within the collaboration.

REFERENCES

Allness DJ. 1997. The Program of Assertive Community Treatment (PACT): The model and its replication. *New Directions for Mental Health Services* 74:17–26.

Altman DG. 1995. Sustaining interventions in community systems: On the relationship between researchers and communities. *Health Psychology* 14:526–536.

APA (American Psychiatric Association). 1996. *American Psychiatric Association: Practice Guidelines*. Washington, DC: American Psychiatric Association Press.

Backer TE. 1991. *Drug Abuse Technology Transfer*. Rockville, MD: National Institute on Drug Abuse.

Backer TE, Liberman RP, Kuehnel T. 1986. Dissemination and adoption of innovative psychosocial interventions. *Journal of Consulting and Clinical Psychology* 1:111–118.

Backer TE, David SL, Soucy G. 1995. Introduction. In: Backer TE, David SL, Soucy G eds. *Reviewing the Behavioral Science Knowledge Base on Technology Transfer*. NIDA Research Monograph 155. Rockville, MD: National Institute on Drug Abuse. Pp. 1–20.

Brown BS. 1995. Reducing impediments to technology transfer in drug abuse. In: Backer TE, David SL, Soucy G eds. *Reviewing the behavioral science knowledge base on technology transfer*. NIDA Research Monograph 155. Rockville, MD: National Institute on Drug Abuse. Pp. 169–185.

Cobau CD. 1994. Clinical trials in the community: The Community Clinical Oncology Program experience. *Cancer Supplement* 74(9):2694–2700.

Coeling HVE, Simms LM. 1993. Facilitating innovation at the nursing unit level through cultural assessment: Part 1, how to keep management ideas from falling on deaf ears. *Journal of Nursing Administration* 23(4):46–53.

Crump CE, Earp JA, Kozma CM, Hertz-Picciotto I. 1996. Effect of organization-level variables on differential employee participation in 10 federal worksite health promotion programs. *Health Education Quarterly* 23(2):204–223.

Czaja R et al. 1997. Preferences of community physicians for cancer screening guidelines. *Annals of Internal Medicine* 120(7):602–608.

Diamond MA. 1995. Organizational change as a human process, not technique. In: Backer TE, David SL, Soucy G eds. *Reviewing the behavioral science knowledge base on technology transfer.* NIDA Research Monograph 155. Rockville, MD: National Institute on Drug Abuse. Pp. 119–132.

Ford L et al. 1987. The effects of patient management guidelines on physician practice patterns: The Community Hospital Oncology Program. *Journal of Clinical Oncology* 5:504–511.

GAO (General Accounting Office). 1995. *Block Grants: Characteristics, Experience and Lessons Learned.* GAO/HEHS-95-74. Washington, DC: General Accounting Office.

Glaser EM, Abelson HH, Garrison KN. 1983. *Putting Knowledge to Use: Facilitating the Diffusion of Knowledge and the Implementation of Planned Change.* San Francisco, CA: Jossey-Bass.

Goldberg HI, Cummings MA, Steinberg EP, Ricci EM, ST, Soumerai SB, Mittman BS, Eisenberg J, Heck DA, Kaplan S, Kenzora JE, Vargus AM, Mulley AG, Rimer BK. 1994. Deliberations on the dissemination of PORT products: Translating research findings into improved patient outcomes. *Medical Care* 32(7):JS90–JS110.

Greco PJ, Eisenberg JM. 1993. Changing physician practices. *New England Journal of Medicine* 329:1271–1273.

Greer AL. 1995. The shape of resistance . . . the shapers of change. *Journal on Quality Improvement* 21(7):328–332.

Gustafson JS, Sheehan K. 1997. Linking substance abuse treatment funding to performance measurement will take time. *Connection* April:1–2, 5.

Hanes PP, Greenlick MR. 1998. The alchemy of accountability: Science and art of consumer scorecards. In: Hanes PP, Greenlick MR eds. *Grading Health Care: The Science and Art of Developing Consumer Scorecards.* San Francisco: Jossey-Bass. Pp. 119–129.

IOM (Institute of Medicine). 1992. *Guidelines for Clinical Practice from Development to Use.* Washington, DC: National Academy Press.

IOM. 1994. *Reducing Risks for Mental Disorders: Frontiers for Preventive Intervention Research.* Washington, DC: National Academy Press.

IOM. 1997. *Managing Managed Care: Quality Improvement in Behavioral Health.* Washington, DC: National Academy Press.

Kaluzny AD, Lacey LM, Warnecke R, Hynes DM, Morrissey J, Ford L, Sondik E. 1993. Predicting the performance of a strategic alliance: An analysis of the Community Clinical Oncology Program. *Health Services Research* 28(2):159–182.

Kaluzny AD, Warnecke RB et al. 1996. *Managing a Health Care Alliance: Improving Community Cancer Care.* San Francisco, CA: Jossey-Bass.

Kavanaugh KH. 1995. Collaboration and diversity in technology transfer. In: Backer TE, David SL, Soucy G eds. *Reviewing the Behavioral Science Knowledge Base on Technology Transfer.*NIDA Research Monograph 155. Rockville, MD: National Institute on Drug Abuse. Pp. 42–64.

Klabunde C, O'Malley M, Kaluzny A. 1997. Physicians' reactions to changing recommendations for mammography screening. *American Journal of Preventive Medicine* 13(6):432–438.

Leshner AI. 1997. Taking drug abuse research to the community. *NIDA Notes* 12(1):3–4.

Mittelmark MB. 1990. Balancing the requirements of research and the needs of communities. In: Bracht N ed. *Health Promotion at the Community Level.* New York: Sage Publications.

NIDA (National Institute on Drug Abuse). 1993. *How Good is Your Drug Abuse Treatment Program? A Guide to Evaluation.* NIH Pub. No. 93-3609. Rockville, MD: National Institute on Drug Abuse.

NIDA. 1996. *National Institute on Drug Abuse Community-Based HIV Prevention Research.* Rockville, MD: National Institute on Drug Abuse.

NRC (National Research Council). 1997. *Assessment of Performance Measures for Public Health, Substance Abuse, and Mental Health.* Washington, DC: National Academy Press.

Nutbeam D. 1996. Improving the fit between research and practice in health promotion: Overcoming structural barriers. *Canadian Journal of Public Health* 87(Suppl 2):S18–S23.

Nurco DN, Hanlon TE. 1996. The linking of research and service. *Substance Use and Misuse* 31(8):1059–1062.

Nystrom PC. 1993. Organizational cultures, strategies, and commitments in health care organizations. *Health Care Management Review* 18(1):43–49.

Office of Quality Assurance, American Medical Association. 1996. *Attributes to Grade the Development of Practice Parameters.* Chicago, IL: American Medical Association.

Orlandi MA. 1996. Health promotion technology transfer: Organizational perspectives. *Canadian Journal of Public Health* 87(Suppl. 2):S28–S33.

Rogers EM. 1995a. *Diffusion of Innovations.* 4th Edition. New York: Free Press.

Rogers EM. 1995b. Lessons for guidelines from the diffusion of innovations. *Joint Commission Journal on Quality Improvement* 21(7):324–328.

Rogers EM et al. 1976. *Extending the Agricultural Extension Model. Preliminary Draft.* Washington, D.C.: National Science Foundation.

Seago JA. 1996. Work group culture, stress, and hostility. Correlations with organizational outcomes. *Journal of Nursing Administration* 26(6):39–47.

Sobell LC. 1996. Bridging the gap between scientists and practitioners: The challenge before us. *Behavior Therapy* 27:297–320.

Sorensen JL, Hall SM, Loeb P, Allen T, Glaser EM, Greenberg PD. 1988. Dissemination of a job seekers' workshop to drug treatment programs. *Behavior Therapy* 19:143–155.

Tenkasi RV, Mohrman SA. 1995. Technology transfer as collaborative learning. In: Backer TE, David SL, Soucy G eds. *Reviewing the Behavioral Science Knowledge Base on Technology Transfer.* NIDA Research Monograph 155. Rockville, MD: National Institute on Drug Abuse. Pp. 262–279.

Weingarten S. 1997. Practice guidelines and prediction rules should be subject to careful clinical testing. *Journal of the American Medical Association* 277(24):1977–1978.

4
Benefits and Challenges of
Research Collaboration for
Community-Based Treatment Providers

Albuquerque's late afternoon sun slanted through the dusty windows of Scholes Hall at the University of New Mexico. Mick Kirby had waited patiently sitting in an uncomfortable chair throughout the morning in early September and now, finally, it was his turn to share the Arapahoe House story with the Committee on Community-Based Drug Abuse Treatment. He stood and, speaking quietly, described a research and practice collaboration that competes successfully for grants and cooperative agreements, improves services for clients, and facilitates the organization's growth and evolution.

Arapahoe House Comprehensive Substance Abuse Treatment Center opened in 1976 to provide alcohol detoxification and halfway house services for Arapahoe County, Colorado. Over two decades, the center grew to become the largest alcohol and drug abuse treatment program in Colorado. Facilities located in Denver and the four adjacent counties serve residents from throughout the state. Today, Arapahoe House supports a continuum of services for prevention, intervention, and treatment of alcohol and drug abuse and dependence—school-based prevention and intervention services in

This chapter was edited by Victor A. Capoccia with contributions by Gaurdia E. Banister, Merwyn R. Greenlick, Emily Jean Hauenstein, Dennis McCarty, and David L. Rosenbloom. Joseph Westermeyer contributed the "Opportunities for Collaboration" in Appendix I.

ten elementary, middle, and high schools in Denver and other contiguous counties, seven outpatient clinics located in six communities, case management services for homeless clients, beds for non-medical detoxification in three facilities, a 32-bed short-term intensive residential treatment program for adults, an 18-bed rehabilitation program for adolescents, and 22 beds of transitional housing for homeless clients in early recovery. Most recently, Arapahoe House entered into a partnership with the University of Colorado Medical School and three additional treatment programs and formed a not-for-profit managed behavioral health care organization that contracts with the State of Colorado and manages drug abuse treatment services for individuals in several geographic areas of the state.

Working with research investigators from the University of Denver, Arapahoe House has participated in research and demonstration programs funded by the National Institute on Alcohol Abuse and Alcoholism, the National Institute on Drug Abuse, the Center for Substance Abuse Treatment, and the Center for Mental Health Services. As chief executive officer, Dr. Kirby guided the development of the non-profit corporation and crafted the research collaborations that contributed to the agency's evolution and expansion. He believes in a team approach. Research questions and study design are negotiated in partnership with the investigators. Researchers challenge and clarify clinical thinking and clinicians add practical perspectives. Together, the team identifies and designs the interventions that are most likely to be feasible. Research funds are used to supplement and expand a core staff of five who are responsible for the center's ongoing evaluation and outcome studies.

Although Arapahoe House prefers to be the applicant and recipient of research funding (the organization has negotiated a federal indirect rate), Dr. Kirby recognizes that universities are more competitive applicants for some funding. Thus, the applicant organization is usually determined by the nature of the proposal. The relationship with the research team is built on 14 years of collaboration, and the researchers and clinicians have developed substantial mutual trust and respect. They recognize that the collaboration is stronger because of the complementary strengths and abilities.

OVERVIEW

Community-based treatment organizations learn and grow in response to personal and professional experience, education, research findings, established standards and guidelines, city, state or federal mandates, evaluation, observation, trial and error, and technological advancements. They also grow by "opportunity taking and opportunity making," in the words used by a workshop participant in describing her program's success in building a research collaboration to address questions of particular interest to them.

This chapter examines the research/practice collaboration from the perspective of the treatment provider. The Arapahoe House story illustrates some of the ways in which this collaboration can contribute both to the scientific basis for drug and alcohol treatment and to the ability of the community-based drug treatment organization (CBO) to deliver treatment.

Not every community-based treatment program will have the desire or capacity to emulate Arapahoe House. This analysis assumes, however, that all organizations want to grow and change and, as they evolve, they may find it beneficial to participate actively in the research enterprise. Accordingly, the chapter discusses how to negotiate specific roles and ensure tangible and less tangible benefits from the collaboration. It also examines how organizational culture and stage of development influence the type of research in which a particular CBO is likely to become involved. Appendix I provides some examples of potential collaborative research opportunities, written in a format that would be useful for preparing a document to begin the discussion of a research project of interest to the treatment program.

The personal experiences of counselors in recovery have shaped and guided many treatment interventions. Skills and practices were developed primarily on personal learning experiences rather than formal research and have been accepted as essential strategies for successful recovery. However, as the organization and financing of drug abuse treatment becomes more complex and resources become more scarce, payers and consumers are demanding—in this field as well as others—that clinical practice be supported by outcomes data. Successful organizations are developing new ways of learning and responding to the changing environment.

BENEFITS AND CHALLENGES OF
RESEARCH/PRACTICE COLLABORATIONS

The gap separating research from practice is evident from both sides. Researchers observe that many practitioners are slow to adopt findings established by rigorous empirical methods. Practitioners, on the other hand, often perceive research findings as irrelevant to their needs or impractical, if

BOX 4.1
The Learning Organization

Drug abuse treatment programs are not the only corporate entities struggling for survival. Demands for change affect large and small organizations in all settings. For the past decade, chief executive officers and managers have found guidance for corporate change in Peter Senge's concept of the learning organization, as described in *The Fifth Discipline: The Art & Practice of the Learning Organization* (Senge, 1990). Senge defines learning in organizations as "the continuous testing of experience, and the transformation of that experience into knowledge—accessible to the whole organization and relevant to its core purpose." The testing of experience is the essence of the experimental method. Treatment programs that follow this model will be comfortable linking research and practice.

not impossible, to implement in their situations. Consequently, bridging the two perspectives by linking research and practice may improve the relevance of research and the effectiveness of treatment and, ultimately, the viability of treatment programs.

This integration of practice and research is not without its own challenges. On the one hand, the linkage between treatment organizations and research institutions is neither uniform (there are different types of linkages possible) nor universal (not all CBOs will benefit from a relationship with the research enterprise). On the other hand, the direct benefits of research participation may include staff enhancement and development, as well as financial support for direct and indirect expenses of the research. In addition, programs and consumers may benefit indirectly from access to "leading edge" services and technologies, consumer empowerment, and support for developing an organizational culture and structure that would enhance long-term competitive position.

As in any partnership, it is important to clarify the expectations of the potential partners (see Box 4.2). As these questions asked by a program director illustrate, a research project has the potential to become a hidden cost to the treatment provider. Costs of research participation should be covered by research funds. There should be additional benefits for program staff such as access to emerging clinical issues, enhanced opportunities for professional training, and improved information and quality assurance systems. In some cases the opportunity for staff education could extend beyond training, to access to a degree or other credentialing programs offered by a research partner organization. Treatment agencies invited to collaborate with academic research centers should explore the possibility of negotiating tuition remission benefits or a specific number of credit hours (equivalent in value to the costs incurred) for staff development. Other

---

BOX 4.2
Chilo Madrid's Ten Questions

The challenges for researchers seeking to work with programs that treat alcohol and drug dependence are evident in these questions used by one program to screen researcher requests. Aliviane is an established drug abuse treatment and prevention program serving Mexican-Americans in the El Paso, Texas area. Executive Director Chilo Madrid shared with the IOM committee these questions he has for researchers when they seek access to Aliviane clients and staff.

1. What funds are available for clinical services? Do all of the grant or contract funds go to research?
2. Are the researchers sensitive to cultural issues?
3. Does the study address questions that are applicable to Aliviane or are the research questions unrelated to our work ?
4. Are the research questions practical? Are hypotheses explained to the program or is the program deceived or unaware of the purpose of the investigation?
5. How does the treatment or prevention program benefit? What technical assistance or treatment benefits are provided?
6. Will the research help clients or put them at risk?
7. What are the long-term benefits for the program and for research theory?
8. Does the investigator express genuine concern for the program and its clients?
9. How much choice does the program have in the selection of a specific investigator with whom to work?
10. If there is to be evaluation, does Aliviane have a say in who is chosen to be evaluator?

These questions frame many of the issues investigators should be prepared to confront and willing to discuss when seeking a treatment partner.

---

benefits might include data analysis skills enhanced by research participation, skills which can also support management information needs and program evaluation.

In addition to covering direct research costs, another financial benefit to the treatment agency could be a contribution to indirect and overhead expenses, similar to that received by universities. The programs should be reimbursed for a portion of overhead, to the extent that the overhead expenses support the research. For example, telephone reception and messaging, intake, parking, and common area spaces, accounting, payroll, security, and advertising all represent some of the indirect costs that support all the functions in the treatment program including research activities. And finally, a program with limited access to capital may benefit from new equipment purchased initially with research funds to support the research.

Linkages between practice and research and program participation in research can enhance staff pride and esteem and foster consumer empowerment. Staff take satisfaction in their organization's contribution to building practice knowledge as well as improving treatment. For the treatment consumers, a program's participation in research symbolizes its effort to provide the most current treatments. Consumers can also take pride in the opportunity to participate in research initiatives when the research is viewed as relevant to improving their treatment—and when research recruitment is conducted within established guidelines for the protection of research subjects (Code of Federal Regulations, Title 45, Part 46, 1991). Under these federal guidelines, drug abusers are considered a vulnerable population and thus the informed consent process and content are carefully examined by the institutional review board (IRB) with jurisdiction. The knowledgeable and respectful explanation of the study and obtaining of true informed consent can form an important bond between participant and the program. There are a number of ways in which research participation may motivate consumers to participate more actively in the treatment process. However, the most enduring potential benefit to the CBO of a linkage with research may be assistance in building or enhancing a culture of learning, which loosens the grip of dogmatic approaches that are sometimes barriers to adopting demonstrated best practices and bringing new ideas into an organization.

FACTORS AFFECTING LINKAGE BETWEEN PRACTICE AND RESEARCH

Linkages between treatment providers and research teams can assume many forms, ranging from simply providing access to subjects to becoming full collaborators in the development of research proposals, implementation of protocols, interpretation of data, and publication of results. Collaboration may eventually result in some CBOs developing free-standing research programs, as happened at Arapahoe House.

Examples abound of treatment programs that have simply "hosted" a particular study. Researchers arrive with a funded research protocol and IRB approval, needing only the subjects. For the clinical site, such experiences can be good or bad, depending substantially on the quality of the communication and consideration shown them in the course of the study. The committee heard examples where both communication and consideration failed, even in the context of established relationships, usually because of the failure to understand and appreciate each other's perspective.

Few examples were cited of investigations where the research questions start as clinical conundrums brought forward by treatment providers, where treatment staff have roles as co-investigators, and where the goal is the

BOX 4.3
Practice-Based Research Networks

Practice-based research networks provide a model of collaborative learning among providers. Models exist in several branches of medicine, including the Pediatric Research in Office Settings (PROS) network of the American Academy of Pediatrics (Wasserman et al., 1992), the Ambulatory Sentinel Practice Network (ASPN) of the American Academy of Family Physicians (Green et al., 1984; Niebauer and Nutting, 1994), and the Practice Research Network (PRN) of the American Psychiatric Association (Zarin et al., 1997). These networks are composed of practicing clinicians who collaborate in collecting data and carrying out research, ranging from multi-site clinical trials to the assessment of service delivery mechanisms.

Each of these networks has a geographically dispersed national sample of between 700 and 1200 physicians who have agreed to collect clinical and demographic data for the purpose of answering questions relevant to their clinical practice, including patients' clinical status, treatments provided, and patient outcomes. Such networks provide a natural laboratory for field trials designed to assess methods of disseminating and encouraging the use of practice guidelines and the subsequent effect of guideline use on the delivery and outcome of patient care.

development of knowledge to guide change in practice patterns. The practice-based research networks developed in some medical specialities (and described in Box 4.3) do have this goal. They provide the opportunity for those who must implement the research to be represented in setting the agenda and to participate in the research. The partnership between Arapahoe House and their university research partners demonstrates that intimate collaborations are feasible, as do the collaboration models described in the next chapter. However, failure to develop such relationships is not surprising given the lack of research institutions in many communities and the commitment and investment required on both sides to make such a partnership work.

University-based treatment researchers are obviously familiar with treatment programs, and they are generally engaged in treatment. But many in CBOs feel that these researchers are often not in touch with the realities of delivering services "on the ground." Some workshop participants suggested that the researchers may ignore the "real clinical issues" when they are not relevant to their research interests as illustrated by the vignette that begins the next chapter.

The committee identified a number of variables that appear to interact to affect potential linkages between clinical programs and academically oriented researchers (including those working in non-academic centers, government, and other applied research settings). These interacting variables—theoretical view of addiction; type of research; research functions and roles, as well as stages of organization—are described below in terms of their influence on the opportunities for research collaboration.

Theoretical View of Addiction

There is no single empirically demonstrated explanation of the cause of drug addiction. Neither is there any single universally accepted theory that explains addiction. Therefore the orientation of the treatment program is the first major determinant of the nature of the relationship between researchers and practitioners. Many treatment professionals view addiction as a biopsychosocial (and perhaps spiritual) condition (Ewing, 1978; IOM, 1990, 1997; Metzger, 1988; Moos et al., 1990; Zucker et al., 1994). This eclectic view has significant implications for theory development and for research. Different weights may be ascribed to the biological, psychological, social, and spiritual dimensions depending on the perspective of the investigator or clinician. If, for example, a researcher is interested in investigating genetic predisposition, then the social-cultural triggers to using drugs, or the psychological and emotional dimensions, will likely remain unexamined.

One or a small combination of particular theories forms the underpinning of each treatment research design. Investigations may test (a) a drug to block a receptor, (b) an incentive to change a behavior, (c) knowledge to change understanding, (d) faith to reinforce volition, or (e) the use of vocational rehabilitation to affirm self-esteem. In a parallel, but often less explicit manner, one or more of these orientations also serve as underpinning to treatment programs. Many residential programs are based on reconstructing self-image. Most counseling is based on some combination of behavior modification and self-awareness. Medications like methadone or naltrexone are used to block specific biologic receptor functions.

Compatibility between the theoretical underpinning of the research and those of the treatment program is one important ingredient to a successful relationship. Investigators must, first of all, be willing to explore and understand the explicit or implicit theory that guides the program's treatment strategies. If novel theoretical concepts are being tested or introduced, the investigators should be prepared to orient and train management and treatment staff so they understand the research question as well as the intervention and can provide consistent support.

Type of Research

Linkages between research and treatment enterprises are often impeded by different understanding of what is meant by research. Many researchers think primarily of experimental designs, while the practitioner is more concerned with the question of whether or not the treatment worked and what difference it makes to the consumer and the program. The researcher tries to narrow or refine the study questions to obtain statistically significant results. This may require reducing the diagnostic and demographic variation in the study population in order to decrease the sample size required. This approach reduces the cost of the study and perhaps increases its fundability. This methodological rigor has also done much to advance the credibility of clinical research in the drug treatment field. At the same time it has decreased the applicability of research findings to general patient populations. Conflicting with the researcher's desire is the practitioner's need to broaden the research question to be more relevant to the CBO and to more closely reflect the complexity and multidimensional nature of the population it serves. Appendix C provides a comprehensive review of the contributions and limitations of addiction treatment research for community-based treatment programs.

At the beginning of the research process, clinicians are uniquely positioned to pose broad questions about the nature of drug and alcohol dependence and the value and variability of different interventions. The questions posed by treatment programs and clinicians may be more directly relevant to treatment personnel than those initiated by an investigator several steps removed from the condition, client, or intervention. As "the research question" is formulated, describing its dimensions becomes a shared domain of the practitioner and researcher. By the time that sufficient understanding is acquired to test hypotheses, the roles may reverse, and the researchers become primary with the treatment personnel taking a more supporting role. Ideally, however, by the time the research study is completed, the treatment providers will have assumed ownership and developed the local expertise necessary to sustain the intervention. Without this "transfer of ownership," a process which works best if it is planned for and programmed into the research phase, there is little likelihood that the research will be adopted into practice (Altman, 1995).

Research Functions and Roles

Regardless of the type of research, the functions that occur in the research process are the same. Defining the question, developing an explanation, designing a study, gathering information, analyzing findings, generalizing to the next stage, and disseminating findings represent the basic steps in the process. Here too the link between research and practice can be fluid and shifting, requiring some team members be able to cross boundaries. The importance of these boundary crossers (or "bridge people") to the building and sustaining of research/practice collaborations was stressed by a number of workshop participants. Such individuals can operate in both the practice and research worlds. In the CBO, the bridge person is the "antenna" of the research endeavor, identifying potential research opportunities in patient trends, service delivery system barriers, and practice needs. In the research setting the bridge person can help ensure that research hypotheses are not too partialized to be relevant to practice, and can facilitate research designs that integrate, not interfere, with the work flow. With the benefit of understanding the treatment context, this person (or two or more people sharing this role) may also help with interpreting findings and facilitating the introduction and adoption of evidence-based approaches to treatment.

Clinical professionals, because of their practical experience, have significant knowledge to bring to the formulation stage of the research endeavor. Research professionals, on the other hand, bring significant knowledge to the design phase of research. Data collection lends itself to both domains, while analysis tends to be the domain of the researcher. When it comes to the critical stage of adoption of findings and dissemination for practice, greater involvement of practitioners and consumers is essential for success.

Thus, the particular role of the treatment program is defined by the requirements of the research, the experience with research activities, and the clinical circumstances. For example, a passive role might be appropriate when the research design is highly controlled and narrowly focused on a treatment variable such as a new drug that is outside of the expertise of the program and its staff. In other cases program staff may become collaborators in the investigation, including being responsible for specific and subcontracted duties. Finally, a treatment provider could be a principal in the research and share responsibility for all aspects of the study. And some may take the path of Arapahoe House and become full and permanent partners with research organizations or develop professional research components within their own organizations. In all cases, the treatment program should expect to receive appropriate recognition and publication credit for their role in the research project.

Stage of Organizational Development and Organizational Culture

Community-based drug and alcohol treatment organizations vary in management complexity and the development of management and clinical systems (see Box 4.4). Most organizations begin with relatively simple organizational structures. Management functions and service or production functions are not strongly differentiated. Over time roles and responsibilities become more defined and more complex. This discussion of factors affecting research collaboration includes an examination of the stages of

---

BOX 4.4
Stages of Organizational Development

Stage I. Rudimentary Stage of Organizational Development

The two major determinants of organizational structure in the initial stage of an organization are the environmental pressures an organization faces and the needs of the population within the organization or served by the organization. A relatively simple system emerges in the cooperative response of participants based on their common needs and expectations.

Stage II. The Development of Stable Organizational Structures

The lack of consistent role performance and effective coordination of roles in a rudimentary organization stimulates the successful organization to create stable organizational structures. This leads to institutionalization of basic roles and the formalization of power structure and organizational hierarchy. The organization's work itself may change as more specialized roles begin to be introduced.

Stage III. Highly Differentiated Organizational Structure

As the organization grows and responds to complex challenges in the environment a more complex and differentiated organizational structure emerges. Roles and functions become relatively highly specialized and organizational units become differentiated, partly as a result of size, but also as a result of increasing complexity of organizational output. A relatively large and complex organizational form develops in a systematic way out of the less-complex forms.

SOURCE: Adapted from Katz and Kahn (1978), pp. 70–76.

---

organizational growth and development because these stages influence the level and type of research in which a CBO might participate.

Treatment providers at the first stage of development may not be eager users of, or participants in, research. For other reasons, more developed organizations, whose knowledge and experience in this field is needed by others, may also be reluctant to embrace research. Most organizations, including CBOs, start because a few individuals are drawn together to address a common problem in their environment. They usually reflect both a spatial and social sense of community in the workers and consumers. (See Bowser, Appendix C, for discussion of what creates a sense of community.) At first, there may be few rules or specialized roles to direct their activities. Individual leadership by the founder with a vision often substitutes for procedures and systems. A substantial majority of the community-based treatment providers started this way and many remain at this stage.

TABLE 4.1 Likely Type of Research Participation of Community-Based Drug Treatment Organizations (CBOs) by Stage of Organizational Development and Nature of Belief System

CBO Belief System	CBO Organizational Development Stage		
	Stage I	Stage II	Stage III
Experience and/or faith	Contribute to research questions Respond to surveys	Passive research sites (services research)	Active research sites (services and treatment research)
Scientific	Interest in research Contribute to research questions Respond to surveys	Active research sites (services research)	Full research partners (services and treatment research)

These relatively simple organizations (referred to as Stage I organizations in Box 4.4 and in Table 4.1) tend to offer one modality of treatment to one type of consumer in one or a few nearby locations. If the organization grows, it does so in ways that minimize risks and uncertainty. While management of such a program matures and roles develop over time, the internal information systems may remain very simple. These organizations are still a very important component of the drug and alcohol abuse treatment community in the United States.

For organizations like this, participation in research is likely to introduce uncertainty and risk that can be destabilizing. They typically do not have specialized management, information or training structures. Counselors working in such organizations may receive very limited in-service training. New knowledge is more likely to come from a peer contact, or from individual study and professional development. Therefore, dissemination of new findings for use in these treatment settings must be targeted to the counselors and the consumer community. Historically, important improvements in treatment for mental illness came from better informed and mobilized patients and families pressuring providers to use research findings in their treatments. While small drug treatment providers are not likely candidates for formal research partnerships, they have accumulated knowledge that could improve treatment, especially knowledge about their particular social and geographic communities.

When programs progress beyond this relatively simple organizational stage, they may branch out in new but related areas. For example, outpatient programs that serve men might also develop services for alcohol- and drug-dependent women with young children. When organizations become more complex they develop systems to control and coordinate the growing number of pieces of their business. Among the most important new capacities they develop is specialized management for dealing with institutional actors like regulators, payers, and training institutions (Shortell and Kaluzny, 1983).

In recent years, some CBOs have expanded through mergers with larger organizations and acquisitions of smaller community-based providers (see Appendix E, Table E-2). These growing entities face financial and management challenges as they absorb and integrate other programs, each of which may have its own culture and community. The information and financial systems often are inadequate, and capital and human resources to fix the problems are lacking. Nevertheless, this emerging group of Stage III community providers are the most likely to be able to absorb research findings and to participate as full partners in the development of new clinical knowledge. However, they may also need special support from regulatory agencies, payers, and even research organizations to realize this potential. For example, Stage III CBOs are likely to be very sensitive to payers' demands for measurable improvements in treatment outcomes. To respond, they may need help in providing staff training and implementing information systems that monitor outcomes. In fact, they may need the same information systems to track their operations that researchers need to follow their clinical interventions. However, without special incentives and support, services will always take precedence over research in clinical settings where management teams are likely to be fully stretched responding to the challenges of growth and change.

Another important dimension that mediates a CBO's willingness and ability to engage in research activities is the cultural model defining their "knowledge" about how to treat drug abuse. There are at least two main types of treatment programs in this regard (see Table 4.1). The first group includes programs whose treatment models are based largely on the experiential knowledge of a staff largely comprising people in recovery from drug abuse problems. An example of this would be the drug abuse treatment program built in the tradition of the twelve step programs following the model of AA. The therapists at these programs have come to "know" what it takes to treat the disorder by living with it and they have confidence in their knowledge because it has been tested in what is to them the most important test—their own recovery.

Included in this first group of programs are some which are identified with religious organizations. These programs bring an element of faith into their treatment approach. Since faith is built into the foundation of their treatment approach, their religious beliefs fuel their organizational culture, including (to some extent) their fundamental "knowledge" about the nature of appropriate treatment for drug abuse problems.

The second group are organizations that are related more closely to the general health care system or to the tradition of the behavioral sciences. These treatment programs share more of the culture of the medical sciences or behavioral sciences, including beliefs and values that could be classified as a "scientific" perspective, one that suggests therapists' knowledge about what is appropriate in treatment is defined by the fruits of medical, social, and behavioral research. This same orientation could derive from a program's close affiliation with academia.

Research roles and activities, therefore, need to be tailored both to the organization's developmental stage and to its organizational culture. Stage I organizations can contribute to the development of research questions and provide an important perspective that would be missing if research examines only the more complex service delivery systems. It is critical that organizations at all stages participate in surveys of treatment practices, assessments of organizational characteristics, and censuses of patient and workforce descriptions. Stage II and Stage III organizations have the capacity to participate in a greater variety of treatment research, especially in multicenter research projects. Quasi-experimental investigations of treatment practices will also benefit from inclusion of all stages of organizations and greater diversity of treatment populations. Health services research can answer important questions about the distribution of drug users across different types of programs, as well as the ways in which organizational and social policy factors influence pathways to service (Weisner and Schmidt, 1995). Services research can also contribute to the development of services and to assessments of patient outcomes in organizations at developmental Stage II and Stage III. Controlled clinical trials, however, will generally require the management and clinical structures found in Stage III organizations—well-developed information systems coupled with clinicians whose skills and training assure fidelity to experimental protocols.

SUMMARY

Unique opportunities exist for community-based drug treatment organizations to participate in research at this time of rapid changes in the research, policy, and treatment environments. In fact, much research that is needed can be done only with the participation of treatment providers in community-based settings. Studies of treatment outcomes in the social model residential programs is one such area (Kaskutas, 1998). Needed research, as well as the strengths and limitations of current research for informing community-based treatment are reviewed in a paper prepared for this committee and included in Appendix D and discussed in Chapter 2.

However, the list of areas where collaboration between treatment and research will improve theory and enhance practice may be almost infinite.

The degree of organizational development, the organization's perspective on the basis of treatment knowledge, the type of research, and the type of research participation interact to shape an organization's potential involvement in a research endeavor. While it is not possible to identify specific roles for all community-based organizations in all research activities, it is anticipated that collaboration among CBOs of all types and theoretical orientations will enhance treatment programs and strengthen research.

The treatment program's role can be a relatively passive one (for example, contributing to surveys, databases and facilitating access to patients) but they should expect respectful treatment and adequate compensation, as well as to gain knowledge from their participation. Active participation in research requires a greater commitment of staff and agency resources. Clinicians will work with researchers in the definition of research questions and the design of data collection. Management should have an advisory role and the opportunity to review research reports to enhance the interpretation of results. The more advanced organizations are the ones likely to become full partners in treatment research. Such programs may have investigators on staff and have the capacity to serve as principal investigators in research. They will usually have established collaborations with academic or other research institutions and applications for grants will acknowledge their partnership. As their research staff and experience grows, they may become the applicant agency for grants where the source of funding and the area of research makes this appropriate. Some opportunities offered by major gaps between what is know and what is practiced in drug abuse treatment are summarized in Appendix I, Table I-1. Examples of research areas where the treatment program may be the appropriate applicant are also included in Appendix I which describes collaboration opportunities in four areas:

1. adolescent outreach and early intervention
2. community reinforcement,
3. outreach strategies for early intervention and follow-up, and
4. researching nontraditional interventions.

In summary, the dimensions described in this chapter interact to shape the linkages that tie a clinical program to a research endeavor. Such linkages between research and practice should not only result in a research product that is more relevant, and adaptable, but should also provide direct benefits to the treatment program, its staff, and its consumers.

REFERENCES

Altman DG. 1995. Sustaining interventions in community systems: On the relationship between researchers and communities. *Health Psychology* 14:526–536.

Code of Federal Regulations, Title 45, Part 46. 1991. Title 45—Public Welfare, Department of Health and Human Services, National Institutes of Health, Office for Protection from Research Risks. Part 46—Protection of Human Subjects. Revised June 18, 1991.

Ewing JA. 1978. Social and psychiatric considerations of drinking. In: Ewing JA, Rouse BA eds. *Drinking: Alcohol in American Society—Issues and Current Research*. Chicago: Nelson-Hall.

Green LA, Wood M, Becker LA, Farley FS Jr., Freeman WL, Froom J, Hames C, Niebauer LJ, Rosser WW, Siefert M. 1984. The Ambulatory Sentinel Practice Network: Purpose, methods, and policies. *Journal of Family Practice* 18(2):275–280.

IOM (Institute of Medicine). 1990. *Broadening the Base of Treatment for Alcohol Problems*. Washington, DC: National Academy Press.

IOM. 1997. *Dispelling the Myths About Addiction: Strategies to Increase Understanding and Strengthen Research*. Washington, DC: National Academy Press.

Kaskutas LA. 1998. Methodology and characteristics of programs and clients in the social model process evaluation. *Journal of Substance Abuse Treatment* 15(1):19–25.

Katz D, Kahn R. 1978. *The Social Psychology of Organizations*. 2nd Edition. New York: Wiley and Sons.

Metzger L. 1988. *From Denial to Recovery: Counseling Problem Drinkers, Alcoholics, and Their Families*. San Francisco: Jossey-Bass.

Moos RH, Finney JW, Cronkite RC. 1990. *Alcoholism Treatment: Context, Process, and Outcome*. New York: Oxford University Press.

Niebauer LJ, Nutting PA. 1994. Primary care practice-based research networks active in North America. *Journal of Family Practice* 38:425–426.

Senge PM. 1990. *The Fifth Discipline: The Art & Practice of the Learning Organization*. New York: Doubleday/Currency.

Shortell, Kaluzny AD, eds. 1983. *Health Care Management*. New York: John Wiley and Son. Pp. 471–479.

Wasserman RC, Croft CA, Brotherton SE. 1992. Preschool vision screening in pediatric practice: A study from the Pediatric Research in Office Settings (PROS) Network. *Pediatrics* 89:834–838.

Weisner C, Schmidt LA. 1995. Expanding the frame of health services research in the drug abuse field. *Health Services Research* 30(5):707–726.

Zarin DA, Pincus HA, West JC, McIntyre JS. 1997. Practice-based research in psychiatry. *American Journal of Psychiatry* 154(9):1199–1208.

Zucker R, Boyd G, Howard J. 1994. *The Development of Alcohol Problems: Exploring the Biopsychosocial Matrix of Risk*. NIH Pub. No. 94-3495. Rockville, MD: National Institute on Alcohol Abuse and Alcoholism.

5

Benefits and Challenges of Community-Based Collaboration for Researchers

A subtle smile, twinkling eyes, and Southern charm helped Selbert Wood, President and Chief Executive Officer of STEP ONE, a North Carolina-based drug and alcohol abuse treatment program, illustrate, the gulf between research and practice in the field of addictions treatment and prevention. He sought advice from friends and colleagues on what he "ought to tell a bunch of Ph.D.s and policy folks" in Washington, DC. His community confidants proposed four tongue-in-cheek recommendations for researchers:

*   *"We don't need no studies with long titles and with words more than three syllables."*
*   *"We don't need no studies about mice or monkeys—we just want to know better how to get drunk people sober and addicted people clean."*
*   *"We don't need no control groups or placebos floating around."*
*   *"We don't need no studies that cost more than you're giving us to take care of people."*

In discussion with the panel, Mr. Wood explained that clinicians needed simple answers. A member probed, "What if the answers

This chapter was edited by Dennis McCarty with contributions by Benjamin P. Bowser and Joseph Westermeyer.

are not simple?" Mr. Wood suggested that investigators should provide practical and relevant studies. Another participant noted that many counselors read the research literature and respond to research findings but they too are looking for practical information.

OVERVIEW

Tensions between research and practice were evident in the testimony presented to the committee. Providers expressed concerns that managed care misused findings from controlled clinical trials to inappropriately justify reductions in the length and intensity of care. Policymakers hinted at discomfort with researcher-directed and -managed interventions. Both clinicians and investigators sought more value from the collaborative relationship. The folk wisdom found in the story above characterizes some of these tensions. Even readers who disagree with sentiments in the story should recognize the pragmatic, underlying attitudes. Practitioners and consumers want concrete results with clear applicability to clinical and personal needs. Investigators who seek to work closely and effectively with practitioners must be prepared to describe their research in straightforward language and must be able to explain the relevance for treatment and recovery. Similarly, because consumers and clinicians may not appreciate the need for experimental controls, researchers must be willing to teach practitioners and consumers about the importance of comparison groups. At the same time, investigators must learn to be sensitive to the treatment environment and to understand the culture of recovery. They should also respect the insights of experiential learning and be willing to explore non-experimental research opportunities.

This chapter examines the benefits and challenges to working in a clinical environment from the perspective of the research investigator. The chapter also examines approaches that have been used successfully to build research/practice partnerships, and the lessons to be learned from prior federally sponsored demonstrations that linked practice and research in the field of drug abuse treatment.

HISTORICAL APPROACHES TO COLLABORATION FOR RESEARCH

Rapid development of community-based drug abuse treatment programs requires partnerships among investigators trained in theory and methods, clinical practitioners schooled in working with clients, administrators oriented toward problem resolution, and policymakers who fund and regulate research, treatment, and prevention activities. Research investigators must embrace the challenge and complexity of working within clinical environments, just as clinical practitioners and consumers must be responsive to the burdens of research participation and become active partners in systematic data collection and investigation (see Chapter 4). Alliances between research and practice are required to develop empirically based clinical protocols and document improvements in clinical effectiveness. These alliances evolve slowly, however, as the theoretical underpinnings for research/practice linkages have evolved slowly in the study of prevention and treatment for alcohol and drug dependence. The origins include Kurt Lewin's formulation of action research, subsequent developments in applied social science and program evaluation methods, and the emergence of health services research.

Action Research

Researchers and practitioners have struggled for at least five decades to develop meaningful collaborations that simultaneously contribute to theory and knowledge development and to effective responses to social and clinical problems. Kurt Lewin was a pioneering and influential thinker on the nexus of application and theory. In the late 1940s, Lewin and his colleagues developed what they called action research to address gang-related anti-Semitism, monitor racial integration of work settings and housing projects, and explore the roots of racial and ethnic prejudices. During World War II, he applied science to management problems in a research partnership with the owners and employees at a furniture factory. This research collaboration documented the value of engaging workers in the design and collection of data, allowing them the opportunity to learn on their own and test the validity of their beliefs (Marrow, 1969). Today, many of these concepts and practices are central to the application of continuous quality improvement strategies: the importance of group participation, the value of self-management, and the use of data to test ideas and strategies.

These early studies demonstrated the feasibility of conducting research in real-world settings and the potential to generate data that both solved problems and informed theory. As early as 1944, Lewin articulated four issues that must be addressed when conducting studies in applied settings: control, influence, education, and the need for theory (Lewin, 1951). He observed that investigators have relatively little control in organizational and community settings; consequently, they must seek active cooperation and must provide some value to the group in order to gain access and to introduce systematic change. Education about scientific methods is also essential in order to reduce resistance and to help participants understand the process. Finally, Lewin noted that effective study of social problems required both theory and application.

[Collaboration can be achieved] if the theorist does not look toward applied problems with high brow aversion or with a fear of social problems, and if the applied psychologist realizes that there is nothing as practical as a good theory.

Kurt Lewin in *Theory in Social Science: Selected Theoretical Papers* (1951), p. 169

Although he never studied treatment programs for alcohol and drug dependence, Lewin's observations remain clearly applicable to the integration of research and practice in substance abuse treatment programs. His exhortation on the value of research in industrial and community environments could have been written about many contemporary community-based substance abuse treatment programs:

> The organizational form of the existing factories, unions, political parties, community centers, associations—in short, of most groups—is based on tradition, on ideas of "a born organizer," on the nonsurvival of the unfit, or at best, on primitive methods of trial and error. Of course, much practical experience has been gathered and systematized to a degree. We know from other fields, however, that the efficiency of this procedure is far below what can be achieved with systematic scientific experimentation (Lewin, 1951).

Applied Social Science

Lewin's legacy is echoed in the work of social psychologist Leonard Bickman, who articulated the distinctions between laboratory and field settings and outlined the opportunities associated with conducting research in clinical environments (Bickman, 1980). His essays assert that investigators have much to gain when they enter clinical environments. For one thing, they are challenged to make a difference: concrete solutions for current problems become a central focus, rather than the more abstract development of knowledge. Research results may have visible influence on policy and practice. Clinical settings also stimulate urgency; timeliness is critical because policymakers and practitioners demand rapid results. Large, observable, and clinically meaningful effects are more valuable than small but statistically significant changes. And demonstrated effectiveness in community treatment settings enhances adoption of clinical techniques and interventions and increases generalization of research findings.

Bickman also recognized that clinical environments are challenging settings for research. Reduced statistical control and rival hypotheses can complicate interpretation of results. Discussion of results with clinicians and clients may be a critical step in the development of a full understanding of the findings and the articulation of subtle but real influences on the observed outcomes. A cadre of clinicians and data collectors is often required to implement investigations, so teamwork is essential to success and the management of the research process and personnel can be as important as the collection and analysis of data. The investigator must also be willing and able to negotiate access and procedures with a full range of stakeholders: clients, clinicians, administrators, policymakers, and funding agencies. Chilo Madrid's ten questions (Box 4.2) illustrate the importance of this negotiation.

Ownership of the data and publication of the findings are issues that often generate controversy. Investigators should recognize that the participating treatment programs have a stake in the data and have claims to the findings. Investigators who make data available to the clinicians for treatment planning and evaluation and invite participation in data interpretation and publication may be encouraged to continue investigations. Those who demand autonomy and control, on the other hand, are likely to find inhibited access to programs and patients. Finally, the complexity of the research initiatives means that investigations that involve clinical settings may require a substantial investment of time and money. Funding should include incentives for patient participants (if primary data collection is required) and for treatment agencies that permit access. These influences and tensions have been apparent in the development of health services research.

Health services research is a multidisciplinary field of inquiry, both basic and applied, that examines the use, costs, quality, accessibility, delivery, organization, financing, and outcomes of health care services to increase knowledge and understanding of the structure, processes and effects of health services for individuals and populations.

Health Services Research: Workforce and Educational Issues, IOM (1995), p. 3.

Health Services Research

The study of health care delivery systems uses social science and economic analysis to span the gulf between research, practice, and policy. Health services research can be characterized in four general categories of investigations:

1. clinical (studies of providers and patients and their influences on the process and outcome of care),
2. institutional (studies that emphasize organizational and administrative aspects of service delivery),
3. systemic (analyses of the interrelation among providers, institutions, and demands for care, including the financing and regulation of service), and
4. environmental (assessments of the influence of social, political, and economic forces on the delivery and effects of health care).

Services research often contributes to the development and implementation of health care policies through (a) documentation (health care indicators and markers specify and describe problems), (b) causal and correlational analyses (relationships are identified and policy influences are assessed often using demonstration programs), and (c) prescriptions (strategic models outline implementation requirements and provide guidelines for policy development) (Brown, 1991).

Although the formal link between services research and policy formation can be traced most directly to the development, implementation, and analysis of Medicaid and Medicare during the 1960s, health services research evolved from descriptive and analytic investigations beginning in the first decade of the twentieth century (Ginzberg, 1991). The complexity of contemporary medical markets increases the importance of health services research and the dependence of policymakers on the data and results from these investigations. This complexity and need for data is strongly felt by community-based drug treatment organizations (CBOs) in their current environment.

Only recently has services research been applied to the study of treatment services for alcohol and drug dependence. The ADAMHA Reorganization Act of 1992 (P.L. 101-321) separated the funding of research and practice in this field. The Act placed the research institutes (National Institute of Alcohol Abuse and Alcoholism, National Institute on Drug Abuse, and National Institute of Mental Health) under the auspices of the National Institutes of Health. At the same time, the service-focused agencies (Office for Treatment Improvement and the Office of Substance Abuse Prevention) were renamed the Center for Substance Abuse Treatment and the Center for Substance Abuse Prevention, respectively, and were located within the Substance Abuse and Mental Health Services Administration (SAMHSA) of the Department of Health and Human Services, along with the newly created Center for Mental Health Services. Concerns about the separation of research and practice led to language in the Act that required the three research institutes to allocate 15 percent of their research portfolio to health services research. The conference committee report on the legislation also requested a national plan for services research from the National Advisory Council on Alcohol Abuse and Alcoholism. The report identified eight areas where health services research was needed (Subcommittee on Health Services Research, 1997):

1. analyses of the organization and financing of treatment for alcohol dependence;
2. studies on the influence of managed care;
3. investigations on access to care and utilization of services;
4. assessments of treatment outcomes, effectiveness and the cost-effectiveness of care;
5. studies of prevention services;
6. development of improved research methods and databases;
7. strategies for the dissemination of research results; and
8. workforce analyses, reviews of training needs, and assessments of the peer review process.

NIAAA's recommendations for health services research should facilitate continued development of research and practice collaborations. Another recent IOM report similarly stresses the importance of collaborative research linkages with managed care and community-based organizations to promote quality improvement in behavioral health care (IOM, 1997b). A similar set of priorities from NIDA would be helpful. Because services research is still emerging on treatment and prevention for alcohol and drug abuse and dependence, influences on policy and practice have been limited and there is much to be learned.

MODELS FOR COLLABORATION

Collaboration between research and practice takes many forms in the substance abuse treatment field and a number of collaboration models that impressed the committee are presented below. Arthur J. Schut, President of the Iowa Substance Abuse Program Director's Association, introduced the committee to the Iowa Consortium that brings together treatment providers, policymakers, and researchers based in each of the state's major universities to collaborate on research initiatives. The consortium facilitates the development, implementation, and interpretation of investigations that examine the need for substance abuse treatment and the effects of major policy initiatives in the state.

Carol Leonard from the Navajo Nation and Philip May, Director of the University of New Mexico's Center on Alcoholism, Substance Abuse and Addictions (CASAA) offered another collaboration strategy. Their partnership illustrates a culturally sensitive approach to the combination of research and community oriented prevention and treatment. Importantly, the collaboration allows academic researchers to study a population (Native Americans) and service system (traditional practices) that would otherwise be difficult to investigate; the Navajo Nation gains through increased support from federal funding authorities and enhanced credibility of the findings from demonstration programs.

The basis for partnerships between research and practice may be strengthened when treatment agencies employ investigators to develop assessment and monitoring protocols. Chestnut Health Systems in Illinois provides an example with its in-house research staff that collaborates with clinical and management staff to develop client information and outcomes monitoring systems. The researchers use the information not only to evaluate specific interventions but also to help practitioners improve the quality of care.

The Community Clinical Oncology Program (CCOP), which has effectively linked cancer research and treatment for almost fifteen years, provides another model of collaboration. As described by Arnold Kaluzny from the University of North Carolina School of Public Health, this network, funded by the National Cancer Institute (NCI) brings together treatment providers and researchers in more than 30 states to get faster answers to research questions and bring state-of-the-art treatment to communities.

Iowa Consortium for Substance Abuse Research and Evaluation

The Iowa Consortium for Substance Abuse Research and Evaluation (the Consortium) provides a structure for communication and cooperation among policymakers, practitioners, and researchers. Representatives from the Iowa Substance Abuse Program Directors Association and investigators from four Iowa universities (University of Iowa, University of Northern Iowa, Iowa State University, and Drake University) joined with policymakers from the state agencies responsible for corrections, education, Medicaid, public safety, and public health to develop a forum to promote the collection of data and the use of research in policy formation and clinical practice. Convened in 1991 by the Governor's Alliance on Substance Abuse, the Consortium has become a vehicle for practical investigations, collaborative design and implementation of studies, multidisciplinary cooperation, and the application of research findings to practice and policy. Current membership includes the directors of community- and hospital-based treatment agencies; researchers trained in education, psychiatry, psychology, social work, and sociology; and women and men responsible for substance abuse treatment and prevention activities in state agencies. The Consortium uses newsletters, reports, meetings, and seminars to communicate and achieve three goals:

1. encourage collaboration in research and evaluation studies,
2. improve prevention and treatment services and contribute to public policy making, and
3. educate students and professionals in substance abuse.

Grants and contracts are the primary source of funding for Consortium activities. A small appropriation from the State of Iowa supports infrastructure and coordination. The Iowa Department of Public Health collaborates with Consortium members to apply for federal awards and state contracts. Funding from the Center for Substance Abuse Treatment and the Center for Substance Abuse Prevention supports needs assessment projects. Funding from NIDA supported investigations of case management strategies. Finally, Consortium affiliated investigators evaluated Iowa's implementation of a managed care approach for publicly funded substance abuse treatment services.

Investigators who work through the Consortium structure may request letters of support from treatment providers and the state substance abuse authority when they apply for services research funds from federal, state, and local governments. The support letters strengthen applications and demonstrate a history of collaboration. The forum empowers treatment programs to participate in the design of investigations and to request support for necessary staff functions related to the research. Programs may also use the Consortium to discourage less clinically useful studies and to promote investigations that meet clinical priorities.

The Consortium's goal of fostering discussion and cooperation among treatment providers, investigators, and policymakers has been difficult to articulate and implement. Individuals trained to conduct scientific research are not initially responsive to policymaker needs to review and comment on reports prior to public release. Practitioners do not always appreciate investigator requests for changes in clinical processes, and they can make demands for information and communication that investigators find intrusive. Policymakers are frustrated by the time required for investigators to collect and analyze data. Control and autonomy remain persistent concerns. Practitioners struggle with the added burdens of data collection and seek clarification around control and ownership of data.

For some participants, the Consortium may be merely a vehicle to access data or clinical populations rather than a venue for collaboration. Nonetheless, the Iowa Consortium for Substance Abuse Research and Evaluation illustrates one way in which investigators, policymakers, and treatment providers can partner in the design and implementation of research. It provides an important example of an alliance between research, policy, and practice, and it suggests mechanisms that can be extended and applied to foster more local partnerships.

Navajo Nation

Community-based research now being undertaken by the Navajo Nation was initiated almost two decades ago by officials of the Navajo Nation (beginning with Mr. Gorman, a former tribal official) and a social science researcher, Philip May. After many years of patience and persistence, the research was finally undertaken with federal moneys, conducted under the aegis of the Navajo Nation with the collaboration of Dr. May and other researchers from the University of New Mexico's Center for Alcohol, Substance Abuse, and Addictions (CASAA), where Dr. May is now the director. CASAA worked with treatment providers in the Navajo Nation to evaluate an alcohol treatment program addressing the underlying cultural conflicts that contribute to high alcoholism rates among the Navajo. The approach was consistent with the high value the Navajo place on achieving balance and harmony with nature, family, and spirits. The collaboration provided the Navajo Nation with increased support from federal funding authorities and enhanced credibility for findings from demonstration programs.

Obstacles to establishing this community-based research program included the following:

- initial suspicions within the tribe that the researchers were only interested in their own ends and did not have a long-lasting commitment to the tribe;
- a lack of familiarity by the tribe in addressing a major problem related to behavior, youth, health, family, law, and other social factors through research;
- absence of collaborative arrangements between nearby universities and the Navajo Nation; and
- insufficient awareness and trust in the funding agencies in working with the Navajo Nation.

Five factors contributed to the eventual success of this community-based research:

- persistence of Tribal leaders and concerned Navajo leaders and community members;
- training and education of younger Navajo community members to participate actively in the administration and operation of a complex research endeavor;
- collaboration of Dr. Phillip May, a researcher with two decades of research experience with substance abuse among Native American people (see for example, May, 1992; May and Dizmang, 1974);
- the interest and flexibility of government officials in working with the tribe and local academics to bring about a funded project; and
- the capability to undertake convincing research across languages and cultures in a largely rural population, many of whom were unfamiliar with research methods or suspicious of the uses to which research might be put.

Academicians, Navajo leaders, and Navajo collaborators in the research project had to cooperate in a variety of complex tasks to establish a state-of-the-art-and-science project. For example, materials had to be translated into Navajo using a standard, yet time-consuming and costly method of initial translation, back-translation, pilot study, renorming and restandardizing, and final acceptance (Brislin, 1986).

Negotiations regarding data access were also important. Data that might result from such a study has the potential for embarrassing tribal officials, leaders, or members at large, while reputable researchers engage in such projects to foster the expansion of knowledge and understanding. Funding organizations wanted assurances that the findings would benefit the people for whom the project was intended, and not languish unused because they were unpalatable to one of the parties involved. After these issues were worked out to each party's satisfaction, projects were undertaken.

Drug Outcome Monitoring System

Two large community-based drug abuse treatment providers in Illinois designed and implemented a performance measurement system to monitor client outcomes and enhance their accountability with purchasers and consumers. Chestnut Health Systems and Interventions, operating 49 facilities, collaborated on a field trial of the Drug Outcome Monitoring System (DOMS). Clinical records, administrative information, and service utilization data are integrated and used for quality improvement and outcome monitoring initiatives. The system includes an assessment tool (Global Appraisal of Individual Needs—GAIN) that facilitates a diagnosis based on

DSM-IV criteria, patient placement using the American Society of Addiction Medicine criteria for level of care, treatment planning consistent with Joint Commission for the Accreditation of Health Care Organizations standards, and compliance with federal and state data reporting requirements (Dennis et al., 1997). This monitoring during and after treatment is expected to enhance clinical processes and improve outcomes. Although still in development and testing, the emphasis on clinical needs and client outcomes increases the potential value for consumers, counselors, management, and payers.

Developed with funding from NIAAA and CSAT, the Drug Outcome Monitoring System illustrates an important strategy for integrating services and research and meeting the needs for both sets of stakeholders. Because the data are of clinical value, counselors are likely to be more careful completing interviews and responding to data elements, thus enhancing data quality for research studies and policy analyses. Client subgroups are developed and benchmarks are established for levels of services and outcomes and postdischarge client tracking. The monitoring system engages clinicians and consumers in the process of tracking and recording clinical status and incorporates early reintervention protocols when postdischarge follow-up suggests that a client is in early relapse. The design of this system to be responsive to consumer and counselor needs contrasts with the top-down development of many administrative data systems that stress payer requirements and management needs.

Community Clinical Oncology Program

Initiated by the National Cancer Institute (NCI) in 1983, the goal of the Community Clinical Oncology Program (CCOP) has been to bring state-of-the-art cancer treatment, prevention, and control research to local communities. This is accomplished by involving community oncologists and community-based primary care physicians in NCI-approved clinical trials (Kaluzny et al., 1996).

CCOP is a strategic alliance among existing organizations. The three main organizations are: (1) NCI, which provides overall direction, funding, and program management; (2) NCI-designated cancer centers and clinical cooperative groups, which develop protocols, analyze data, and provide quality assurance; and (3) the community oncology programs composed of community oncologists, primary care physicians, and their clinical staff who are involved with the accrual of patients to approved treatment, prevention, and control protocols.

As of 1997, there were 51 CCOPs located in 30 states, with 300 participating hospitals where some 2000 physicians cooperate to enter patients and individuals at risk for cancer on NCI-approved clinical trials. An additional 8 minority-based CCOPs are funded to enhance participation of minority populations in clinical trials research. This group adds 42 hospitals and 350 participating physicians to the alliance (NCI, 1997).

The CCOP experience demonstrates certain general principles regarding community-based care. As well-described by Ann Greer (1988) some years ago, "There are no magic signatories or formats which will cause knowledge to jump off the page and into practice." In CCOP, however, the creation of an infrastructure provided an opportunity to close the gap between state-of-the-art care and community practice patterns. For example, in the care of breast cancer, patients treated by CCOP physicians were the ones most consistently receiving state-of-the-art care as defined by current protocols. Moreover, changes in referral patterns among non-CCOP physicians within the community increased the likelihood that patients would receive appropriate adjuvant therapy—an important indicator of CCOP impact on quality of care delivered in participating institutions (Kaluzny et al., 1996).

This approach has also demonstrated the necessity for protocols not only to be available but to be "user friendly," "feasible," and "relevant" in the local context. Moreover, it is necessary that data managers, nursing personnel, and other support personnel be involved in the effort and that CCOP physicians be able to link to primary care providers in the community. The role of support personnel is especially critical to the successful completion of day-to-day tasks involved in patient recruitment, protocol assignment, data collection, and follow-up (Kaluzny et al., 1993).

CCOPs are not inexpensive and present a significant managerial challenge. The infrastructure alone at each clinical site can exceed $200,000. Interactions among community providers are often uneasy, and there is a need to maintain a working relationship between the cancer center (or university), the cooperative groups, and the community physicians.

Local leadership of the CCOP is a particularly critical element. To be a clinician leader requires a commitment to a research perspective with a particular emphasis or at least an orientation to epidemiology and the social behavioral sciences. To meet the realities of a changing health care delivery system, partnerships with managed care organizations must be developed (Kaluzny, 1997). Such partnerships are in the process of development. For example, the American Association of Health Plans has recently adopted a new policy intended to encourage their member HMOs to participate in clinical trials sponsored by NIH, and there appear to be an increasing number of research partnerships between managed care organizations and cancer centers (Glass and Greenlick, 1989; Myers et al., 1997), as well as new partnerships for research developing among managed care organizations (Durham, 1998).

The critical point is to close the gap between policy, research, and treatment and thereby assure "institutional learning" at the community level. This requires an infrastructure among a set of relevant organizations. The CCOP provides this infrastructure, permitting NCI, cancer centers, cooperative groups, and community-based physicians to achieve strategic objectives that were not possible for any single organization.

LESSONS FROM DEMONSTRATION INITIATIVES

The National Institute on Alcohol Abuse and Alcoholism (NIAAA) and the National Institute on Drug Abuse (NIDA) have long traditions of supporting demonstrations to develop and evaluate treatment and prevention interventions. The institutes used a variety of funding and management mechanisms to promote prevention programs, develop services for homeless men and women, and test strategies to reduce the risk of HIV infection among drug users. Three sets of demonstration initiatives are examined to identify lessons for research-practice collaborations in community-based drug treatment.

Prevention Demonstrations

NIAAA and NIDA prevention initiatives began in the 1970s. State Prevention Coordinators were supported to facilitate state planning, provide prevention training, manage state prevention contracts, and serve as liaisons with the federal Institutes (Williams and Vejnoska, 1981). NIAAA funded the development of prevention curriculum for children, adolescents, and college students. After the models were implemented, NIAAA used a demonstration replication program to test the generalizability of the three prevention models. Eight local communities and State Alcoholism Authorities were funded to replicate and evaluate one of the prevention programs. The replication highlighted the need for systematic documentation and illustrated the variations encountered as communities deviated from model frameworks (NIAAA, 1981). The two formal school-based curricula (Here's Looking at You and CASPAR) have evolved during more than 20 years of use and remain cornerstones of prevention activities in many school systems. The university-based model, however, faded as neither the original campus nor the replication campuses maintained the initiative for long after the termination of federal funding.

Based on these experiences, NIAAA designed subsequent prevention projects to be "conceptually tighter, more skeptical, and careful in statements of objectives and intentions, more modest in whom they mean to reach and what they mean to do with people, and more deliberate in how they plan to go about it" (NIAAA, 1981). There was more emphasis on theory, and projects were more likely to be funded in public health departments and research centers than in community-based schools and organizations. The prevention strategies evolved from an emphasis on individual change to an emphasis on policy and environmental interventions. These demonstrations illustrate both the value of building system capacity (there was a substantial need for educational curricula) and the challenges of collaborating with community groups to test applications. The replications enhanced curriculum development but appear to have contributed little to science.

Projects for Homeless Individuals

The 1987 Stewart B. Mckinney Homeless Assistance Act (P. L. 100-77) authorized initiatives to address the national problem of widespread homelessness. NIAAA and NIDA collaborated to support demonstration projects that implemented and evaluated interventions for homeless men and women with alcohol- and drug-related problems. Initially, nine projects were funded in eight cities. Each project was required to allocate at least 25 percent of the award for process and outcome evaluation. A separate contract was awarded for cross-site evaluation, coordination, assistance, and data analysis (Lubran, 1990; Orwin et al., 1993). A diversity of interventions was encouraged because there was little empirical data on effective services for alcohol and drug involved homeless individuals (Huebner and Crosse, 1991). The applicants tended to be community organizations or state or local health departments. The community organizations subcontracted with academic-based investigators for the evaluation research. Each site was unique. A special issue of the *Alcoholism Treatment Quarterly* (McCarty, 1990) and reports from NIAAA (Murray, 1993; Shane et al., 1993) provide more details.

The evaluation report on the first round of demonstrations drew lessons, noted key findings, and made recommendations (Orwin et al., 1993). An obvious but often overlooked finding was that when working with homeless men and women, issues related to food, shelter, and security must be addressed before treatment can be initiated. Programs also learned that both program structure and flexible responses were necessary to engage and retain homeless participants. Start-up required substantial resources and persistence, especially when there was resistance to siting services in specific locations. Overall improvements in client functioning were modest. Generally, the services led to reductions in alcohol and drug use. Composite scores from the Addiction Severity Index suggested improvements in employment and economic security in some of the study sites. Housing stability was increased in a project that facilitated access to alcohol- and drug-free housing; psychiatric status improved in a different city.

Substantial project variation made cross-site comparisons difficult, and only five of the nine sites provided useful outcome data (Huebner and Crosse, 1991; Orwin et al., 1993). The quality of the data submitted for cross-site analysis varied because the study sites tended to be community-based organizations with little research experience. Low follow-up rates compromised the integrity of the evaluation designs and threatened the validity of the findings. Finally, variability among the nine study sites and the relatively small number of study sites limited the ability to identify robust interventions and to generalize study findings.

Based on these lessons and limitations, the cross-site evaluation has general implications for collaboration between community-based organizations and researchers (Huebner and Crosse, 1991; Orwin et al., 1993). The ability of seven of the nine sites to collect and submit standardized data suggested that research is feasible in community settings even when the population is difficult to serve. The evaluators also recommended longer funding periods, larger sample sizes, more rigorous evaluation designs, standardization of research tools and interventions, and more emphasis on follow-up data collection. First, research demonstrations require at least five years of funding for implementation, maturation, and the development of a sufficient sample. Second, programs should receive technical assistance as needed on evaluation design, data collection, and analysis. Finally, adequate follow-up rates are essential to provide scientifically valid data on the effects of the interventions.

NIAAA applied these lessons to the design of a second round of community demonstration programs. Significantly, the funding mechanism was changed from grants to cooperative agreements to give NIAAA staff and its subcontractors more control and influence over development and implementation (Huebner et al., 1993). NIAAA provided guidelines for service interventions and site-level evaluations and mandated a core set of instruments. NIAAA also attempted to increase the consistency of the data collection and improve the potential for meaningful cross-site analyses. As a result of these modifications, the second round projects were primarily awarded to universities and research centers which subcontracted with community organizations for services. Details on the study sites are provided in a special issue of the *Alcoholism Treatment Quarterly* (Conrad et al., 1993) and an issue of *New Directions for Program Evaluation* (Conrad, 1994).

The evolution of the Community Demonstration Project between the first set of grants to community organizations and the second set of cooperative agreements with academic research centers illustrates the challenges of building effective collaborations among practitioners, researchers, and policymakers. The funding agency and the external (cross-site) evaluators were disappointed with the level of control and influence in the initial investigations. In the subsequent awards, research expertise was emphasized and specific research instruments were required. This was designed to improve the quality of the science, but changing the rules also changed the roles of the participants: service providers tended to be less directly involved, and investigators had a more dominant influence.

National AIDS Demonstration Research Project

The spread of HIV infection led Congress to ask NIDA to develop interventions that encouraged injection drug users to reduce HIV risk behaviors and enter treatment. During 1987 and 1988, the National AIDS Demonstration Research (NADR) Program funded demonstration outreach and intervention services in 47 cities (NIDA, 1996). These programs combined research and services to gather data on drug use and to test the efficacy of behavior change strategies.

Individually and collectively, the study sites demonstrated that injection drug users were responsive to education and outreach interventions (NIDA, 1996; Needle and Coyle, 1997). NIDA encouraged state substance abuse prevention and treatment authorities to promote the adoption and continuation of the outreach and educational models that appeared to be most effective (NIDA, 1996). Three strategies for behavior change among injection drug users were disseminated: (1) a two-session risk reduction education intervention (Coyle, 1993); (2) a four-session psychoeducational intervention using behavioral counseling techniques (Rhodes, 1993); and (3) an outreach and community change strategy where recovering drug users provide education and support for behavior change (Wiebel, 1993).

NIDA also used a cooperative agreement mechanism to support multi-site studies to monitor HIV risk behaviors and test outreach interventions among out-of-treatment drug users. Collaboration among the 23 study sites permitted more rapid data collection on infrequent behaviors and small populations (NIDA, 1996). The Cooperative Agreement for AIDS Community-Based Outreach/Intervention Research Program appears to have been an effective approach to multisite research collaborations with community-based services.

These programs demonstrated that out-of-treatment drug users could be found and educated, and they also illustrated the value of collaborations between research and services. Involvement of multiple sites and varied teams of investigators increased the generalizability of the findings, and policymakers were able to be more confident in their programming recommendations. There appears to have been substantial teamwork among the outreach workers, counselors, and investigators. The initiatives document the feasibility of developing structures that support partnerships among consumers, clinicians, and researchers.

GUIDANCE FOR GRANT REVIEW

To participate in research, evaluation, and demonstration opportunities, treatment programs and investigators usually must respond to program announcements and requests for applications from the NIH research institutes and the SAMHSA service centers. The committee heard much apprehension about the application and review process—the competition is great, the review process is biased against clinically useful investigations, community-based agencies are not strong applicants, and controlled clinical trials are more likely to be funded than services research. Similar concerns were voiced in another IOM Committee report, *Dispelling the Myths About Addiction: Strategies to Increase Understanding and Strengthen Research,* (IOM, 1997a). The relatively small proportion of applications that are approved and funded attests to the difficulty of the process. But the widespread misgivings also suggest basic misunderstandings about the review process. More education and guidance about the application and review process may be useful, especially if it is pragmatic.

An experienced perspective on the review process is provided by the former chair of a NIDA initial review group, who identifies ten common mistakes in grant writing (Oetting, 1990). Applicants should recognize their weaknesses and build a team that strengthens the proposal. Sufficient detail is required to convince reviewers that the study can be completed. If the proposal has been previously reviewed, the resubmission should respond to the prior critiques. The aims of the study must be important and address real needs and issues. Methods must be used appropriately and applicants should not make excuses for inadequate procedures.

Three of Oetting's list of ten mistakes seem directly applicable to the challenge of research and practice collaborations. First, applications that seek research funds primarily to enhance treatment capacity are usually a mistake. While services can be funded through research applications (if the service is necessary to test specific hypotheses), reviewers evaluate the quality of the research plan and the potential for knowledge generation not the need for more treatment. In research applications, the quality of the research is the major determinant of the application score. Another common grant writing mistake is to attach analyses of drug use and abuse to programs and investigations with a different primary interest. Although drug abuse affects many facets of life, applications that fail to address drug use and abuse directly tend to be weak. Applicants must demonstrate a comprehensive understanding of the connections to drug abuse and not merely seek additional funding. Finally, Oetting (1990) suggests that the most critical mistake is not to apply. The process is difficult and the probability of funding is low. Agencies that never apply, however, can never be funded and can not benefit from the literature review and thinking required to develop an application and from the opportunity to receive reviewer feedback, revise and submit revised applications which have a higher probability of funding.

Because community-based organizations receive few research grants, it appears to some observers that nonacademic applicants are disadvantaged in the application and review process. Significant changes may be required in the application and review process in order to increase awards to community-based applicants. If, however, the goal is research that is of high quality and applicable to treatment programs, the application and review process should stress the importance and quality of the proposed research. Applications with strong partnerships between practitioners and investigators should be encouraged and should be competitive in the current review process. Ultimately, the committee determined it was not appropriate to recommend changes in the general process for applying for and reviewing research applications. The committee felt strongly, however, that mechanisms must be created to stimulate and support effective alliances between research teams and treatment providers, and recommended a special grant program with a unique review process to achieve this end.

SUMMARY

The review of applied research and health services research suggests that research in clinical settings is not easy and has many unique aspects, views tht were supported by many who spoke to the committee. Environmental control is reduced. Research teams are required. Access and funding issues must be negotiated. Data and results must be shared. Special skills and training are necessary for research collaboration in a community-based setting, but there are few, if any, programs that provide such training. Professional development programs are needed, similar to the NIH training programs and Robert Wood Johnson clinical scholars program. Services research in community-based substance abuse treatment settings requires investigators who can build meaningful partnerships with drug abuse treatment programs and who have the skills to design and implement high quality research studies that will contribute to the evolution and refinement of community-based treatment interventions.

There is no single best approach to promoting collaborations. Strategies will vary depending on participant personalities, the issues and policies of interest, and the resources available. The Iowa Consortium works, in part, because policymakers help support the research infrastructure and provide a forum for communication. Chestnut Health Systems Drug Outcomes Monitoring System illustrates the advantages of working closely with investigators based in the treatment agency. CCOP also provides research infrastructure support and has the added benefit of having been developed and tested by NCI. The promise of enhanced consumer access to treatment innovations suggests an intriguing potential for application of the CCOP model within community-based drug abuse treatment services. Finally, the collaboration between CASAA and the Navajo Nation shows the importance of long-term relationships. This partnership promotes systematic study of populations and procedures that are often not open to research investigation.

The culture of treatment and recovery requires investigators who are sensitive to its nuances. Demonstration programs funded through NIDA and NIAAA document that research collaborations with treatment programs, consumers, and investigators are feasible. The funding requirements appear to influence the nature of the collaborations: the homeless demonstrations and the HIV demonstrations were more service oriented when funding went to community-based providers who subcontracted for research and evaluation services, however, there was more emphasis on science when academic research centers controlled the funding and subcontracted for services. Both research and service must have adequate and specific funds. Adequate funding for both will empower services researchers and treatment providers alike. Practitioners and researchers must have a mutual understanding and appreciation for the other's role. Ultimately, research and practice alliances must balance scientific control and rigor with the realities of clinical environments.

REFERENCES

Bickman L. 1980. Applied Social Psychology, SPSSI, and Kurt Lewin. In: Bickman L ed. *Applied Social Psychology Annual : 1.* Vol. 1. Beverly Hills, CA: Sage Publications. Pp. 7–18.

Brislin RW. 1986. The wording and translation of research instruments. In: Lonner JW, Berry JW eds. *Field Methods in Cross-Cultural Research.* Beverly Hills, CA: Sage.

Brown LD. 1991. Knowledge and power: Health services research as a political resource. In: Ginzberg E, ed. *Health Services Research: Key to Health Policy.* Cambridge, MA: Harvard University Press. Pp. 20–45.

Conrad KJ, ed. 1994. *Critically Evaluating the Role of Experiments, Vol. 63.* San Francisco, CA: Jossey-Bass.

Conrad KJ, Hultman CI, Lyons JS, eds. 1993. *Treatment of the Chemically Dependent Homeless: Theory and Implementation in Fourteen American Projects* (10)3/4.

Coyle SL. 1993. *The NIDA HIV Counseling and Education Intervention Model: Intervention Manual.* NIH Pub. No. 93-3580. Rockville, MD: National Institute on Drug Abuse.

Dennis ML, Godley SH, Scott C, Foss M, Godley MD, Hagan R, Senay EC, Bailey J, Bokos PJ. 1997. *Drug Outcome Monitoring Systems (DOMS): Developing a New Biopsychosocial Paradigm for Health Services Research.* Bloomington, IL: Chestnut Health Systems.

Durham ML. 1998. Partnerships for research among managed care organizations. *Health Affairs* 17(1):111–122.

Ginzberg E. 1991. Health services research and health policy. In: Ginzberg E ed. *Health Services Research: Key to Health Policy*. Cambridge, MA: Harvard University Press. Pp. 1–19.

Glass AG, Greenlick MR. 1989. Opportunities for cancer research in a Health Maintenance Organization. *Cancer Investigation* 7(3):283–286.

Greer AL. 1988. The state of the art vs the state of the science. *International Journal of Technology Assessment in Health Care* 4:5–26.

Huebner RB, Crosse SB. 1991. Challenges in evaluating a national demonstration program for homeless persons with alcohol and other drug problems. *New Directions for Program Evaluation* :33–46.

Huebner RB, Perl HI, Murray PM, Scott JE, Tantunjian BA. 1993. The NIAAA cooperative agreement program for homeless persons with alcohol and other drug problems: An overview. *Alcoholism Treatment Quarterly* 10(3/4):5–20.

IOM (Institute of Medicine). 1995. *Health Services Research: Workforce and Educational Issues*. Washington, DC: National Academy Press.

IOM. 1997a. *Dispelling the Myths About Addiction: Strategies to Increase Understanding and Strengthen Research*. Washington, DC: National Academy Press.

IOM. 1997b. *Managing Managed Care: Quality Improvement in Behavioral Health*. Washington, DC: National Academy Press.

Kaluzny A. 1997. Cancer prevention and control research in a changing health services system. *Preventive Medicine* 26:31–35.

Kaluzny AD et al. 1993. Cancer prevention and control with the National Cancer Institute's Clinical Trial Network: Lessons from the Community Clinical Oncology Program. *Journal of the National Cancer Institute* 85(22):1807–1811.

Kaluzny AD, Warnecke RB et al. 1996. *Managing a Health Care Alliance: Improving Community Cancer Care*. San Francisco, CA: Jossey-Bass.

Lewin K. 1951. *Theory in Social Science: Selected Theoretical Papers*. New York: Harper & Brothers Publishers.

Lubran B. 1990. Alcohol and drug abuse among the homeless population: A national response. *Alcoholism Treatment Quarterly* 7(1):11–23.

Marrow A. 1969. *The Practical Theorist: The Life and Work of Kurt Lewin*. New York: Basic Books.

May PA. 1992. Alcohol policy considerations for Indian reservations and bordertown communities. *American Indian Alaska Native Mental Health Research* 4(3):5–59.

May PA, Dizmang LH. 1974. Suicide and the American Indian. *Psychiatric Annals* 4:22–28.

McCarty D. 1990. Nine demonstration grants: Nine approaches. *Alcoholism Treatment Quarterly* 7(1):1–9.

Murray MM. 1993. *Community Demonstration Grant Projects for Alcohol and Drug Abuse Treatment of Homeless Individuals: Innovative Strategies for Treating Alcohol and Drug Abuse Problems Among Homeless Men and Women*. NIH Pub. No. 93-3540. Rockville, MD: National Institute on Alcohol Abuse and Alcoholism.

Myers RE, Schlackman N, Kaluzny AD. 1997. A promising process for creating an AHC—Managed care organization alliance for research and care. *Academic Medicine* 72(5): 321–322.

NCI (National Cancer Institute). 1997. *The Nation's Investment in Cancer Research: A Budget Proposal for Fiscal Year 1999*. Rockville, MD: National Cancer Institute, National Institutes of Health.

NIAAA (National Institute on Alcohol Abuse and Alcoholism). 1981. *Fourth Special Report to the U.S. Congress on Alcohol and Health*. DHHS Pub. No. ADM 81-1080. Rockville, MD: National Institue on Alcohol Abuse and Alcoholism.

NIDA (National Institute on Drug Abuse). 1996. *National Institute on Drug Abuse Community-Based HIV Prevention Research.* Rockville, MD: National Institute on Drug Abuse.

Needle RH, Coyle SL. 1997. *Community-Based Outreach Risk Reduction Strategy to Prevent HIV Risk Behaviors in Out-of-Treatment Injection Drug Users.* Rockville, MD: National Institute on Drug Abuse.

Oetting ER. 1990. Ten fatal mistakes in grant writing. In: Kazdin AE ed. *Methodological Issues and Strategies in Clinical Research.* Washington, DC: American Psychological Association. Pp. 739–748.

Orwin RG, Goldman HH, Sonnefeld LJ, Smith NG, Ridgely MS, Garrison-Morgren R, O'Neill E, Luchese J, Sherman A, O'Connell ME. 1993. *Community Demonstration Grant Projects for Alcohol and Drug Abuse Treatment of Homeless Individuals: Final Evaluation Report.* NIH Pub. No. 92-3541. Rockville, MD: National Institute on Alcohol Abuse and Alcoholism.

Rhodes F. 1993. *The Behavioral Counseling Model for Injection Drug Users: Intervention Manual.* NIH Pub. No. 93-3579. Rockville, MD: National Institute on Drug Abuse.

Shane P, Ridgely MS, Sherman A, O'Neill E, Goldman HH, Wittman F, Smith NG. 1993. *Community Demonstration Grants Projects for Alcohol and Drug Abuse Treatment of Homeless Individuals: Case Studies of Nine Community Demonstration Grants.* NIH Pub. No. 93-3539. Rockville, MD: National Institute on Alcohol Abuse and Alcoholism.

Subcommittee on Health Services Research, National Advisory Council on Alcohol Abuse and Alcoholism. 1997. *Improving the Delivery of Alcohol Treatment and Prevention Services: Executive Summary.* Rockville, MD: National Institute on Alcohol Abuse and Alcoholism.

Wiebel W. 1993. *The Indigenous Leader Outreach Model: Intervention Manual.* NIH Pub. No. 93-3581. Rockville, MD: National Institute on Drug Abuse.

Williams M, Vejnoska J. 1981. Alcohol and youth: State prevention approaches. *Alcohol Health & Research World* 6(1):2–13.

6

Findings and Recommendations

The committee's review of current research, models for collaboration between research and practice, community-based organizations, and dissemination strategies led to findings and recommendations in six areas: (1) strategies for linking research and practice, (2) strategies for linking research findings, policy development, and implementation, (3) strategies for knowledge development, (4) strategies for dissemination and knowledge transfer, (5) strategies for consumer participation, and (6) training strategies for community-based research collaboration. The committee believes that attention to its recommendations will lead to improvements in clinical practices and will enhance the value of treatment research to clinicians, investigators, policymakers, clients, and to the general public.

STRATEGIES FOR LINKING RESEARCH AND PRACTICE

The committee found some striking examples of strong collaborations between community-based drug and alcohol abuse treatment programs and academic research institutions. It was apparent, however, that relatively few investigators work closely with community treatment programs and even fewer programs participate actively in research.

Treatment programs benefit from being part of a learning culture that, among other characteristics, values knowledge development and hypothesis testing. Research collaboration can provide tangible and intangible benefits that improve an agency's competitive position—enhanced information systems, education and mentoring for clinical staff, contributions to overhead costs, access to state-of-the-art treatment interventions, staff pride, and more informed consumers.

Research participation becomes a possibility for treatment providers when community-based organizations are compensated for the true costs of research participation, and when program staff and investigators collaborate in construction of hypotheses, research design, and data collection, analysis, and interpretation.

Only a small proportion of community-based agencies currently have the capacity to participate fully in long-term partnerships with teams of investigators. The level of participation in research collaborations depends on an agency's stage of organizational development, the compatibility of the studies with the organization's mission and culture, and its financial stability. Thus, participation may vary from relatively passive participation (completing surveys and submitting data to state databases) to involvement as a partner in the development of research questions, data collection, and data interpretation. However, incentives must change for all parties if real progress is to be made.

The trust necessary for long-term collaboration is generally based on a history of increasing involvement. Successful collaborative programs from other health fields include support for a permanent infrastructure that facilitates long-term development. The National Cancer Institute's Community Clinical Oncology Program (CCOP) uses this strategy to bring state-of-the-art oncology research to community-based cancer treatment programs. CCOP facilitates research collaborations and enhances the ability of treatment programs to apply research findings to the general patient population. Development of a similar mechanism for use in community-based drug abuse treatment programs could catalyze research/practice collaborations and stimulate improvements in practice. The CCOPs are not inexpensive and they present a significant managerial challenge. The infrastructure alone at each clinical site can exceed $200,000. However, the infrastructure recommendation that follows does not necessarily require a model with that complexity. It could begin as a demonstration project involving a basic infrastructure enhancement of perhaps one full-time equivalent staff person and some computer support to a small set of diverse treatment sites. This level of support would be the target, whichever of the various network collaboration models is finally implemented.

Based on these findings, the committee offers two recommendations and identifies certain key characteristics that will facilitate their successful implementation.

RECOMMENDATION 1. The National Institute on Drug Abuse and the Center for Substance Abuse Treatment should support the development of an infrastructure to facilitate research within a network of community-based treatment programs, similar to the National Cancer Institute's Community Clinical Oncology Program (CCOP) networks.

To be successful, the infrastructure and network development will depend on commitment from the community-based treatment programs and researchers. Certain key areas will need to be addressed to foster partnership. For the community-based treatment programs, these include:

- encouraging and, when appropriate, participating in biomedical, social-behavioral, treatment effectiveness, and services research;
- seeking collaboration with researchers to build information systems that enhance the delivery of clinical services, improve program management and operations, and contribute to research databases;
- enhancing quality improvement strategies and fostering the development of organizational learning; and
- promoting staff education on current research and creating strategies to encourage adoption of clinical protocols that hold promise to improve treatment services.

Likewise, for treatment researchers, the following approaches are suggested:

- encouraging and, when appropriate, seeking collaborative opportunities with community-based drug treatment organizations (CBOs);
- recognizing the burdens of research on programs and consumers and providing fair compensation for the time and resources required to participate in studies;
- remaining sensitive to any potential their work has to harm consumers or treatment programs;
- guarding against the misuse of their research findings and the findings of other researchers in the development of funding and regulatory policies and the design of clinical protocols;
- supporting, through their work and their policy participation, consumer education on state-of-the-art clinical services; and
- recognizing the value of consumer participation by providing information accessible to consumers about the benefits of research, by including consumers on study advisory groups and by integrating informed consumer opinion in research proposals and study designs.

RECOMMENDATION 2.   The National Institute on Drug Abuse and the National Institute on Alcohol Abuse and Alcoholism should develop research initiatives to foster studies that include community-based treatment programs as full partners.

Issues to be addressed by these initiatives are:

- including representatives from the treatment community in the development of the research initiative and in the review of proposals;
- showing sensitivity to the needs and constraints of community-based programs;
- requiring, in the proposal, an assessment of the study's burden and impact on the treatment program and its clients, as well as its potential relevance and practicality for CBO implementation;
- requiring active, early, and permanent participation of treatment staff in the development, implementation, and interpretation of the study;
- emphasizing the consideration of gender, gender identity, race, and urban/rural issues in research priorities; and
- providing a rapid funding mechanism to promote small research projects on emerging issues affecting treatment (e.g., managed care, welfare reform, performance measurement).

STRATEGIES FOR LINKING RESEARCH FINDINGS, POLICY DEVELOPMENT, AND TREATMENT IMPLEMENTATION

State and federal policies sometimes hinder the diffusion of knowledge flowing from research relevant to drug abuse treatment. Selective prohibitions on the use of state and federal funds can inhibit the application of proven research findings. Language in the Substance Abuse Prevention and Treatment Block Grant, for example, prohibits the use of federal funds for needle exchange, despite studies demonstrating this improves the effectiveness of outreach to the population at highest risk for HIV infection. A similar restriction on the use of funds for client payments inhibits the implementation of behavioral reinforcement strategies. Local laws and policies restrict the development and operation of methadone services. Moreover, state and federal officials have generally not used funding mechanisms to facilitate collaboration between treatment programs and researchers, to foster adoption of new and effective treatments, or to improve the design of clinical research.

The committee believes that the coordination of state and federal programs is important to facilitate active collaboration and improvement of drug and alcohol treatment. Two recommendations are offered emphasizing the role of states in this collaboration, accompanied by approaches to undergird needed support.

RECOMMENDATION 3. State authorities should provide financial incentives for collaborative investigations between CBOs and academically oriented research centers; and should support structures to foster broad participation among researchers, practitioners, consumers, and payers in the development of a treatment research agenda, including studies to measure outcomes and program operations.

RECOMMENDATION 4. CSAT and the states need to cooperate in the development of financial incentives that encourage the inclusion of proven treatment approaches into community-based treatment programs. This approach should include making additional funds available for implementing targeted treatment approaches.

To improve treatment, the following are considered critical areas to address:

- Creating mechanisms to ensure the adoption of treatments proven to be effective and development of requests for proposals that support implementations of specific treatments within local community-based settings.
- Supporting the development of management information systems within community-based drug treatment programs, including consultation for system planning. These data systems should not be a one-way conduit to a state database but should also provide information to the treatment programs in a usable format and become the basis of public reports on outcomes.
- Expanding researcher, provider, and consumer participation in the development of licensing standards, staff development requirements, and initiatives to enhance consumer participation. State licensing standards provide the basis for monitoring treatment outcomes and processes and for managing progress toward desired patient outcomes. The best staff development standards require ongoing staff training and education (e.g., through publications, seminars, enrollment in continuing education, and attendance at training sessions that disseminate information on emerging developments in clinical care). Consumer participation standards provide consumers with information on state-of-the-art treatment techniques, and outcomes measurement systems are best developed with input from families and patients.

STRATEGIES FOR KNOWLEDGE DEVELOPMENT

Drug and alcohol abuse treatment providers were often critical of treatment research. At the same time, there was considerable support for collaborating on research projects that had immediate application to problems faced in patient care. Practitioners and policymakers requested more research on treatment effectiveness—studies that help programs operate more effectively and identify interventions that serve clients more effectively.

The committee's findings suggest that expanding the range of studied treatment settings, treatment modalities, and treatment populations may result in more broadly applicable treatment research findings. These observations led the committee to make two specific recommendations in this area.

RECOMMENDATION 5. CSAT and NIDA should develop mechanisms to enable state policymakers to monitor service delivery in community-based treatment programs and to determine if consumers receive services empirically demonstrated as effective and to ascertain if the treatment dosage and intensity are sufficient to be effective.

RECOMMENDATION 6. NIDA and NIAAA should continue to support "real world" services research and cost-effectiveness studies and include the development of services research in their strategic plans.

STRATEGIES FOR DISSEMINATION AND KNOWLEDGE TRANSFER

The committee found at least four factors that inhibit diffusion of drug abuse treatment knowledge: (1) the structure of treatment delivery systems; (2) the diversity of the clients, providers, and other stakeholders; (3) the stigmatization of people who are dependent on alcohol and other drugs; and (4) an inadequate base of knowledge about technology transfer specific to the field. Differences in perspective among consumers, clinicians, researchers, and policymakers also inhibit knowledge dissemination and use.

While there is a general knowledge base about technology transfer, there has been little research on information exchange in the drug abuse treatment field. Research findings about technology transfer specific to drug abuse treatment are needed to help overcome the critical barriers to information exchange and reduce the knowledge gaps in this field.

Treatment programs are underutilizing research findings in the area of psychosocial interventions, pharmacotherapy, and integrated service delivery approaches. Several approaches have been shown in other fields to successfully close the gaps between treatment, research, and policy and there are models that could be applied more widely in the future.

Because providers and payers are often unaware of the latests research, the committee found a pressing need to create consensus in the field about which treatments have been proven to be effective and which have been proven to be ineffective. Further, the research agendas of the federal agencies should continue to be fueled by agreement in the field on which models have not received adequate study. The fruits of this consensus process should be widely distributed.

Key to improving knowledge dissemination will be cooperation and collaboration across federal agencies, states, professional organizations, and consumer groups, among others. The committee recommends two general approaches to establish the needed collaboration.

RECOMMENDATION 7. CSAT, NIDA, NIAAA, and AHCPR are the federal agencies that should develop formal collaborations, where appropriate, to synthesize research, reduce the barriers to knowledge transfer, and provide updated information about drug and alcohol treatment strategies to purchasers of health care.

A variety of approaches could be utilized to accomplish these goals. For example, expert panels of investigators, practitioners, program administrators, policymakers, and consumers could be convened by NIDA, NIAAA, and CSAT to generate up-to-date consensus recommendations for community-based drug and alcohol treatment programs based on current research. NIDA-, NIAAA-, and AHCPR-sponsored research on drug treatment knowledge dissemination would help to reduce barriers to the transfer of treatment knowledge and encourage treatment programs and policymakers to adopt proven treatments. Research findings need to be prepared in a form, and disseminated within channels, that enhance availability and acceptability to community-based treatment programs—especially frontline treatment staff. Continued support for and improvement of electronic and print publications directed to treatment programs and consumers is necessary; and other media, such as public access television, should be considered.

CSAT, NIDA, and NIAAA also have an important role in the development of information to enable purchasers of care to take research findings into account explicitly in making purchasing decisions. At the same time, purchasers should develop treatment criteria that ensure treatments of proven effectiveness are adequately funded and should consider withholding funding when the science base shows the treatment to be unequivocally ineffective.

RECOMMENDATION 8. CSAT, in collaboration with state substance abuse authorities, professional organizations, and consumer organizations in the addiction field, should continue the development of evidence-based treatment recommendations for use by clinicians of all disciplines involved in the treatment of drug and alcohol use disorders.

To ensure that these treatment recommendations have a positive impact on health care, these agencies and groups should work to encourage their use. Measurement of the impact of guidelines on clinical care delivery will optimally include short-, intermediate-, and long-term treatment outcomes.

STRATEGIES FOR CONSUMER PARTICIPATION

Consumers are rarely involved in the issues of how drug abuse treatment research is supported and conducted. Although many community-based treatment programs were founded by men and women in recovery and counselors in recovery make up a significant portion of the workforce, there are few advocacy groups for patients and their families. In view of the stigma and legal hazards attached to illicit drug abuse, the reluctance to advocate is understandable but unfortunate. Consumer advocacy for state-of-the-art services has improved care for individuals with cancer and with HIV/AIDS. Drug abuse treatment may enjoy similar benefits if drug treatment consumers become informed consumer advocates.

RECOMMENDATION 9. CSAT and NIDA, in collaboration with state substance abuse authorities, should develop public awareness programs to encourage consumers and their families to recognize high-quality treatment programs so they will begin to demand that treatment programs include research-proven treatment approaches within their treatment models.

There are a variety of approaches that can be considered by these groups to accomplish this goal. These include:

- Encouraging provider quality scorecard development to assure that consumer-oriented quality and satisfaction data, including short- and long-term data, are available to the public. Scorecard development is an early stage but growing movement in health care generally and could provide useful information about community-based treatment programs.
- Reviewing and updating the formats and content of communication vehicles to assure that treatment and research information is accessible to consumers and to the community-based treatment organizations.

It is also critically important that representatives of consumers and their families, with the support and assistance of the research, treatment, and policy communities, promote local as well as national advocacy groups to work with state funding agencies, insurers, managed care organizations, and self-insured employers to encourage the use of valid and reliable measures of treatment outcomes. Such measures serve as a basis for evaluating the efficacy of specific treatment modalities and the cost effectiveness of treatment programs, individual treatment providers and networks of care. State and federal government and employers and purchasing alliances could then be encouraged to use these data to inform their health care purchasing and contracting decisions. Consumer groups should also advocate for the development of standards of care in community-based clinics, treatment networks, integrated delivery systems, and managed care networks. Such standards could be used in accreditation of treatment programs and are best if based on findings from clinical research as well as broadly accepted clinical consensus.

TRAINING STRATEGIES FOR
COMMUNITY-BASED RESEARCH COLLABORATION

Research collaboration, especially collaboration in services research, requires skills and knowledge not generally provided in most graduate training programs. In order to foster collaborative research, it is necessary to enhance these skills in the next generation of drug abuse researchers. At the same time, despite the plethora of prior recommendations for addressing this problem, clinical training programs often fail to provide the background and orientation for treatment research. Thus, both clinical and research training programs need to be more attentive to the need for collaboration to improve treatment in this field.

The committee made three recommendations specific to preparing trainees for active participation in clinical research studies.

RECOMMENDATION 10. NIDA and other research funding agencies should support predoctoral and postdoctoral research training programs that provide experience in drug abuse treatment research and health services research within community-based treatment programs. Programs funded should have the full and active participation of community-based treatment programs and should include resources to fund the costs of participation for the treatment programs.

RECOMMENDATION 11.   University training programs in the health professions should:

- enhance exposure of students to didactic teaching about substance abuse and dependence;
- require didactic teaching as well as supervised clinical experiences in community-based treatment settings;
- teach students to interpret substance abuse treatment research and apply research findings in their clinical practices;
- work with professional organizations to enhance continuing education about the addictions within the residency training curriculum of the various health professions; and
- support researchers seeking to enhance collaborative relationships with treatment programs by offering tuition credit for CBO staff involved in funded collaborative research.

RECOMMENDATION 12.   NIDA, CSAT, and other appropriate funding agencies should create research training programs for staff members of community-based treatment programs to strengthen the ability of the treatment programs to include research activities and to adopt the findings of research into their treatment approaches. Training programs should promote research training for clinical staff through fellowships and tuition remission, and incentives for attending professional meetings.

To enhance the likelihood that these recommendations are given serious consideration by the agencies to which they are addressed, the assistance of foundations is also needed. Foundations could play an important role by developing grant programs to:

- Support training in clinical and services research in the addiction disorders. These grants should emphasize skills needed for participating in collaborative research and in the translation and implementation of treatment research into local community settings.
- Support training for consumers and their families in becoming effective advocates and in the development of advocacy organizations to promote state-of-the-art treatment and treatment research, as well as consumer participation in policy areas such as the development of standards of care.

Appendixes

A

Statement of Task

The broad objectives of this Institute of Medicine project will be to determine mechanisms for the effective transfer of information from the research communities to community-based drug treatment centers. Additionally, it will explore mechanisms for transfer of information from the treatment community back to the researchers. The committee will explore barriers that might hinder this transfer and integration of knowledge, and develop strategies for increasing technology transfer in this bidirectional manner. The committee will seek input through a variety of mechanisms, such as a review of the relevant literature; site visits to geographically dispersed community treatment programs; commissioned papers; and two workshops. Individuals involved in the research and treatment communities will be invited to participate in the workshops, including clinical researchers, health services researchers, experts in program evaluation, clinicians from a range of drug abuse treatment modalities, state and local health department personnel, administrators of community-based treatment programs, and experts in management information and decision support systems. The committee will:

- identify relevant treatment strategies and promising research approaches, including the development of a typology linking specific treatment strategies with amenable research approaches;
- identify mechanisms by which community-based treatment programs are participating in research, including subsequent use of that research;

- identify mechanisms for technology transfer (review model programs, e.g., AIDS, cancer);
- identify barriers that may hinder conduct of research within or the application of research results in the treatment setting;
- identify barriers that hinder the communication of treatment practices back to the researchers; and
- identify innovative yet practical strategies for overcoming those barriers.

Upon synthesizing and analyzing the results of the above review, and input received during the committee workshops, and other mechanisms (e.g., site visits, commissioned papers) the committee will produce a consensus report with recommendations to the Center for Substance Abuse Treatment and the National Institute on Drug Abuse.

B

Workshops and Roundtable: Agendas and Participants

INSTITUTE OF MEDICINE
NATIONAL ACADEMY OF SCIENCES

Committee on Community-Based Drug Treatment
Roundtable on Community-Based Drug Treatment:
*The Need for Partnership Among Providers,
Policymakers, and Researchers*

Tuesday, July 29, 1997
Lecture Room, National Academy of Sciences
2101 Constitution Avenue, N.W., Washington, D.C.

WORKSHOP AGENDA

10:00 a.m.   Welcome and Introductions—Overview of Objectives
for the Day and Review of Open Meetings Policy*
Merwyn R. Greenlick, Committee Chair

---

*The meeting is being held to gather information to help the committee conduct its study. This committee will examine the information and material obtained during this, and other public meetings, in an effort to inform its work. Although opinions may be stated and lively discussion may ensue, no conclusions are being drawn at this time. In fact, the committee will deliberate thoroughly over the next few months before writing its draft report. Moreover, once the draft report is written, it must go through a rigorous review by experts who are anonymous to the committee, and the committee then must respond to this review with appropriate revisions that adequately satisfy the Academy's Report Review Committee and the chair of the NRC before it is considered an NRC report. Therefore, observers who draw conclusions about the committee's work based on today's discussions will be doing so prematurely.

Furthermore, individual committee members often engage in discussion and questioning for the specific purpose of probing an issue and sharpening an argument. The comments of any given committee member may not necessarily reflect the position he or she may actually hold on the subject under discussion, to say nothing of that person's future position as it may evolve in the course of the project. Any inference about an individual's position regarding findings or recommendations in the final report are therefore also premature.

10:25   Provider Panelists—*Robert Fullilove, Panel Host*
                 Arthur Schut,* President, Iowa Substance Abuse
                     Program Director's Association
                 Anne Tafe,* Executive Director, Massachusetts
                     Drug Abuse Association
                 Robert Kahn,* President, California Organization
                     of Methadone Providers
                 Robert G. Newman,* President and CEO, Beth
                     Israel Medical Center
                 Selbert Wood,* President and CEO, STEP ONE, Inc.
                 Gaurdia Banister, Director of Behavioral Health
                     Services, Seton House
                 Beny J. Primm, Executive Director, Addiction
                     Research and Treatment Corporation
                 Mark Publickler, Chief of Addiction Medicine,
                     Kaiser Permanente MidAtlantic Region
                 Discussion: Question and Answer

11:35   Policy Panelists—*Steven Mirin, Panel Host*
                 Marsha Lillie-Blanton, Associate Director, U.S.
                     General Accounting Office
                 Rosalind Brannigan, Vice President, Drug Strategies
                 June Osborn, President, Josiah Macy Jr. Foundation
                 Hernando Posada, Assistant Director, Ohio
                     Department of Alcohol and Drug Addiction
                     Services
                 Richard Suchinsky, Addictive Disorders, Department
                     of Veterans Affairs
                 Discussion: Question and Answer

12:45 p.m.   LUNCH—Provided for panelists and registered observers
                 outside the Lecture Room

1:30   Research Panelists—*James Sorenson, Panel Host*
                 Lisa Borg, Rockefeller University
                 Alec Cristoff, Alexandria, VA
                 Jeffrey Hoffman, President and CEO, Danya
                     International, Inc.

---

*Members, National Coalition of State Alcohol and Drug Treatment and Prevention Associations.

> David Nurco, Social Research Center, University of
> Maryland at Baltimore
> Harold Shinitzky, Department of Pediatrics,
> Johns Hopkins University School of Medicine
> Maxine Stitzer, Principal Investigator, Behavioral
> Biology Research Center, Johns Hopkins University
> School of Medicine
> George Woody, Department of Psychiatry,
> University of Pennsylvania
> Discussion: Question and Answer

2:40   General Discussion

3:30   Summary Recommendations and Wrap-up

4:00–5:00   RECEPTION for Roundtable participants in the
              Rotunda

LIST OF TOPICS TO BE ADDRESSED BY PARTICIPANTS

- Perspectives of providers and policy makers on the value of participating in research.
- Examples of successful and unsuccessful efforts to do collaborative
research.
- Examples of successful and unsuccessful efforts to implement new
research findings.
- Examples of successful and unsuccessful efforts to incorporate new
information into management practice and service delivery.
- Availability of funding for research in a community treatment setting.
- Incentives and disincentives for doing research and implementing
new treatments in community treatment settings.
- Experiences with successful models for research/practice interaction in other fields.
- Changes in the current environment that impact community-based
treatment organizations.
- Suggestions for ways to "market" research findings and shorten
time from "bench to trench."
- What policy makers need from researchers to support implementation of research findings.

PARTICIPANT LIST

Gaurdia E. Banister
Director of Behavioral Health
   Services
Seton House
Washington, DC

Lisa Borg
Laboratory of the Biology of
   Addictive Diseases
Rockefeller University
New York, NY

Joseph V. Brady
Professor of Behavioral Biology
The Johns Hopkins University
   School of Medicine
Baltimore, MD

Rosalind Brannigan
Vice President
Drug Strategies
Washington, DC

Mady Chalk
Director, Managed Care Initiatives
Center for Substance Abuse
   Treatment
Rockville, MD

Alec Christoff
Alexandria, VA

Dorynne Czechowicz
Division of Clinical and Services
   Research
National Institute on Drug Abuse
Rockville, MD

Deborah Haller
Associate Chair
Division of Substance Abuse
   Medicine
Medical College of Virginia
Virginia Commonwealth University
Richmond, VA

Vincent G. Hodge
Employee Assistance Consultant
COPE, Inc.
Washington, DC

Jeffrey A. Hoffman
President and CEO
Danya International, Inc.
Silver Spring, MD

Robin Huffman
Regional Director of Business
   Development/Charter Behavioral
North Carolina Association for
   Behavioral Health Care
Greensboro, NC

Robert B. Kahn
President, California Organization
   of Methadone Providers
San Diego, CA

Andrea Kamargo
Health Services Quality and Public
   Health Issues
U.S. General Accounting Office
Washington, DC

Linda Kaplan
Executive Director
The National Association of
   Alcoholism and Drug Abuse
   Counselors
Arlington, VA

Marsha Lillie-Blanton
Associate Director
Health Services Quality and Public
   Health Issues
U.S. General Accounting Office
Washington, DC

James O. McClyde
Assistant Director
Health Services Quality and Public
   Health Issues
U.S. General Accounting Office
Washington, DC

Robert G. Newman
President and CEO
Beth Israel Medical Center
New York, NY

David N. Nurco
Research Professor
Department of Psychiatry
University of Maryland at
   Baltimore
Baltimore, MD

June Osborn
President
Josiah Macy Jr. Foundation
New York, NY

Nina Peyser
Executive Director
Grants Management and Research
   Support
Beth Israel Medical Center
New York, NY

Harold Alan Pincus
Deputy Medical Director and
Director, Office of Research
American Psychiatric Association
Washington, DC

Hernando J. Posada
Assistant Director
Ohio Department of Alcohol and
   Drug Addiction Services
Columbus, OH

Beny J. Primm
Executive Director
Addiction Research and Treatment
   Corporation
Brooklyn, NY

Mark Publicker
Chief of Addiction Medicine
Kaiser Permanente MidAtlantic
   Region
Merrifield, VA

Gwen Rubinstein
Deputy Director of National Policy
Legal Action Center
Washington, DC

Arthur Schut
President, Iowa Substance Abuse
   Program Directors' Association
c/o Mid-Eastern Council on
   Chemical Abuse
Iowa City, IA

Harold Shinitzky
Psychology Instructor
Department of Pediatrics
Johns Hopkins University
School of Medicine
Baltimore, MD

Maxine L. Stitzer
Professor of Psychiatry and
   Behavioral Sciences
Johns Hopkins University
School of Medicine
Baltimore, MD

Richard T. Suchinsky
Associate Chief for Addictive
   Disorders
Department of Veterans Affairs
Washington, DC

Anne Tafe
Executive Director
Massachusetts Alcoholism and
   Drug Abuse Association
Boston, MA

Selbert M. Wood, Jr.
President and CEO
STEP ONE, Inc.
Winston-Salem, NC

INSTITUTE OF MEDICINE
NATIONAL ACADEMY OF SCIENCES

Committee on Committee-Based Drug Treatment
Workshop on Community-Based Drug Treatment:
The Need for Partnership Among Providers, Policymakers, and Researchers

September 8, 1997
Scholes Hall—Roberts Room
University of New Mexico Campus
Albuquerque, NM

WORKSHOP AGENDA

10:30 a.m.	Welcome and Introductions **Merwyn R. Greenlick**, Committee Chair **Philip A. May**, Director, CASAA
	Review of IOM Open Meeting Policy Overview of Objectives for the Day
11:00	Overview of the community-based drug abuse treatment system in New Mexico, including diverse cultures and special populations (e.g., community corrections, adolescents, pregnant women)
12:30 p.m.	Break to pick up box lunches
12:45	Examples of research carried out in community-based programs with providers as partners from the beginning
1:30	Examples of successes and failures in dissemination of research findings and utilization of relevant clinical experience in the design of research
2:15	Perspectives of community providers on the pros and cons of participating in research. What research is needed and why?
3:00	Wrap-up and Summary
3:30	Adjourn workshop

PARTICIPANT LIST

Patrick Abbott
Center on Alcoholism, Substance
   Abuse and Addiction
Albuquerque, NM

Lynn Brady
Behavioral Health Services Division
Department of Health
Santa Fe, NM

Robert Fiorentine
Drug Abuse Research Center
University of California at Los
   Angeles
Los Angeles, CA

Jan Gossage
Center on Alcoholism, Substance
   Abuse and Addictions
Albuquerque, NM

Valerie L. Graber
Student Support Services
Albuquerque, NM

Linda Grant
Washington Association of
   Alcoholism and Addictions
   Programs
Kirkland, WA

Brian Greenberg
Walden House
San Francisco, CA

James Hall
Sante Fe County District Court
Sante Fe, NM

Constance Horgan
Institute for Health Policy
Brandeis University
Waltham, MA

Arnold Kaluzny
University of North Carolina
School of Public Health
Cecil G. Sheps Center
Chapel Hill, NC

Michael W. Kirby
Arapahoe House, Inc.
Thorton, CO

Patricia Knox
The Center for Alcohol and Drug
   Treatment
Wenatchee, WA

Walter Lang
New Mexico State Probation and
   Parole
Albuquerque, NM

Francesca G. Lanier
Grant Management and
   Accountability
Albuquerque Public Schools
Albuquerque, NM

Carol Leonard
The Navajo Nation
Dine'Center for Substance Abuse
   Treatment
Window Rock, AZ

Chilo Madrid
Aliviane, Inc.
El Paso, TX

Philip A. May
University of New Mexico
Center on Alcoholism, Substance
  Abuse and Addictions
Albuquerque, NM

Robert Meyers
Center on Alcoholism, Substance
  Abuse and Addictions
Albuquerque, NM

Rick Miera
Bernalillo County Juvenile
  Detention Center and New
  Mexico State Legislature
Albuquerque, NM

Joseph "Bo" Miller
Center on Alcoholism, Substance
  Abuse and Addictions
Albuquerque, NM

Josi Noyes
EAP Public Service Co. of New
  Mexico
(Retired)
Sandia Park, NM

Carole Otero
Albuquerque Metropolitan Central
  Intake
Albuquerque, NM

Michael M. Passi
Family and Community Services
  Department
Albuquerque, NM

Robert Phillips
Eastern New Mexico University-
  Roswell
Roswell, NM

Fernando Rodriquez
Aliviane, Inc.
El Paso, TX

Everett Rogers
Department of Communication
  and Journalism
University of New Mexico
Albuquerque, NM

Mary E. Steil
City of Albuquerque, Family and
  Community Services Department
Albuquerque, NM

Scott Wallace
San Juan County DWI Treatment
  Facility
Farmington, NM

Verner Westerberg
Center on Alcoholism, Substance
  Abuse and Addictions
Albuquerque, NM

W. Gill Woodall
Center on Alcoholism, Substance
  Abuse and Addictions
Albuquerque, NM

Carolina E. Yahne
Center on Alcoholism, Substance
  Abuse and Addictions
Albuquerque, NM

INSTITUTE OF MEDICINE
NATIONAL ACADEMY OF SCIENCES

Committee on Committee-Based Drug Treatment
Roundtable Discussion with Local Providers

October 23, 1997
Seton House at Providence Hospital
Washington, DC

PARTICIPANT LIST

Darryl Colbert
Program Administrator
Substance Abuse Network
Catholic Charities
Washington, DC

Diane Lewis
Consultant
Marshall Heights Community
  Development Organization
Washington, DC

Arthur Melvin
Clinic Manager
Umoja Treatment Center
Washington, DC

Betty Palmer
Nurse Manager
Seton House at Providence
  Hospital
Washington, DC

Gale Saler
Executive Deputy Director
Second Genesis
Bethesda, MD

Steve Wright
Center Manager
Addiction, Prevention, and
  Recovery Administration
Washington, DC

Ronald D. Wynne
Director
Washington Assessment and
  Therapy Services
Washington, DC

C

Drug Treatment Programs and Research: The Challenge of Bidirectionality

Benjamin P. Bowser
California State University at Hayward

INTRODUCTION

The charge of this committee is to recommend ways to increase the bidirectional flow of information and science between drug treatment providers and drug treatment researchers. The first major difficulty we had with this charge is defining the term "community" in community-based drug treatment. A subcommittee was formed to address the problem. Our response was to study the sociological and anthropological literatures on community and members of the overall committee talked at length with directors and staff in "community-based" programs that do drug treatment.

Based on treatment program interviews and presentations before the committee, a sense emerged of the challenge before us. The non-utilization of research findings by community-based practitioners is not simply a problem of more efficient technical transfer of information between professional communities. There is a continuum among all drug treatment programs. At one end are programs that are vigorous consumers of research, and at the other are programs that do not use nor understand research, and are suspicious of researchers' intent. Programs are not evenly distributed across the continuum. The vast majority are nonresearch consumers. There is also a similar continuum among treatment researchers. Some have experience working with community-based treatment programs that are not research consumers, while most others have little experience with programs not affiliated with universities, hospitals, and now health maintenance organi-

zations. The majority of drug treatment providers and researchers are organized into vastly different worlds, have different missions, cultures, histories, and information needs. With some exceptions, each has distinct ways
of formulating, assessing, processing, and disseminating information. What
both groups have in common are: (a) drug abuse and treatment are issues of
primary concern, and (b) reducing drug abuse is their primary goal. Bidirectionality must be built on these two common points.

We have come to realize the relationship between drug treatment providers and drug treatment researchers is more problematic than we thought.
To call for bidirectionality between treatment providers and researchers has
at least four requirements. First, treatment research has to be produced for
practitioners and must be useful to them. Second, practitioners must want
to work with and provide information to researchers. Third, researchers
must be interested in what practitioners know and want to know. And
fourth, we assume that better information exchanges between practitioners
and researchers will improve client outcomes. The testimony from practitioners and researchers before our overall committee challenged all of these
assumptions. The exception is the current attempt of NIDA and CSAT to
bridge the gap between drug treatment practitioners and researchers. This
is because the context for mutuality between practice and research has yet
to be achieved. The work of this committee and the necessity to bridge the
gap between practice and research are made all the more timely by congressional and public criticism of the perceived ineffectiveness of drug treatment. This criticism threatens funding for practitioners and researchers
alike, and provides motivation for collaboration.

In this paper, we do three things. First, we review how community has
been defined in the sociological and anthropological literatures. Second, we
define what is meant by "community-based" drug treatment as distinct
from other treatment contexts. Third, we discuss strategies for bridging the
gap between practice and research.

WHAT IS COMMUNITY AND
WHAT DIFFERENCE DOES IT MAKE?

Community Defined

There is an extensive literature on community that is useful to our
committee's problems with defining community-based drug treatment. The
two most commonly repeated descriptors of community are: (1) social land
use—those who share common residence within specific geographic boundaries; and (2) social identity—those who identity with one another regardless of shared land use. Shared land use without social identity is not
sufficient to define community, while shared identity is. Social identity is

the essential factor in working definitions of community. George Murdock (1949) gave us one of the earliest definitions of community. Social land is combined with social identity as "groups of people who normally reside together in face-to-face association." Community is both place and identity. A third descriptor of community is social identity through temporal periods. In this third definition, community consists of a social identity unfolding through time (Arensberg and Kimball, 1965). Examples are secret societies, age cohorts with distinct life courses, or people who share a decisive historic event such as war, the Great Depression, the "Sixties." There are two variations of social identity defined in time. The first is with a shared place and the second is without. A fourth descriptor defining community is function. Community is having a specific basis for a shared identity such as an occupation, a profession, common mission or common craft.

In sum, the classic definitions of community are social identities bound (a) by place; (b) by time; (c) by time and place; (d) by function; (e) by function and time; and (f) by function, time, and place (Arensberg and Kimball, 1965). These types of community are not mutually exclusive, nor are they single dimensions. Different kinds of communities can coexist simultaneously, and of course, individuals can be members of multiple communities at the same time. We are all in some community—our clients come from community, our programs regardless of sponsorship are set up in community, and drug treatment researchers are a "community" as well. At first, the definitions of community appear to have little to do with this committee's deliberations. But in fact they have a lot to do with our mission and highlight the major challenge to bidirectional communication between drug treatment practitioners and researchers. Professionals who work in institutional settings are more apt to define community by function as did our full committee at our first meeting. We defined eight descriptors of community with regard to drug treatment. "Community-based" treatment programs were defined by (1) treatment modality, (2) setting, (3) service units in large organizations, (4) accountability, (5) profit–nonprofit, (6) residential or outpatient treatment, (7) source of funding, and (8) client catchment area. Furthermore, treatment programs are sponsored by hospitals, universities, health departments, corporations, and prisons. These descriptors corresponded with only two classical definitions of community—place (setting) and function. We have not considered temporal period nor have we addressed the most common of all descriptor of community, social identity. Essentially, we have taken the legal and formal organization of treatment programs as bases for community. By focusing on only setting and function, we miss what is "community" for most drug treatment programs. Given our review of community definitions, what then does "community-based" mean?

The Meaning of Community-Based

In 1929 Congress recognized that drug addiction was primarily a medical and social problem and that treatment of addiction by incarceration was illogical (NIH, 1995). The Lexington, Kentucky, and Forth Worth, Texas "narcotic farms" were set up by Congress to confine and treat persons addicted to habit-forming drugs. After congressional recognition of drug abuse as a social and medical problem, alcohol rather than drug treatment and support programs were started all across the country by community-based social service programs and by ex-alcoholics through organizations such as Alcoholics Anonymous (Bill W, 1967). The alcohol drug problem was much more pervasive until the 1960s. Then the epidemic of heroin use sparked a second community response. The "narcotic farms" and a few drug treatment programs expanded rapidly as an adjunct to community social services, and with government financial support (Musto, 1973). The expansion of alcohol and drug treatment into community settings was very much in keeping with popular institution building social movements. Local schools, health clinics, community policing, and cooperative grocery stores (Cox, 1994) are a few examples of an ongoing movement in American life (Anner, 1996; Fisher, 1994; Hoffman, 1989; McCarthy and Zalder, 1973). The establishment of needle exchange programs is an example a recent movement among community-based AIDS activists (Bowser, 1993).

Local agencies that provided housing, children, and food services in residential neighborhoods started drug treatment programs. Churches with social missions started drug treatment programs. People who were themselves in recovery, started programs. All of these programs have come out of specific racial, social class, ideological, and residential social identities and places. Despite the fact that drug abuse is a chronic relapsing disease, the movement has had visible successes. There are many people who are now clean and sober due to these programs. What is particularly important for our purpose is that their successes have come without a scientific basis. With government funding and regulation of drug treatment, the distinct histories and missions of community-based drug treatment has been obscured. At the same time the Department of Veterans Affairs, county hospitals, university medical centers, and now health maintenance organizations have also rapidly expanded their own drug treatment programs. These are "institutionally based" treatment efforts. The following table gives a sense of the scope of each type of treatment base. In the SAMHSA (1996) survey, "community-based" programs are called "free-standing outpatient" programs.

Table C-1 shows that "community-based" or free-standing programs treat 53 percent of all drug abusers seeking recovery. Clearly, university based treatment programs exist to advance research and knowledge about drug abuse. The hospital programs are responding to local public health

TABLE C-1 Estimated Clients in Specialty Substance Abuse Treatment by Institutional Setting, 1994

Institutional Setting	24-Hour Care	Outpatient	Total	Percent
Free-standing outpatient	1,460	501,853	503,313	53.3
Community mental health center	4,178	136,420	140,598	14.9
General hospital (includes VA)	13,937	81,830	95,767	10.1
Specialized hospitals	8,714	14,045	22,759	2.4
Halfway house/recovery home	18,912	5,416	24,328	2.6
Other residential facilities	47,214	23,140	70,354	7.5
Correctional facilities	18,369	19,960	38,329	4.1
Other/unknown types	7,855	40,320	48,175	5.1
All types	120,639	822,984	943,623	100.0

SOURCE: SAMHSA (1996).

needs. Corporations have started programs to address employee's drug abuse. But in comparison, there are many more community-based programs that have arisen in response to the drug treatment needs of people with specific area or residential race, ethnic, and social class bound identities.

In the mission of community-based drug treatment, people come to abuse drugs not simply as individuals, but as members of some constellation of social identities. How they became addicted, what sustains them in their addiction, and the major source of motivation for "recovery" lies in their relationships and changing relationships with communities of people having similar social identities. The assumption of people who start programs within a community framework is that their specific social community is the best agent to address the cultural content of the abuser's drug abuse problem, treatment and recovery (Joe et al., 1977; Peyrot, 1982). For example, firefighters who became addicted to drugs as firefighters and who are going to remain firefighters are best treated by those most familiar with firefighting and who have respect among firefighters. Chinese-American heroin abusers are best treated by people who share the same social identity, are from the same regional and provincial culture, and who have the same generational immigrant experience—time- and place-bound. The same is true for business executives, and celebrities who go to discrete "retreat" programs, for New York Puerto Ricans ("NewYorRicans") and for African Americans from the South, who are culturally distinct from African Americans from southern Louisiana and the Caribbean. People and organizations emerge in varied communities to address drug abuse within their community (DHHS, 1989; Smith et al., 1971). What makes these programs "community-based" are their history, mission, focus on location, social identity around neighborhood, service to people in the neighborhood, and accountability to local residents and institutions. Whether one agrees or not with the centrality of community in treatment, community is central to their mission and treatment efforts.

An example of the most successful model of community-based drug treatment are Alcohol and Narcotics Anonymous Twelve Step programs. They began as community-based treatment, and continue as such. The legal and formal organizational structure of Twelve Step programs is only part of what makes them "community-based." What is more important to their identity and what they do is their worldview that values locality, their method for the social support of recovery, and their social identity as part of the twelve step recovery movement (Stephens, 1991). The same is true for drug treatment programs started by churches, Afrocentric organizations, woman's recovery groups, labor unions, and university-based treatment programs with missions to advance teaching and research. They define themselves by their mission and location, social identity and place.

Program accountability comes closest to capturing the essence of social identity in the definition of community-based. Accountability tells us what interests, mission, and social setting the program serves. Drug treatment programs accountable to health maintenance organizations (HMOs) serve HMO clients and the profit or not-for-profit (time and function) mission of the HMO. Drug treatment programs accountable to university hospitals also serve teaching and research missions (time and function). Drug treatment programs accountable to local citizens (place) with a particular residential allegiance (identity) exist primarily to serve people in the local area. In other words, there are university-based, health department-based, hospital-based, HMO-based, and community-based drug treatment programs. If we investigate all bases of accountability, there are, undoubtedly, additional ones. It is likely that each of these types of drug treatment outposts have both common and unique informational needs, interests, and priorities based on their differing identities and accountabilities.

As we have already seen; however, the community-based programs are the most numerous, and the most diverse. They are also as a group furthest from science and the use of science. The core of our committee's expressed mission is to address the problems of these community-based programs in utilizing science. But the definition what is "community-based" is not without relevance to their openness to using research in the future.

WHITHER COMMUNITY?

One of the reasons why community-based drug treatment is unrecognized as a social movement and as having a distinct identity is the fact of its overwhelming government funding and regulation. Any program that is going to treat more than a few individuals with a paid staff must have a source of regular funding. Private foundations avoid funding direct services, leaving drug treatment to city, state, or federal governments. But the money comes with regulations and guidelines that make community-based programs virtual adjuncts to government social services. Funding has obscured differences and standardized programs in how they are reported. Anyone who has worked in local government to fund community-based drug treatment programs knows of the tension and the potential for conflict in the annual funding process. What is at stake is not simply funding to run generic services. Programs want to treat clients in ways that they feel will work best and are most effective, in line with their mission and purpose. But more often, they are not able to because of funding regulations. For example, there are some community-based programs that offer methadone treatment, but would prefer not to. The idea of maintaining drug abusers on an alternative drug is against their specific view of drug abuse and their mission to reduce drug use, regardless of the drug. But methadone maintenance is a source of funding that can bring more drug abusers into their services and cannot be easily overlooked.

In recent years, drug treatment dollars are in decline and there are increasing calls for evaluation and demonstrations of effectiveness. An undetermined numbers of community-based programs are in crisis. They do not have the human resources to conduct their own evaluations, nor do they have the fiscal resources to hire someone else to do so. Institutionally based programs in hospitals, universities, and HMOs have vastly more human and fiscal resources to meet the new demands for program accountability and evaluation. So larger and more successful community-based as well as institutionally based programs are more than happy to absorb smaller, well managed community-based programs and their support dollars. The rest will simply wither. We are now witnessing a consolidation and shaking out of community-based drug treatment.

Community-based drug treatment programs are not the only community institutions shrinking in number and influence. The possibilities and resources of residential and neighborhood institutions are themselves in transition (Southworth and Owens, 1993; Wellman and Wortley, 1990). The historic centrality of residential community is itself in decline as is evident from a century of community studies (Abu-Lughod, 1994; Seeley et al., 1956; Spectorsky, 1958; Stein, 1960; Vidich and Bensman, 1958). We are now in the third generation of community research in the United States. The first and classic period was in the 1920s and 1930s, when teams of investigators spent years in the field studying Chicago, Illinois, Newburyport, Connecticut, and Natchez, Mississippi, as representative small cities. The post-World War II period was the second period, where smaller and shorter community studies were conducted because of the rapid expansion of survey and marketing research techniques (Stein, 1960). The third period began in the 1960s with a focus on understanding specific social problems in community context.

Part of the reason for renewed interest in community studies today is because of drug abuse and AIDS prevention. NIDA realized in the mid-1980s that large-scale AIDS intervention efforts could not be mounted among injection drug users (IDUs) to slow the spread of HIV without qualitative knowledge of drug abusers and their communities. To reach IDUs would require accessing them where they congregated. Knowledge of IDUs in their social context was literally "a black box." In addition, AIDS activists argued that one could not mount a community-wide AIDS prevention effort if you knew little about community in the first place. Gay and bisexual activists insisted that their successful effort to reduce HIV infections in their communities was based on knowledge of the community and sensitivity to its cultural differences. As a result, NIDA's National AIDS Demonstration Research Projects required presurvey ethnography to "ground" the research in community.

Despite the methodological and theoretical differences over three generations of community research, analysis of almost 80 years of work have noted consistent trends:

1. Residential communities have become increasingly dependent upon outside institutions to sustain their existence and quality of life (Clark, 1993; Stein, 1960).

2. The industrialization of work and the bureaucratization of institutions have reduced community autonomy and distinctiveness (Stein, 1960; Wellman and Wortley, 1990) .

3. Social affiliations based upon kinship, ethnic ties, and proximity (neighboring) are being replaced by affiliations based on friendship, work, and social class, diffused in locality and marked in time (Fischer, 1982; Pilisuk and Parks, 1986).

4. Self-identification by residential community is increasingly temporary as more and more Americans move. Residential communities are becoming increasingly segregated by social class, and multiclass communities are declining rapidly (Fischer, 1982).

5. Despite continuing racial segregation, residential communities are becoming more ethnically diverse and economically homogeneous (Clark, 1993; Lynn and McGeary, 1990).

6. People's inability to define and shape their local living space, and their dependency on outside institutions, largely account for mounting alien-

ation in American life (Bellah et al., 1985; Harrell and Peterson, 1992; Stouffer et al., 1949).

Based upon these trends, there is an emerging view that residential community is increasingly problematic and in decline in the United States. There is a sense that most Americans have fewer, weaker, and more conditional social affiliations today than at the turn of the century (Stein, 1960). Evidence from drug treatment research shows the importance of social support while in treatment as well as supportive social relationships to sustain recovery. If these trends in community are accurate, they must heavily impact drug abuse and the prospects for successful treatment.

An alternative view of the very same evidence is that community is not in decline, but is only in transition (Fischer, 1982; Wellman and Wortley, 1990). In this alternate interpretation, there are many people trying to maintain the older and now outmoded form of folk community, a point missed in the research on black poverty (Williams, 1992), drug abuse, and crime in the United States (Harrell and Peterson, 1992). Where residents are able to maintain control over their public space, violent crime is lower (Simpson et al., 1997). Community based upon kinship, neighbors who hopefully will not move, a clear residential area social identity, local autonomy and decision making, and same ethnicity and race may be waning. There is a declining economic and cultural basis for such community (Anner, 1996). A young urban professional can live in the very same area in decline for traditional residents. This new resident may experience a community in emergence, because his social relationships are based upon friends and work associates, and are diffused rather than local. This new social identity is not defined by physical neighborhood and community (Fischer, 1982).

In the alternative view of community, we can hypothesize that community-based drug treatment serves drug abuse clients from traditional racial, ethnic, and social class communities in transition. Communities in transition have compromised employment bases, are heavily dependent upon social services, are centers of drug dealing and trafficking, and are heavily policed (Lynn and McGeary, 1990). In these communities, drug abuse is conditioned by poverty, and successful recovery from drug abuse is conditioned by efforts to achieve freedom from poverty. Alternatively, recovery from drug abuse among people with the appropriate education, skills, and employment is now more likely to take place in HMO-, union-, professional, and private hospital-based drug treatment programs. For clients from new communities, drug use is likely to be initiated from experimentation and curiosity, and sustained by background trauma, and personal and professional stress rather than poverty.

DISCUSSION

With the sorting out of community-based drug treatment, the first open question is: Who will respond to the growing need in traditional communities for drug treatment? It is questionable whether institutionally based programs in universities and hospitals, and the few community-based programs that make the transition to the new community, can meet the need. The continuing need for drug treatment will not go away because there is less government funding and fewer treatment programs. The consequence for neglect of drug and alcohol abuse through prevention and treatment costs the nation an estimated $77.6 billion per year in federal entitlements (CASA, 1996). This does not include the costs to the nation of drug-related crimes and criminal justice costs for using jail and prisons for drug treatment. The second open question is whether there is the capacity in communities in decline or transition to continue to produce new drug treatment programs. General social movements have uncanny abilities to continue generating organizations to address community needs and to rise anew when they are least expected (McCarthy and Zalder, 1973) and even attempt to affect expressed needs through invention (Abbott, 1987). When the current generation of drug treatment programs declines far enough, we may very well witness the emergence of another generation of drug treatment initiatives which may not be so ready to compromise their missions for government funding (Frye, 1991).

Despite the problems and open questions, bidirectionality between community-based treatment practitioners and drug treatment researchers is possible. But it will require researchers to see the community-based research movement and mission as a source of new theory, as people with potentially useful insights about drug abuse and treatment, and as a well of experience waiting to be tested that can benefit both clients, practitioners, and science. Community-based practitioners can also benefit from alliances with researchers sensitive to community-based issues. Practitioners want to know the outcomes of their best efforts and improve outcomes for clients. Many want their ideas tested and improved upon. They want to know why some clients recover and others do not. They also want to be able to learn from research, and to show specifically where their work has value. For these reasons collaborative research is crucial. Community-based drug treatment is not simply an attempt to treat individual addicts in their community. Whether one takes the view that community is in decline or in transition, community-based drug treatment is part of a larger effort to struggle with neighborhood decline or transition. It is an effort to maintain residential community as a vital human institution for the majority of people who do not have a place in the postmodern world.

REFERENCES

Abbott P. 1987. *Seeking Many Inventions: The Idea of Community in America*. Nashville: The University of Tennessee Press.

Abu-Lughod J. 1994. *From Urban Village to East Village: The Battle for New York's Lower East Side*. Cambridge: Blackwell.

Anner J, ed. 1996. *Beyond Identity Politics: Emerging Social Justice Movements in Communities of Color*. Boston: South End Press.

Arensberg C, Kimball S. 1965. *Culture and Community*. New York: Harcourt, Brace, and World.

Bellah RN et al. 1985. *Habits of the Heart: Individualism and Commitment in American Life*. Berkeley: The University of California Press.

Bowser BP. 1993. What are the community responses to needle exchange programs? In Lurie P and Reingold A, eds. *The Public Health Impact of Needle Exchange Programs in the United States and Abroad*. Rockville: CDC National Clearing House.

CASA (National Center on Addiction and Substance Abuse at Columbia University). 1996. Costs of Substance Abuse [WWW Document]. URL http://www.casacolumbia.org/costs.

Clark W. 1993. Neighborhood transition in multiethnic/racial contexts. *Journal of Urban Affairs* 15(2): 161–172.

Cox, C. 1994. *Storefront Revolution: Food Co-ops and the Counter-Culture*. New Brunswick: Rutgers University Press.

DHHS (U.S. Dept. Health and Human Services). 1989. *Drug Abuse Treatment: A Community Solution*. DHHS Publication (ADM) 89-1633. Rockville: U.S. Department of Health and Human Services.

Fischer C. 1982. *To Dwell Among Friends: Personal Networks in Town and City*. Chicago: The University of Chicago Press.

Fisher R. 1994. *Let the People Decide: Neighborhood Organizing in America*. New York: Twayne Publishers.

Frye H. 1991. Changing the black inner city: Black urban reorganization. In Bowser BP, ed. *Black Male Adolescents: Parenting and Education in Community Context*. Lanham, MD: University Press of America.

Harrell A, Peterson G, eds. 1992. *Drugs, Crime, and Social Isolation: Barriers to Urban Opportunity*. Washington: The Urban Institute Press.

Hoffman E. 1989. *The Politics of Knowledge: Activists Movements in Medicine and Planning*. Albany: State University of New York Press.

Joe GW et al. 1977. *Community Factors and Racial Composition of Drug Abuse Treatment Programs and Outcomes*. DHEW Publication (ADM) 78-573. Rockville: U.S. Department of Health, Education, and Welfare.

Lynn L, McGeary MGH, eds. 1990. *Inner City Poverty in the United States*. Washington: National Academy Press.

McCarthy J, Zalder M. 1973. *The Trend of Social Movements in America: Professionalization and Resource Mobilization*. Morristown, NJ: General Learning Press.

Murdock GP. 1949. *Social Structure*. New York: MacMillan.

Musto D. 1973. *The American Disease: Origins of Narcotic Control*. New Haven: Yale University Press.

NIH (National Institutes of Health). 1995. Images From the History of the Public Health Service. NLM HyperDOC [WWW Document]. URL http://public.nlm.nih.gov/exhibition/phs_history/130.html.

Peyrot M. 1982. *The Social Organization of Community Based Drug Abuse Treatment*. Doctoral Dissertation. Department of Sociology, University of California, Los Angeles.

Pilisuk M, Parks SH. 1986. *The Healing Web: Social Networks and Human Survival.* Hanover, NH: University Press of New England.

SAMHSA (Substance Abuse and Mental Health Services Administration). 1996. National Drug and Alcoholism Treatment Unit Survey (NDATUS): Data for 1994 and 1980–1994. Advance Report Number 13. Rockville: Substance Abuse and Mental Health Services Administration.

Seeley J, Sim RA, Loosley E. 1956. *Crestwood Heights.* New York: Basic Books.

Simpson R, Raudenbush S, Earls F. 1997. Neighborhoods and violent crime: A multilevel study of collective efficacy. *Science* 277:918–924

Smith D, Bentel D, Schwartz J, eds. 1971. *The Free Clinic: A Community Approach to Health Care and Drug Abuse.* Beloit, WI: Stash Press.

Southworth M, Owens P. 1993. The evolving metropolis: studies of community, neighborhood, and street from at the urban edge. *Journal of The American Planning Association* 59(3):271–287.

Spectorsky AC. 1958. *The Exurbanites.* New York: Berkeley Publishing.

Stein M. 1960. *The Eclipse of Community: An Interpretation of American Studies.* New York: Harper and Row.

Stephens RC. 1991. *The Street Addict Role: A Theory of Heroin Addiction.* Albany, NY: State University of New York Press.

Stouffer S et al. 1949. *The American Soldier.* New York: John Wiley and Sons.

Vidich A, Bensman J. 1958. *Small Town in Mass Society.* Princeton: Princeton University Press.

W Bill. 1967. *Alcohol Anonymous: A Brief History of Alcohol Anonymous.* New York: Alcohol Anonymous World Services.

Wellman B, Wortley S. 1990. Different strokes from different folks: Community ties and social support. *American Journal of Sociology* 96(3):558–588.

Williams B. 1992. Poverty among African Americans in the urban United States. *Human Organization* 51(2):164–173.

D

The Treatment of Addiction: What Can Research Offer Practice?

A. Thomas McLellan and James R. McKay
Penn-VA Center for Studies of Addiction and The Treatment
Research Institute at the University of Pennsylvania

INTRODUCTION

Problems of substance dependence produce dramatic costs to society in terms of lost productivity, social disorder and of course health care utilization (NIDA, 1991; Merrill, 1993). Over the past twenty years many of the traditional forms of substance abuse treatment (e.g., methadone maintenance, therapeutic communities, outpatient drug free and others) have been evaluated multiple times and shown to be effective (Ball and Ross, 1991; DATOS, 1992; Hubbard et al., 1986, 1997; IOM, 1989, 1990b; McLellan et al., 1980; Simpson, 1981, 1997; Simpson et al., 1997a,b). Importantly, this research has shown that the benefits obtained from addiction treatments typically extend beyond the reduction of substance use, to areas that are important to society such as reduced crime, reduced risk of infectious diseases, and improved social function (Ball and Ross, 1991; Institute of Medicine, 1989, 1990b; McLellan et al., 1980). Finally, research findings indicate that the costs associated with the provision of substance abuse treatment provide 3- to 7-fold returns to the employer, the health insurer, and to society within approximately three years following treatment (Everingham and Rydell, 1994; Gerstein et al., 1994; Holder et al., 1991; IOM, 1990b; OTA, 1983; State of Oregon, 1996).

Supported by grants from the National Institute on Drug Abuse, the Center for Substance Abuse Treatment, and the Robert Wood Johnson Foundation. Parts of this paper appear in McKay and McLellan, 1997 and an earlier IOM report on Managing Managed Care, 1997.

How Do These Research Results Translate into Recommendations that Can Be Useful for Treatment Providers?—Although the conclusions from reviews of the recent treatment research literature are important and gratifying, they are not adequate to inform important clinical questions regarding the delivery of substance abuse treatment services. Simply knowing that those who stay in treatment longer have better outcomes does not help when the funding and duration of treatment in "real world" settings is regularly reduced (McLellan et al., 1996a). Further, research demonstrating that highly specialized and resource-intensive treatments "work" with highly selected samples of patients may not be helpful to "real world" treatment providers who have no prospects of accessing those treatments and whose caseloads contain very few of the patients on whom the specialized treatment was tested. This is particularly true at the level of the "community-based" public sector treatment programs that have been forced to operate under limited budgets with little access to sophisticated services. How can research in the treatment setting inform these providers? How can these providers use information from research studies to upgrade or expand their treatment efforts—within the practical constraints of budget and personnel available?

Parameters of the Literature Review—In response to these questions, we have reviewed the existing treatment outcome literature to summarize the available knowledge regarding the important patient and treatment factors that have been shown to influence the outcomes of addiction rehabilitation treatments. We felt this was an important first step in recognizing and recommending proven, practical, and cost-effective treatment strategies that can be implemented by community behavioral treatment programs. In this regard, we have elected not to review literature on detoxification methods in order to better focus on standard rehabilitation treatments for drug and alcohol dependence—typically following detoxification. Our review does not include the adolescent drug abuse treatment literature since it is still a developing field and there is a paucity of pertinent outcome studies in this area. In addition, we elected not to include a review of the smoking cessation literature as there have been excellent recent reviews of this entire field (see Fiore et al., 1996).

From a methodological perspective, we included only those clinical trials, treatment matching, or health services studies where the patients were alcohol or drug dependent by contemporary criteria (e.g., DSM); where the treatment provided was a conventional form of rehabilitation (any setting or modality); and where there were measures of either treatment processes or patient change during the course of treatment as well as posttreatment measures of outcome as defined later in the chapter. We have elected to include methadone maintenance (as well as its long acting form, *levo*-alpha-acetylmethadol [LAAM]) as part of the general category of out-patient rehabilitation treatments, rather than create a special category.

In the review that follows we first discuss some of the basic assumptions underlying rehabilitation forms of addiction treatment since they set the stage for the clinical methods currently in use and for the types of studies that are in the research literature. Next we discuss some of our considerations regarding definitions of "outcome." With these assumptions and considerations in mind, we then review the most significant patient and treatment process contributors to the outcomes of addiction treatment.

REHABILITATION TREATMENTS IN ADDICTION: WHO ARE THEY FOR, WHAT SHOULD THEY DO?

What Is Addiction Rehabilitation Designed to Do?—In contrast to "detoxification," which is a relatively brief, usually medical procedure designed to stabilize the acute physical and emotional distress and instability caused by recent termination of heavy alcohol and/or drug use, "rehabilitation" is a much longer process, usually involving multiple types of medical and social services, that is designed to help recently stabilized patients achieve sustained periods of drug-free living and stable personal and social function.

There are clear physical signs and symptoms associated with the cessation of most addictive substances and there are standard medications and withdrawal procedures that are very effective in ameliorating these acute "detoxification" symptoms and restoring physiological and emotional stability. Despite the efficacy of these detoxification methods, there is uniform agreement among professionals that detoxification by itself—regardless of the type or the duration—is rarely associated with sustained periods of abstinence or even improved function. Well after the return of physiological and emotional stability, most patients continue to experience regular periods of intense craving for alcohol and drugs and this can lead to "loss of control" in situations where these drugs of abuse are (or have been) present. There has been substantial research showing that among former addicts who have been abstinent for up to a year, even the sight or sound of stimuli associated with former periods of drug use can produce (through learned association) measurable changes in brain chemistry that mimic the actual use of the drug and the withdrawal symptoms produced by those drugs (see Childress et al., 1985, 1986, 1992; O'Brien et al., 1991).

Rehabilitation Methods—While there is universal agreement that some form of rehabilitation is necessary, there has been a very wide range of professional opinion regarding the nature or amount of rehabilitation necessary to produce sustained benefits. In part this is due to disagreement regarding the etiology and course of the addiction syndrome. These etiological theories include a genetic predisposition, an acquired metabolic abnormality, learned negative behavioral patterns, self medication of underlying psychiatric or physical medical problems, and lack of family and community support for positive function. For this reason, there is an equally wide range of treatment methods that have been applied to address these etiological and predisposing factors and to provide continuing support for the targeted behavioral changes. These have included such diverse elements as psychotropic medications to relieve underlying psychiatric problems, "anti-craving" medications to relieve alcohol and drug craving, acupuncture to correct acquired metabolic imbalances, educational seminars, films and group sessions to correct false impressions about alcohol and drug use, group and individual counseling and therapy sessions to provide insight, guidance and support for behavioral changes, and peer help groups (AA/NA/CA) to provide continued support for the behavioral changes thought to be important for sustaining improvement.

These rehabilitation methods have been traditionally provided in two types of settings—inpatient and outpatient. At this writing, inpatient rehabilitation programs can be divided into three general categories (Hubbard et al., 1989, 1997):

1. Inpatient hospital-based treatment (now very rare)—from 7 to 11 days.
2. Nonhospital "residential rehabilitation"—from 30 to 90 days.
3. Therapeutic Communities—from 6 months to 2 years.

Outpatient forms of treatment (at least abstinence oriented treatments) range from 30 to 120 days (Hubbard et al., 1989, 1997). Many of the more intensive forms of outpatient treatment (Intensive Outpatient, Day-Hospital) begin with full or half-day sessions, five or more times per week for approximately one month. As the rehabilitation progresses the intensity of the treatment reduces to shorter duration sessions (one to two hours) delivered twice weekly to semi-monthly.

Regardless of whether the rehabilitation process is initiated in an inpatient or outpatient setting, most rehabilitation programs recognize the need for some level of continuing involvement with the rehabilitation process. Thus the final part of outpatient rehabilitation is typically called "Continuing Care" or "Aftercare" and includes weekly to monthly group support meetings continuing (in association with parallel activity in self-help groups) for as long as two years (McKay et al., 1998).

A Special Note on Maintenance Forms of Treatment. The opiate dependence treatment field has had the availability of orally administered, long-acting agonist medications. Three forms of opiate maintenance medications are currently available, Methadone, Levo-alpha-acetyl methadol (LAAM) and Buprenorphine. While each is different in nature and duration of action, they provide 24–72 hours of continuing relief from opiate withdrawal and craving; and serve as the basis for adjunctive social supportive therapy and medical care. This maintenance modality is quite similar in purpose and practice to the combined regimens of pharmacotherapy and supportive therapy now provided for depressed, diabetic, hypertensive, asthmatic, and other chronic illness patients. Like most forms of pharmacotherapy for patients with chronic illnesses, opiate maintenance treatments are designed with an indeterminate length—possibly continuing throughout the life of the patient.

Outcomes Expected from Addiction Rehabilitation Treatments—We have argued in earlier work (McLellan et al., 1996b, 1997a) that outcome expectations for substance abuse treatment should not be confined simply to reduction of alcohol and drug use since the public, the payers of treatment, and even the patients themselves are interested in a broader definition of "rehabilitation." Further, we have argued that for substance abuse treatments to be "worth it" to the multiple stakeholders who are involved in treatment, the positive effects of addiction treatment should be sustained beyond the end of the treatment period and carry on at least six to twelve months. Most researchers in the addiction field have taken a similar, broad view of outcome expectations in the addiction treatment field (See Anglin et al., 1989; Babor et al., 1988; Ball and Ross, 1991; De Leon, 1984; Hubbard et al., 1989, 1997; Simpson, 1981, 1997; Simpson et al., 1997a,b).

Thus in the review that follows we have given greater attention to studies where multiple outcomes were measured six to twelve months following inpatient discharge or at the same points during the course of the outpatient period of care. Further, we have considered three domains that we feel are relevant to the rehabilitative goals of the patient and to the public health and safety goals of those societal stakeholders that support treatment:

1. *Sustained reduction of alcohol and drug use.* This is the foremost goal of substance dependence treatments and we consider it as the *primary outcome domain.* Within the review, we accepted as operational evidence for improvement in this domain both objective data from urinalysis and breathalyzer readings as well as patients' self reports of alcohol and drug use when those reports were recorded by independent interviewers under conditions of privacy and impartiality.

2. *Sustained increases in personal health and social function.* Improvements in the medical/psychiatric health and social function of addicted patients are important from a societal perspective in that these improvements reduce the problems and expenses produced by the addiction. In addition, improvements in these areas are important for maintaining reductions in substance use. Within the review, we accepted evidence from measures such as general health status inventories, psychological symptom inventories, family function measures, and simple measures of days worked and dollars earned, collected either directly from the patient via confidential self report or from independent medical/psychiatric evaluations and employment records.

3. *Sustained reductions in public health and public safety threats.* The threats to public health and safety from substance abusing individuals come from behaviors that spread infectious diseases and from behaviors associated with personal and property crimes. With regard to infectious disease, the sharing of needles, unprotected sex, and trading sex for drugs are serious behaviors that have clearly been linked to addiction and are significant threats to public health. Within the review, we accepted evidence of improved public health from confidential self reporting techniques or (rarely) through laboratory tests. Public safety threats were measured in the studies reviewed either by confidential interviews and questionnaires or by objective records of arrests and incarcerations.

In our view, the first two domains are quite consistent with the "primary and secondary measures of effectiveness" typically used by the Food and Drug Administration to evaluate new drug or device applications in controlled clinical trials (FDA) and quite consistent with the mainstream of thought regarding the evaluation of other forms of health care (Stewart and Ware, 1989). The final outcome dimension we believe is more specific to the treatment of substance use disorders since it acknowledges the significant public health and public safety concerns associated with addiction.

RESEARCH ON PATIENT FACTORS
RELATED TO TREATMENT OUTCOME

Demographic Factors—While demographic factors are typically important predictors of the development of drug abuse problems (IOM, 1990b; Wilsnack and Wilsnack, 1993) there is little evidence that race, gender, age, or educational level are consistent predictors of treatment outcome—among those who begin a treatment episode. An inspection of a wide range of treatment outcome studies in the substance abuse rehabilitation field suggests that demographic factors such as age, education, race, and even treatment history are relatively poorly related to the three outcome domains defined above in any of the major rehabilitation modalities (see Ball and Ross, 1991; Finney and Moos, 1992; McLellan et al., 1994; Rounsaville et al., 1987). For example, a study of 649 patients entering 22 treatment programs (seven inpatient, eight outpatient, seven methadone maintenance) for treatment of primary alcohol, opiate, or cocaine dependence evaluated the contribution of demographic variables including age, ethnicity, gender, marital status, years of education, and years of problematic substance abuse (McLellan et al., 1994). Results showed that none of the demographic measures was a significant predictor of either posttreatment substance use or posttreatment social adjustment. Similarly, studies by Simpson and Savage (1980) showed no significant effect of demographic and social indicators in predicting multiple outcome domains among heroin addicts treated in methadone maintenance and outpatient drug free treatment.

Though less studied at this time, there may be some important exceptions to this conclusion. For example, pregnant and parenting women are an important subgroup of the larger patient population who require different features to permit access to treatment as well as different constellations of treatment to address their often significant treatment problems (see Gomberg and Nirenberg, 1993; Wilsnack and Wilsnack, 1993). There has been indication that these patients have been reluctant to get into "standard" treatments because of stigma and because of the absence of services for their children. There have been experimental programs created to meet the needs of this important subgroup—and some excellent evaluations have followed these groups posttreatment (see Hagan et al., 1994). There have been very few longer term outcome studies of specialized treatments for pregnant and parenting women and only the most obvious conclusions can be drawn regarding the factors that appear to be important for attraction, retention, and improved outcomes for these patients. These factors would include but not be restricted to:

1. *The availability of care for children—and sometimes a residence that will accommodate the patients and their children.* Many of the addicted women who could benefit from treatment are responsible for the care of children and facilities that will provide respite care are likely to be necessary for these women to be able to enter outpatient treatment. Other women will not have the resources to be self supporting and may need temporary accommodations for themselves and their children. Still others may require a facility that will offer protection from aggressive and/or drug involved partners. Problems of safety from physical and sexual abuse and separation from drug involved relationships are common in a large proportion of these women (Hagan et al., 1994; Wilsnack and Wilsnack, 1993;

Schmidt and Weisner, 1995; Weisner and Schmidt, 1992). Residential settings are potentially important to address these problems.

2. *The availability of general medical, OB/GYN, and psychiatric services*. Disproportionately high numbers of these women have shown significant medical and psychiatric problems (Finnegan, 1991; Hagan et al., 1994; Schmidt and Weisner, 1995; Weisner and Schmidt, 1992; Wilsnack and Wilsnack, 1993). Therefore, it is important for programs that treat women substance abusers to provide adjunctive services in these areas.

Severity of Substance Use—Various measures of higher levels of severity and greater chronicity of patients' substance use patterns have been reliably associated with poorer retention in treatment and more rapid relapse to substance use following treatment. This has been true of both alcohol dependent patients (Babor et al., 1988; Finney and Moos, 1992); opiate dependent patients in therapeutic communities and in methadone maintenance (Ball and Ross, 1991; De Leon et al., 1984, 1994; Simpson, 1981, 1997a); and cocaine dependent patients treated in outpatient and inpatient settings (Alterman et al., 1994; Carroll et al., 1991; McLellan et al., 1994). The uniform nature of these predictive relationships across different types of drug dependence and treatment modalities suggests a pervasive trend toward poorer performance across all forms of treatment among those with longer durations and/or more intensive use patterns. This relationship is strongest between severity of substance use at treatment admission and posttreatment substance use. It is less clear whether the severity of alcohol and drug use at treatment admission is predictive of the other domains of personal health and social function, or public health and safety (McLellan et al., 1981b, 1992b, 1994). Thus, while the severity of substance use prior to treatment admission (measured in terms of amount, duration, and intensity of alcohol and drug use) is negatively related to posttreatment substance use—accounting for perhaps 10%–15% of outcome variance in that measure—it is less related to outcome in the other outcome domains (Babor et al., 1988; McLellan et al., 1994).

Severity of Psychiatric Problems—After the severity of the substance abuse problem, perhaps the most robust general patient variable predicting treatment response and posttreatment outcome has been the chronicity and severity of the psychiatric problems presented by the patient at the start of treatment (Carroll et al., 1993; Kadden et al., 1990; McLellan et al., 1983a,b, 1994; Powell et al., 1982; Project MATCH, 1997; Rounsaville et al., 1987; Woody et al., 1984, 1987). It is important to note that psychiatric problems have been measured using many scales and interviews in these studies, and all have attempted to distinguish more enduring or chronic psychiatric symptoms from the acute and temporary effects of alcohol and drug withdrawal. In the case of methadone maintained, opiate dependent patients, studies by McLellan and colleagues (1983a,b) indicated that the psychiatric severity scale from the Addiction Severity Index was the single best predictor of six month substance use, personal health, and social adjustment. Similar findings have been shown by Ball and Ross (1991) and by Kosten and colleagues (1987) and Rounsaville and colleagues (1983, 1987) with methadone maintained patients.

Measures of psychiatric severity have also been shown to be predictive of outcome in studies of opiate and multiple drug dependent patients entering an inpatient therapeutic community setting. For example, De Leon (1984) showed that opiate and non-opiate dependent patients with MMPI profiles indicative of high levels of psychopathology entering a therapeutic community were more likely to drop out of treatment and showed significantly less improvement on all outcome measures at discharge and at subsequent twelve month follow-up evaluations. In an earlier study of mixed opiate and non-opiate dependent male veterans entering into a therapeutic community McLellan and colleagues (1984) found that patients with the highest scores on the ASI psychiatric severity scale were most likely to drop out prematurely and actually showed 20%–40% less improvement than other patients who entered treatment at the same time. In that study, the "high psychiatric severity" patients who stayed in treatment longest actually showed the worst posttreatment status—suggesting that the therapeutic environment that had been demonstrably effective for patients with lower levels of psychiatric severity, was actually *counter* therapeutic for the high severity patients.

In the case of cocaine dependent patients, Carroll et al. (1991) also found poorer outcomes for patients with greater psychiatric pathology, as defined by scores on the Addiction Severity Index (ASI) psychiatric problem scale. Her findings were obtained in an outpatient rehabilitation setting. Similar results were found among cocaine dependent patients by Alterman et al. (1994) for patients treated in both a day-hospital and an inpatient rehabilitation setting.

Finally, there has been a great deal of evidence for the predictive power of general psychiatric symptomatology among alcohol dependent patients. Rounsaville and colleagues showed that psychiatric severity as measured by the ASI psychiatric scale was the best predictor of overall adjustment among previously treated alcohol dependent patients at a 2.5 year posttreatment follow-up (Rounsaville et al., 1987). Other authors have found that severity of depression (Powell et al., 1982; Schuckit et al., 1990) and anxiety (Brown et al., 1991; Schuckit et al., 1990) have been predictive of posttreatment drinking and posttreatment social adjustment among various samples of alcohol dependent patients. More recently, findings from the NIAAA sponsored, multisite study of patient treatment matching (Project MATCH,

1997) showed that the ASI psychiatric scale was a significant general predictor of posttreatment drinking and posttreatment social adjustment in a sample of more than 1200 alcohol dependent patients in three types of outpatient treatment.

Note: While there are a number of studies relating severity of psychopathology to posttreatment outcome, it should be noted that Schuckit and his colleagues have argued cogently against "over diagnosing" psychiatric symptoms, especially among alcohol dependent patients (Brown et al., 1991; Schuckit and Monteiro, 1988). These authors have shown that much of the serious psychopathology seen among alcohol dependent patients at treatment admission is reduced following even four weeks of abstinence. There is also evidence for rapid dissipation of psychiatric symptoms following abstinence from cocaine (Satel et al., 1991; Weddington, 1992). This proviso suggests that care should be taken to distinguish acute alcohol and/or drug related psychopathology from more enduring and chronic psychiatric symptoms.

Patient Motivation and Stage of Change—Evidence for patient "motivation for treatment" has traditionally been measured as the extent to which patients have freely entered into treatment. Conversely, patients who have been coerced into treatment based on pressure from legal, family, or employment sources, have been considered "treatment resistant." While this is a face valid measure of motivation—and presumably a good predictor of patient performance during and following treatment—the large literature on coerced treatment indicates the opposite of what would be expected. That is, patients who have been forced to enter a substance abuse treatment have shown during and posttreatment results that are quite similar to those shown by supposedly "internally motivated" patients (Inciardi, 1988; Lawental et al., 1996; Roman, 1988). This rather broad literature has led to the conclusion that when "motivation" is conceptualized and measured in terms of the degree to which the patient has been coerced into treatment, it is *not* an important predictor of treatment response.

However, there is rapidly growing body of research indicating that when motivation is defined as "readiness for change" and is conceptualized and measured in stages as suggested by Prochaska, DiClemente and their associates (e.g., Prochaska and DiClemente, 1984; Prochaska et al., 1992), "stage of change" motivation can be a very important predictor of treatment response and treatment outcome. According to the stage of change model, the process of behavior change occurs in a progression of five distinct stages, each characterized by a different constellation of attitudes and behaviors. An individual in the "precontemplation stage" has no awareness of a problem and no desire to change. A patient in the "preparation stage" has made the decision to change and is already taking steps to do so. A patient in the "maintenance stage" has shown change and is maintaining the changed behavior (see Prochaska and DiClemente, 1984).

The power of the model comes from two sets of findings. First, a relatively simple measure of stage of change such as the University of Rhode Island Change Assessment (URICA) (Prochaska and DiClemente, 1984; Prochaska et al., 1992) can apparently identify individuals in the precontemplation stage of change for whom traditional forms of rehabilitation treatment (most of which assume desire and ability to change as a precondition of admission) will *not* be effective. Specifically, there are several studies showing failure of traditional forms of counseling and therapy in patients identified as "precontemplators" on the URICA (DiClemente et al., 1991; Heather et al., 1993; Marlatt, 1988). The second important finding from work with this measure is that the "stage of change" is apparently an important predictor of treatment response and treatment outcome across all types of substance dependent patient samples (especially alcohol and nicotine dependent patients, but it is less studied among cocaine and opiate dependent patients), even those who are not in treatment (DiClemente et al., 1991).

The model provides a way of identifying patients with different levels of motivation and outlines a way of tailoring interventions to match their stage of change. It makes sense that those patients who consciously intend to change are more likely to succeed in treatment than those who do not. In this regard, the majority of the predictive power of the stage of change model has been the identification of precontemplators. Additional research is warranted to determine the extent to which the remaining stages of change can predict response to standard rehabilitation treatments.

Employment—There is ample indication from research with methadone maintained patients that employment, employability, and self support skills are a significant problem for this population; and that unemployed patients are more likely to drop out of treatment prematurely and to relapse to substance use early following treatment (Dennis et al., 1993; Hubbard et al., 1989; Platt, 1995). This was illustrated in a study of male veterans in methadone maintenance treatment by McLellan and colleagues (1981a). These authors found that patients who derived most of their income from employment showed more improvement and better six-month outcomes in several outcome domains including drug use, legal, and psychiatric problems and of course employment, than similar patients who derived the majority of their income from unemployment or welfare.

Hubbard and his colleagues (1989) showed that the development of employable skills and the capacity for self support were among the most important requirements for sustained reductions in drug use among a large cohort of drug dependent patients in treatment. Similar findings were shown by De Leon among opiate dependent patients in a therapeutic community setting (1984). Finally, Hall and her colleagues showed that unemployment was a significant predictor of early relapse to opiate use among detoxified heroin dependent males (1981). Similarly, in a sample of primarily employed, multiple substance abusers entering private inpatient or outpatient, abstinence oriented treatment programs, McLellan and colleagues showed that employment problems (getting along with supervisor, dissatisfaction with present job and salary, etc.) were one of the most significant predictors of both posttreatment substance use as well as posttreatment personal health and social function, measured at six-month follow-up (McLellan et al., 1994).

Family and Social Supports—Social supports have been widely studied in the field of alcohol and drug dependence. Social support has been conceptualized variously as the active participation in peer-supported treatments such as AA/NA; as the availability of relationships that are not conflict producing (McLellan et al., 1980, 1984) and in more detailed models, as the level of support for abstinence from those relationships (Longabough et al., 1993, 1995). Among alcohol dependent patients, there is often indication of significant "dysfunction" among the families, and in turn, the level of this disruption has been associated with earlier drop out from outpatient treatment (McLellan et al., 1983a, 1994), earlier relapse to drinking following treatment (Moos and Moos, 1984) and generally worse posttreatment function (McKay et al., 1994; McCrady et al., 1986; Moos and Moos, 1984).

Among opiate dependent patients there has been very little work associated with family and social supports as they relate to outcome. One prominent exception has been the work of Stanton and colleagues who showed both significant disruption and social pathology among families of methadone maintained patients; and a significant relationship between level of social pathology in the family of origin (typically also the posttreatment family environment in these patients) and use of heroin during methadone treatment (Stanton 1979; Stanton and Todd, 1982). McLellan et al. (1983a,b) found that the family relationship scale on the ASI was one of three significant predictors of posttreatment drug use and general personal and social function among opiate dependent patients in either inpatient therapeutic community or outpatient methadone maintenance treatment. In a subsequent study, this group also found that the family relationship scale was a significant predictor of posttreatment social function and relapse to cocaine and alcohol use among insured, working patients referred to substance abuse treatment through their employee assistance program (McLellan et al., 1993a, 1997a). An interesting, paradoxical finding in this area was reported by Havassy and her colleagues (1991). Among primarily

African-American cocaine dependent patients, these authors found a paradoxically negative relationship between the reported number of available family and friends of the patient and relapse to cocaine use following treatment: the more friends and family available to the patient, the earlier the return to cocaine use. The authors' hypothesize that in this severely affected cohort of patients, the only available sources of social support may have been associates with whom the patients had previously used drugs.

RESEARCH ON TREATMENT PROCESS FACTORS RELATED TO REHABILITATION OUTCOME

Patient factors have been much more widely studied than treatment setting, modality, process, and service factors as predictors of outcome from addiction rehabilitation treatments. Perhaps the major reason for this is that while there have been many reliable and valid measures of various patient characteristics, there are still very few measures of treatment setting (Moos, 1974; Moos et al., 1990) or treatment services (McLellan et al., 1992a; Widman et al., 1997).

There is good news however, regarding the study of treatment factors in the substance abuse field. Recent developments in the psychotherapy field have led to the creation of manual-based treatments and with them, appropriate measures of treatment fidelity and integrity. Following on this progress, the multisite NIAAA study of patient treatment matching (Project MATCH, 1997) has provided the field with new manuals for the three Project MATCH treatments as well as additional measures of the nature and fidelity of each treatment. These are likely to improve the study of addiction treatment process in the years to come. Below we review several dimensions or characteristics of treatment that have been studied and that have shown some relationship with outcome following treatment.

Setting of Treatment—There have now been many studies investigating potential differences in outcome between various forms of inpatient and outpatient rehabilitation. For example, studies by McCrady et al. (1986) and Alterman et al. (1994) randomly assigned alcohol dependent patients to an equal length (28–30 days) of either inpatient or day-hospital rehabilitation, where the treatment elements were also designed to be similar. Both studies showed very similar findings. Patients in both the inpatient and outpatient arms of both these studies showed substantial and significant reductions in alcohol use, as well as improvements in many other areas of personal health and social function—suggesting that both settings of care were able to produce substantial benefits. At the same time, a wide range of outcome measures collected at six-month follow-up in both studies, showed essentially no statistically significant or clinically important differences between the two settings of care—suggesting that the setting of care might not be an important contributor to outcome. A further analysis of data from the Alterman et al. study (McKay et al., 1995) indicated that 12-month outcomes in the day hospital group were generally at least equal to outcomes following inpatient care, and pertained to both randomized and nonrandomized subjects.

Consistent with the results of these two studies, reviews of the literature on inpatient and outpatient alcohol rehabilitation by Miller and Hester (1986) and Holder et al. (1991) also concluded that across a range of study designs and patient populations there was no significant advantage provided by inpatient care over outpatient care in the rehabilitation of alcohol dependence, despite the substantial difference in costs. In contrast, a widely cited study by Walsh et al. (1991) did find a significant difference in outcome favoring an inpatient program. However, this difference was shown among employed alcohol dependent patients who were assigned to either an inpatient program plus Alcoholics Anonymous (AA) or to AA meetings only (rather than to formal outpatient treatment). One recent review of the alcohol inpatient–outpatient literature did conclude that in studies that found an advantage to inpatient care over outpatient treatment, outpatients did not receive inpatient detoxification and the studies tended to not have social stability inclusion criteria or to require randomization (Finney et al., 1996). This review points to the need to consider "real world" factors when evaluating the effectiveness of different treatment settings.

In the field of cocaine dependence treatment, there have also been several studies examining the role of treatment setting. Again, while there is evidence for high attrition rates (e.g., Kang et al., 1991), there is still evidence indicting that outpatient treatments for cocaine dependence can be effective, even for patients with relatively limited social resources. In a recent study, Alterman and his colleagues followed up a prior comparison study of inpatient and day-hospital treatment of alcohol dependence (1994) with an identical examination comparing the effectiveness of four weeks of intensive, highly structured day hospital treatment (27 hours weekly) with that of inpatient treatment (48 hours weekly) for cocaine dependence. The subjects were primarily inner city, male African Americans treated at a Veterans Administration Medical Center. The inpatient treatment completion rate of 89% was significantly higher than the day-hospital completion rate of 54%. However, at seven months posttreatment entry self reported outcomes indicated considerable improvements for both groups in drug and alcohol use, family/social, legal, employment, and psychiatric problems. The finding of reduced self reported cocaine use was supported by urine screening results. Both self report and urine data indicated 50%–60% abstinence for both groups at the follow-up assessment. The comparability of both treatment settings was also evident in 12-month outcomes in both randomized and self-selecting patients (McKay et al., 1994).

Similar findings have been shown in field studies of private substance abuse treatment programs treating primarily cocaine and cocaine-plus-alcohol-dependent patients (McLellan et al., 1993a; Pettinati et al., 1998). In all of these studies, patients who were assigned to one of several outpatient treatment programs, were less likely to complete treatment than those assigned to the inpatient programs; but those who did complete treatment showed equal levels of improvement and outcome in the inpatient and outpatient settings. It is important to note that virtually all studies of this type have shown greater engagement and retention of patients in inpatient settings.

There have been at least two attempts to formalize clinical decision processes regarding who should, and should not be assigned to inpatient and outpatient settings of care (Cleveland Criteria; American Society of Addiction Medicine [ASAM] Criteria). McKay et al. (1992) failed to show evidence for the predictive validity of the Cleveland placement criteria at least when applied to the assignment of alcohol and drug dependent patients to day hospital or inpatient care. That is, patients who met the Cleveland Criteria for inpatient treatment did not have worse outcomes than those who met criteria for day hospital only when both groups received day hospital treatment. If the Cleveland Criteria had been valid, those who "needed inpatient treatment" but did not receive it should have had poorer outcomes than those who were appropriately "matched" to day hospital. In a similar study evaluating the psychosocial predictors from the ASAM criteria, McKay et al. (1997b) did find at least partial support for the predictive validity of these placement variables. That is, among patients who "needed inpatient treatment" as defined by the *psychosocial elements* of the ASAM criteria, those who were randomly assigned to outpatient care did show somewhat worse abstinence rates and generally poorer social outcomes than those who were randomly assigned to inpatient rehabilitation. The retrospective nature of this study made it impossible to complete a full evaluation of these criteria.

The most recent versions of the ASAM criteria have attempted to make very fine grained decisions regarding placements to levels of care defined by the amount and quality of medical supervision and monitoring. Research is needed to determine the predictive validity of these finer distinctions and whether placements to settings and modalities with "more medical supervision" actually receive more medical contact or services than placements that are not expected to receive such services.

Length of Treatment/Compliance with Treatment—Perhaps the most robust and pervasive indicator of favorable posttreatment outcome in all forms of substance abuse rehabilitation has been length of stay in treatment. Virtually all studies of rehabilitation have shown that patients who stay in treatment longer and/or attend more treatment sessions, have better posttreatment outcomes (Ball and Ross, 1991; De Leon, 1984, 1994; Hubbard et al., 1997; Simpson 1981, 1997; Simpson et al., 1997a,b). Specifically, several studies have suggested that outpatient treatments of less than 90 days are more likely to result in early return to drug use and generally poorer response than treatments of longer duration (Ball and Ross, 1991; Simpson, 1981, 1997; Simpson et al., 1997a,b).

Though length of stay is a very robust, positive predictor of treatment outcome, the nature of this relationship is still ambiguous. Clearly, one possibility is that patients who enter treatment gradually acquire new motivation, skills, attitudes, knowledge, and supports over the course of their stay in treatment; that those who stay longer acquire more of these favorable attributes and qualities; and that the gradual acquisition of these qualities or services is the reason for the favorable outcomes. An equally plausible possibility is that "better motivated and better adjusted patients" come into treatment ready and able to change; that the decisions they made to "change their lives" were made in advance of their admission and because of this greater motivation and "treatment readiness" they are likely to stay longer in treatment and to do more of what is recommended. These two interpretations of the same facts have very different implications for treatment practice. If treatment gradually produces positive changes over time, it is obviously clinically sound practice to retain patients longer—perhaps even through coercion—and to provide them with more services during treatment. On the other hand, if well motivated, high functioning, compliant patients enter treatment with the requisite skills and supports necessary to do well, then efforts to provide more services or to coerce patients into longer stays may not add to the effectiveness of more streamlined and less expensive rehabilitation efforts.

Participation in AA/NA—AA is of course recognized as a self-help or mutual support organization and not a formal treatment. For this reason, and because of the anonymous quality of the group, not much research has been done to evaluate this important part of substance abuse rehabilitation until recently (McLatchie and Lomp, 1988; McCrady and Miller, 1993; Nowinsky and Baker, 1992; Project MATCH, 1997). While there has always been consensual validation for the value of AA and other peer support forms of treatment, the past few years have witnessed new evidence showing that patients who have an AA sponsor, or who have participated in the fellowship activities—have much better abstinence records than patients who have received rehabilitation treatments but have not continued in AA. McKay and his colleagues (1997a) found that participation in posttreatment self-help groups predicted better outcome among a group of cocaine or alcohol dependent veterans in a day hospital rehabilitation program. Timko et al., (1994) found that more AA attendance was associated with better 1-year outcomes among previously untreated problem drinkers regardless of whether they received inpatient, outpatient, or no other treatment. Finally, a recent review of the literature on the impact of self-help programs concluded that greater participation was generally associated with better alcohol and psychosocial outcomes, although the magnitude of the effects tended to vary as a function of the quality of the study and whether patients were treated in inpatient or outpatient settings (Tonigan et al., 1996).

There has been less research in the use of self-help organizations among cocaine and/or opiate dependent patients. However, a recent study of cocaine patients participating in outpatient counseling and psychotherapy showed that while only 34% attended a cocaine anonymous (CA) meeting, 55% of those who did became abstinent as compared with only 38% of those who did not attend CA.

In contemporary addiction treatment, AA has become synonymous with the last part of rehabilitation—aftercare. Virtually all alcohol dependence rehabilitation programs and most cocaine dependence rehabilitation programs refer patients to AA programs with instructions to get a sponsor, "share and chair" at meetings, and to attend 90 meetings in 90 days as a continued commitment to sobriety. Thus, while the research studies done to date have generally suggested that the peer support component of rehabilitation is valuable, it is also difficult to sort out the extent to which AA attendance constitutes an active ingredient of successful treatment and/or the extent to which it is simply a marker of general treatment compliance and commitment to abstinence.

In this regard, several investigators have studied the relationship of completing various 12-step processes during the course of rehabilitation, to relapse following treatment. Morgenstern and colleagues reported that patients who adopted more of the attitudinal and behavioral tenets of the 12-step model of rehabilitation such as admission of powerlessness, acceptance of a higher power, commitment to AA, and agreement that alcoholism is a disease, were no more (or less) likely to relapse following treatment than patients who had adopted very few of the 12-step tenets by the end of the rehabilitation treatment (Morgenstern et al., 1997). At the same time, two general tenets found in all rehabilitation models—greater commitment to abstinence and greater intention to avoid high risk situations—did predict a lower likelihood of relapse (Morgenstern et al., 1997). In another analysis from the same study, greater affiliation with AA following treatment predicted better outcomes. AA affiliation was in turn positively associated with self-efficacy, motivation, and coping efforts, which were themselves significant predictors of outcome (Morgenstern et al., 1997). Thus, more research in this area is warranted to determine how participation in AA exerts its positive effects.

The Therapist or Counselor—There is a growing body of research suggesting that having access to regular drug/alcohol counseling can make an important contribution to the engagement and participation of the patient in treatment and to the posttreatment outcome. Perhaps the clearest example of the role of the counselor and at least individual counseling was shown in a study of methadone maintained patients, all within the same treatment program and all receiving the same methadone dose, who were randomly assigned to receive counseling or no counseling in addition to the methadone (McLellan et al., 1993b). Results were unequivocal showing that 68% of patients assigned to the no counseling condition failed to reduce drug use (confirmed by urinalysis) and 34% of these patients required at least one episode of emergency medical care. In contrast, no patient in the counseling groups required emergency medical care, 63% showed sustained elimination of opiate use, and 41% showed sustained elimination of cocaine use over the six months of the trial.

A study by Fiorentine and Anglin (1997) as part of a larger "Target Cities" evaluation also showed the contribution of counseling in drug rehabilitation. Group counseling was the most common modality (averaging 9.5 sessions per month) followed by 12-step meetings (average 7.5 times per month) and individual counseling (average 4.7 times per month). Greater frequency of both group and individual counseling sessions were shown to decrease the likelihood of relapse over the subsequent six months. One important contribution of this study, given the above cautions regarding the role of simple length of stay in determining treatment outcome (see above), is that the relationships shown between more counseling and lower likelihood of relapse to cocaine use were seen even among patients who completed treatment—that is, having approximately the same tenure in the programs. Thus, it may be that beyond the simple effects of attending a program, more involvement with the counseling activities is important for improved outcome.

At least four studies of substance abuse treatment have documented between-therapist differences in patient outcomes. These differences have emerged both among professional psychotherapists with doctoral level training and among paraprofessional counselors. Luborsky et al. (1985) found outcome differences in a variety of areas among nine professional therapists providing ancillary psychotherapy to methadone maintenance patients. McLellan et al. (1988) found that assignment to one of five methadone maintenance counselors resulted in significant differences in treatment progress over the following six months. Specifically, patients transferred to one counselor achieved significant reductions in illicit drug use, unemployment, and arrests while concurrently reducing their average methadone dose. In contrast, patients transferred to another counselor evidenced increased unemployment and illicit drug use while their average methadone dose went up. In a study of two different interventions for problem drinkers, Miller, Taylor, and West (1980) found significant differences between paraprofessional therapists in the percentage of their patients who improved by six-month follow-up. These percentages varied from 25% for the least effective therapist to 100% for the most effective therapist. Finally, McCaul and Svikis (1991) reported significant differences in posttreatment drinking rates and several other outcomes among alcohol dependent patients assigned to different individual counselors within an alcohol treatment program.

There is much research that needs to be done in this area. Although it is relatively clear that therapists and counselors differ considerably in the extent to which they are able to help their patients achieve positive outcomes, it is less clear what distinguishes more effective from less effective therapists. In an experimental study of two different therapist styles, Miller, Benefield, and Tonigan (1993) found that a client centered approach emphasizing reflective listening was more effective for problem drinkers than a directive, confrontational approach. In a review of the literature on therapist differences in substance abuse treatment, Najavits and Weiss (1994) concluded, "The only consistent finding has been that therapists' in-session interpersonal functioning is positively associated with greater effectiveness" (p. 683). Among indicators of interpersonal functioning were the ability to form a helping alliance (Luborsky et al., 1985), measures of the level of accurate empathy (Miller et al., 1980; Valle, 1981), and a measure of "genuineness," "concreteness," and "respect" (Valle, 1981).

It should be noted that there are a variety of certification programs for counselors (Committee on Addiction Rehabilitation [CARF] and Certified Addictions Counselor [CAC]) as well as other professions treating substance dependent patients (American Society of Addiction Medicine; American Academy of Psychiatrists in Addiction; recent added certification for psychologists through the American Psychological Association). These "added qualification certificates" are offered throughout the country, usually by professional organizations. Although the efforts of these professional organizations to bring needed training and proficiency to the treatment of addicted persons are commendable, we were unable to find any studies validating whether patients treated by "certified" addictions counselors, physicians, or psychologists have better outcomes than patients treated by noncertified individuals. This is an important gap in the existing literature and results from such studies would be quite important for the licensing efforts and health policy decisions of many states and health care organizations.

Medications—At this writing, there is a great deal of research spon-sored by both the National Institute on Alcoholism and Alcohol Abuse and the National Institute on Drug Abuse aimed at developing useful medica-tions for the treatment of substance dependent persons. Great progress has been made over the past ten years in the development of new medications and in the application of existing medications for the treatment of particu-lar conditions associated with substance dependence and for particular types of substance dependent patients (see IOM, 1995; O'Brien, 1996; O'Brien and McKay, in press). Here we have only summarized some of the clearest results from the use of agonist and antagonist medications in the treatment of substance dependence and have provided citations for more comprehensive medication reviews for interested readers.

Agonist Medications—Methadone has been an approved agonist medi-cation for the maintenance treatment of opiate dependence for more than 25 years. The long-acting form of methadone (48- to 72-hour duration), LAAM has recently received FDA approval and has been accepted by 16 states for prescription only at methadone maintenance programs. Buprenorphine is a partial opiate agonist that has been widely used in Europe and in the United States. It is thought to have some advantages over methadone in that it produces far fewer (often none) withdrawal symptoms (see Bickel et al., 1997). At this writing, it is not yet approved for use.

Among the most robust findings in the treatment literature is the rela-tionship between dose of methadone and general outcome in methadone treatment (Ball and Ross, 1991; D'Aunno and Vaughn, 1992, 1995; Insti-tute of Medicine, 1995). Higher doses are more effective than lower doses. In a well controlled double blind multisite VA study, Ling et al. (1976) found that 100 mg per day was superior to 50 mg as indicated by staff ratings of global improvement and by a drug use index comprised of weighted results of opiate urine tests. In a more recent randomized, double-blind study, Strain et al. (1993) compared 50 mg and 20 mg with a 0 mg placebo-only group. They found orderly dose-response effects on treatment retention, and they found that 50 mg was more effective than 20 mg or 0 mg at decreasing opiate and cocaine use as measured by urinalysis results. In a randomized double blind comparison of moderate (40–50 mg) and high (80–100 mg) dose methadone, Strain and his colleagues (1996) found a significantly lower rate of opiate positive urine specimens among patients receiving the high dose of methadone (53% vs. 62%). There are many other studies of opiate agonist medications, but space limitations do not permit more detail here (see IOM, 1995 for additional information).

Antagonist and Blocking Agents—Naltrexone has been used for more than 20 years in the treatment of opiate dependence (see Greenstein et al., 1981; O'Brien et al., 1984). It is an orally administered opiate antagonist that blocks actions of externally administered opiates such as heroin by competitive binding to opiate receptors. It has been particularly effective as an adjunct to probation in opiate addicted federal probationers (see Cornish et al., 1997). More recently, naltrexone (marketed under the trade name Revia®) has been found to be effective in the treatment of alcohol dependence (O'Malley et al., 1992; Volpicelli et al., 1992). Naltrexone at 50mg/day has been approved by the FDA for use with alcohol dependent patients since independent studies have shown it to be a safe, effective pharmacological adjunct for reducing heavy alcohol use among alcohol dependent patients. Its mechanism of action appears to be the blocking of at least some of the "high" produced by alcohol consumption, again through competitive binding with the mu opiate receptors (O'Malley et al., 1992; Volpicelli et al., 1992).

With regard to other medications designed to block the effects of an abused drug, disulfiram (Antabuse ®) has been used the longest and most pervasively in the treatment of alcohol dependence (see Fuller et al., 1986). However, disulfiram seems to be most effective under certain conditions, such as when the patient contracts to having a significant other witness him or her take the medication each day. More recently, European researchers have found encouraging results with acamprosate as a treatment for alcoholism (Ladewig et al., 1993; Lhuintre et al., 1990). While acamprosate acts on different receptor systems than naltrexone, the clinical results are remarkably similar (Anton, 1995; Ladewig et al., 1993; Lhuintre et al., 1990). Alcohol dependent patients who take acamprosate have shown 30% greater posttreatment abstinence rates at six-month follow-up than those randomly assigned to placebo. Further, those who have returned to drinking while taking acamprosate report less heavy drinking (greater than five drinks per day) than those who returned to drinking while prescribed placebo (Anton, 1995). While both of these medications can be used for extended periods, in practice they are generally prescribed for about one to three months as part of a more general rehabilitation program that includes behavioral change strategies (see review by Anton, 1995).

There have been many agents tried as blocking agents in the treatment of cocaine dependence and while this literature is quite large, it has been disappointing (see Institute of Medicine, 1995; O'Brien, 1996; O'Brien and McKay, in press). At this writing, there is no convincing evidence that any of the various types of cocaine blocking agents are truly effective for even brief periods of time or for even a significant minority of affected patients. Research continues in this important area and there have been indications of a potentially successful "vaccine" that may be able to immediately metabolize and inactivate active metabolites of cocaine (see Fox, 1997). This promising work is currently being tested in animal models, but there are no treatment relevant medications available for cocaine rehabilitation at this time.

Although the use of opiate and alcohol antagonists or blocking agents is increasing as addiction physicians are more comfortable with the prescription of adjunctive medications and as more substance dependence is treated by primary care physicians in office settings (see Fleming and Barry, 1992), there are still relatively few patients that receive—or practitioners that prescribe—these medications (Institute of Medicine, 1995). Furthermore, the available literature in this area still does not provide an unambiguous conclusion regarding the parameters that are most effective when using antagonist or "blocking" pharmacotherapy. For example, a recent cautionary article by Moitto and colleagues warned about an unusually high rate of deaths (particularly suicides) among opiate dependent individuals who were transferred to naltrexone (Moitto et al., 1997). The appropriate use of these antagonist or blocking medications in "real world" treatment of substance dependence disorders may be among the most important topics for future research in the treatment field. These medications are often expensive and managed care companies have been slow to permit these medications to reach formularies (see Institute of Medicine, 1995; O'Brien, 1996; O'Brien and McKay, in press). In addition, there is a need for long term studies of patients who have been prescribed these medications as well as studies examining the most appropriate and efficient mix of psychosocial and pharmacological services to maximize rehabilitation for various types of substance dependent patients.

Provision of Specialized Services—The majority of patients admitted to substance abuse treatment have significant "addiction related" problems in one or more areas such as medical status, employment, family relations, and/or psychiatric function (McLellan and Weisner, 1996). As has been indicated above, the severity of these problems at the time of treatment admission is generally a good *negative* predictor of posttreatment outcome. Studies have documented that strategies designed to direct and focus specialized services to these "addiction related" problems can be applied in standard clinical settings and can be effective in improving the results of substance abuse treatment. Again, this conclusion follows more than a decade of research showing that the addition of professional marital counseling (Fals-Stewart et al., 1996; McCrady et al., 1986; O'Farrell et al., in press; Stanton and Todd, 1982), psychotherapy (Carroll et al., 1991, 1993, 1994a,b; Woody et al., 1983, 1984, 1987, 1995) and medical care (Fleming and Barry, 1992) produces clinically and significantly better outcomes from substance abuse treatment.

It should be noted that in some cases, these adjunctive forms of therapy and services have been most clearly associated with improved personal health and social function following treatment but not as well related to reduced alcohol and drug use. In addition, and not surprisingly, these treatments have only been shown to be effective with those patients having more severe problems in the target area (matching effect)—that is, if there has been no indication of a relatively severe problem in the target area, there has typically been no evidence that the provision of the target therapy is effective or worthwhile (see Woody et al., 1984). One exception to this appears to be behavioral marital or couples therapy, which has typically demonstrated a "main effect" for all couples in the studies. This might be because most marriages in which one or both partners are actively abusing alcohol or drugs could be characterized by fairly severe marital problems. However, even in the case of marital therapy, some matching effects have been found. One study found that the effectiveness of couples therapy for alcoholics varied as a function of complex interactions involving the patient's degree of investment in relationships, degree of support for abstinence from significant others, and planned number of conjoint sessions (Longabaugh et al., 1995).

Community Reinforcement and Contingency Contracting—Azrin and colleagues initially developed the "Community Reinforcement Approach" (CRA) and tested it against other "standard" treatment interventions (Azrin et al., 1982). CRA includes conjoint therapy, job finding training, counseling focused on alcohol-free social and recreational activities, monitored disulfiram, and an alcohol-free social club. The goal of CRA is to make abstinence more rewarding than continued use (Meyers and Smith, 1995). In a study in which patients were randomly assigned to CRA or to a standard hospital treatment program, those getting CRA drank less, spent fewer days away from home, worked more days, and were institutionalized less over a 24-month follow-up (Azrin et al., 1982).

A more recent set of studies by Higgins et al. (Higgins et al., 1991, 1993, 1994, 1995) has used the CRA approach with cocaine dependent patients. Here, cocaine dependent patients seeking outpatient treatment were randomly assigned to receive either standard drug counseling and referral to AA, or a multicomponent behavioral treatment integrating contingency managed counseling, community-based incentives, and family therapy comparable to the CRA model (Higgins et al., 1991). The CRA model retained more patients in treatment, produced more abstinent patients and longer periods of abstinence, and produced greater improvements in personal function than the standard counseling approach. Following the overall findings, this group of investigators systematically "disassembled" the CRA model and examined the individual "ingredients" of family therapy (Higgins et al., 1993), incentives (Higgins et al., 1994), and the contingency based counseling (Higgins et al., 1995) as compared against groups who received comparable amounts of all components except the target ingredient. In each case, these systematic and controlled examinations indicated that these individual components made a significant contribution to the outcomes observed, thus proving their added value in the rehabilitation effort. Extending this work on the use of positive reinforcement and behavioral contracting, Silverman and colleagues (Silverman et al., 1996) used essentially the same reinforcement contingencies and contracting procedures that had been applied by Azrin and Higgins to improve the performance of methadone maintained patients.

"Matching" Patients and Treatments—The past two decades have witnessed a great number of research studies attempting to "match" patients with specific types, modalities or settings of treatment. The approach to patient-treatment "matching" that has received the greatest attention from substance abuse treatment researchers involves attempting to identify the characteristics of individual patients that predict the best response to different forms of addiction treatments (e.g., cognitive-behavioral vs. 12-Step, or inpatient vs. outpatient) (Mattson et al., 1994; Project MATCH Research Group, 1997). In general, the majority of these "patient-to-treatment" matching studies have *not* shown robust or generalizable findings (see Gastfriend and McLellan, 1997). Another approach to matching has been to assess patients' problem severity in a range of areas at intake and then "match" the specific and necessary services to the particular problems presented at the assessment. This has been called "problem-to-service" matching (McLellan et al., 1997b). This approach may have more practical application as it is consonant with the "individually tailored treatment" philosophy that has been espoused by most practitioners.

Substance abusers with comorbid psychiatric problems may be particularly good candidates for the "problem-to-service" matching approach; especially the addition of specialized psychiatric services for those most severely affected by psychiatric problems. For example, recent studies suggest that tricyclic antidepressants and the selective serotonergic medication fluoxetine may reduce both drinking and depression levels in alcoholics with major depression (Cornelius et al., 1997; Mason et al., 1996; McGrath et al., 1996). Similarly, the anxiolytic buspirone may reduce drinking in alcoholics with a comorbid anxiety disorder (Kranzler et al., 1994). Highly structured relapse prevention interventions may also be more effective in decreasing cocaine use, as compared to less structured interventions, in cocaine abusers with comorbid depression (Carroll et al., 1995).

Woody and colleagues have evaluated the value of individual psychotherapy when added to paraprofessional counseling services in the course of methadone maintenance treatment (Woody et al., 1983). In that study patients were randomly assigned to receive standard drug counseling alone (DC group) or drug counseling plus one of two forms of professional therapy: supportive-expressive psychotherapy (SE) or cognitive-behavioral psychotherapy (CB) over a six month period. Results showed that patients receiving psychotherapy showed greater reductions in drug use, more improvements in health and personal function, and greater reductions in crime than those receiving counseling alone. Stratification of patients according to their levels of psychiatric symptoms at intake showed that the main psychotherapy effect was seen in those with greater than average levels of psychiatric symptoms. Specifically, patients with low symptom levels made considerable gains with counseling alone and there were no differences between types of treatment. However, patients with more severe psychiatric problems showed few gains with counseling alone but substantial improvements with the addition of the professional psychotherapy.

Another type of substance abuser that can pose particular problems for outpatient treatment is the cocaine dependent patient who is unable to achieve remission from cocaine dependence early in outpatient treatment. Several randomized studies suggest that highly structured cognitive-behavioral treatment is particularly efficacious with such individuals. In two outpatient studies with cocaine abusers, those with more severe cocaine problems at intake had significantly better cocaine use outcomes if they received structured relapse prevention rather than interpersonal or clinical management treatments (Carroll et al., 1991, 1994b). In a third study, cocaine dependent patients who continued to use cocaine during a four-week intensive outpatient treatment program (IOP) had much better cocaine use outcomes if they subsequently received aftercare that included a combination of group therapy and a structured relapse prevention protocol delivered through individual sessions rather than aftercare that consisted of group therapy alone (McKay et al., 1998).

The impact of adding additional, professionally delivered treatment services to a basic methadone program was investigated by McLellan and colleagues (McLellan et al., 1993b). In this study, patients were randomly assigned to receive (a) methadone only; (b) methadone plus standard counseling; or (c) methadone and counseling plus on-site medical, psychiatric, employment, and family therapy services (the "enhanced" condition). Although these additional services were not "matched" to patients on an individual basis, most of the patients in the study were polydrug abusers with relatively high problem levels in other areas. On most outcome measures, the best results were obtained in the enhanced condition, followed by methadone plus counseling, and methadone alone. Improvements in the enhanced condition were significantly better than those in the methadone plus counseling condition in the areas of employment, alcohol use, criminal activity, and psychiatric status. These results demonstrate the value of providing additional professional treatment services to polyproblem substance abusers, even when these services are not "matched" to specific problems at the level of the individual patient.

McLellan and colleagues recently attempted a different type of "problems to services" matching research in two inpatient and two outpatient private treatment programs (McLellan et al., 1997b). Patients in the study (N = 130) were assessed with the ASI at intake and placed in a program that was acceptable to both the Employee Assistance Program referral source and the patient. At intake, patients were also randomized to either the standard or "matched" services conditions. In the standard condition, the treatment program received information from the intake ASI, and personnel were instructed to treat the patient in the "standard manner, as though there were no evaluation study ongoing." The programs were instructed to not withhold any services from patients in the standard condition. Patients who were randomly assigned to the matched services condition were also placed in one of the four treatment programs and ASI information was forwarded to that program. However, the programs agreed to provide at least three individual sessions in the areas of employment, family/social relations, or psychiatric health delivered by a professionally trained staff person to improve functioning in those areas when a patient evidenced a significant degree of impairment in one or more of these areas at intake. For example, a patient whose intake ASI revealed significant impairments in the areas of social and psychiatric functioning would receive at least six individual sessions, three by a psychiatrist and three by a social worker.

The standard and matched patients were compared on a number of measures, including number of services received while in treatment, treatment completion rates, intake to six-month improvements in the seven problem areas assessed by the ASI, and other key outcomes at six months. Matched patients received significantly more psychiatric and employment services than standard patients, but not more family/social services or alcohol and drug services. Second, matched patients were more likely to complete treatment (93% vs. 81%), and showed more improvement in the areas of employment and psychiatric functioning than the standard patients. Third, while matched and standard patients had sizable and equivalent improvements on most measures of alcohol and drug use, matched patients were less likely to be retreated for substance abuse problems during the six-month follow-up. These findings suggest that matching treatment services to adjunctive problems can improve outcomes in key areas and may also be cost-effective by reducing the need for subsequent treatment due to relapse.

Limitations of the Matching Services to Problems Approach—It is difficult to argue against the face validity of a treatment approach for polyproblem substance abusers that stresses the importance of providing additional services to address co-occurring medical, economic, psychiatric, family, and legal problems. After all, effective substance abuse focused interventions such a Cognitive Behavioral Therapy or Twelve Step Facilitation (Project MATCH, 1997), no matter how well delivered, are not designed to address serious problems in other areas. If left untreated, co-occurring problems can increase risk for poor treatment response and poor posttreatment outcome. And in some cases, it may be impossible to even initiate treatment for a substance abuse problem until treatment for a severe co-occurring problem has been provided. In addition to benefits for the patients, the matching services to problems approach can also reduce stress levels in clinicians who treat polyproblem individuals, provided that a team approach to treatment is taken and regular lines of communication are established between clinicians involved with a case.

The primary limitation of this approach concerns the potential lack of resources in a time of health care cost containment. Funding may not be available to substance abuse treatment providers for adjunctive services in areas such as medical and psychiatric care, unless the level of problem severity is high enough that these co-occurring disorders can be considered as "primary." Recent research has shown that substance abuse programs vary widely in the number and frequency of adjunctive services they provide (D'Aunno and Vaughn, 1995; McLellan et al., 1993a; Widman et al., 1997), which may reflect differences between programs in the funding available for such services. Obviously, it is impossible to match services to problems if the appropriate services are not available. The scarcity of resources underlies the need for accurate assessment and diagnosis of co-occurring problems, so as to ensure that patients who are more in need of such services will stand a better chance of receiving them. Also, not all services may be potent enough to make a significant impact on the target problem area. For example, despite the importance of employment related problems in predicting treatment outcome, and the range of interventions that have been developed to improve employment and self-support among substance dependent patients (see French et al., 1992), there is little evidence that this type of specialized service is effective in improving the employment of the patients or in improving abstinence from drugs (Hall et al., 1981 is an exception).

Another potential problem with the matching services-to-problems approach is that even when adjunctive services are available in the community, they may not be offered at the clinic or agency in which the patient is receiving substance abuse focused treatment. In cases where patients have to go to other agencies to obtain additional services, there is a greater chance of attrition due to logistical problems or flagging motivation. This is a strong argument for combining substance abuse treatment with a broader array of services, which is sometimes referred to as "one-stop shopping," in settings where a more interdisciplinary approach can be taken for the treatment of the polyproblem individual.

SUMMARY AND DISCUSSION

In the text above we have attempted to review the substance abuse treatment research literature to identify patient and treatment process variables that have been shown to be important in determining outcome from addiction rehabilitation efforts; and in this way to contribute to the discussion of what treatment research may offer to practitioners in the field. While it is true that many of the research studies reviewed employed highly selected patient samples and/or sophisticated, resource-intensive interventions that would not be practical in "real world" community treatment programs, it is also true that this literature offers some important starting points for our larger effort to fill the gaps between what is known and what needs to be known at the level of the treatment program. This in turn is important for identifying clinical and policy issues that should be the focus of future research. Our review of this research has suggested the following three points:

1. *The existing literature on treatment outcomes has been disappointing with regard to informing treatment practice at the level of the community treatment program.* Most of the outcome studies in the current literature were conducted by clinical researchers, typically in controlled trials. The purpose of these studies was generally to determine whether the index treatment, *when delivered under specified conditions to rather highly selected samples of patients,* could effect the expected changes relative to standard or minimal treatment conditions. Many of the clinical trials reviewed here excluded important classes of patients (e.g., polysubstance users) that are most prevalent in community treatment agencies. In addition, many of these studies used very specific, resource-intensive interventions studied under rarefied conditions for fixed periods of time. In most clinical practice settings, when a patient fails to respond to one type of intervention, the sensitive clinician will alter the approach. Thus the interventions that are compared in experiments may not reflect what happens in practice.

2. *Despite these caveats, there are important findings from controlled clinical research that suggest important directions for treatment practice in the "real world"*—Given a definition of good outcome from rehabilitation treatment as "lasting improvements in those problems that led to the treatment admission and that were important to the patient and to society," the

APPENDIX D 175

following patient and treatment process factors have been significantly and repeatedly related to favorable outcomes.

Patient variables associated with better outcome from rehabilitation included:

a. low severity of dependence,
b. few psychiatric symptoms at admission,
c. motivation beyond the precontemplation stage of change,
d. being employed or self supporting, and
e. having family and social supports for sobriety.

Treatment variables associated with better outcome from rehabilitation included:

a. staying longer in/ being more compliant with treatment—especially through behavioral contracting for positive reinforcement;
b. having an individual counselor or therapist;
c. having specialized services provided for associated medical, psychiatric, and/or family problem;
d. receiving proper medications—both for psychiatric conditions and anticraving medications; and
e. participating in AA or NA following treatment.

In contrast to the above findings, it was surprising that some of the treatment elements that are most widely provided in substance abuse treat ment have *not* been associated with better outcome. For example, our review of the literature has shown little indication that any of the following lead to better or longer lasting outcomes following treatment:

a. alcohol/drug education sessions;
b. general group therapy sessions, especially "confrontation" sessions;
c. acupuncture sessions;
d. patient relaxation techniques; and
e. treatment program accreditation or professional practice certification criteria.

For the sake of brevity, studies of these five interventions were not described above. These findings are generally in accordance with a review of the alcohol rehabilitation field by Miller and Holder (1994), which concluded that there are a number of therapeutic practices and procedures that remain prevalent in the field that have not *yet* shown indication of success. It is important to note that "the absence of evidence" does not prove a treatment element is ineffective. Some of the treatment practices or conventions cited may actually have benefits for some patients or under some circumstances but we have found little support for these in the existing literature.

3. *A reviewer of this field will get substantially different views about the "outcome" of an addiction treatment depending upon the perspective taken regarding what "outcome" is; and when, how, and by whom it is measured.* Consider three common perspectives on the evaluation of an outpatient addiction treatment program. A quality assurance or service delivery evaluation of that treatment might conclude that the program "had very good outcomes" since there was no waiting for treatment entry and at discharge, more than 80% of the patients were "highly satisfied" with their counselor and physician. A clinical researcher, having interviewed a sample of patients at admission to the program, and again six months following discharge, might conclude that the program "had mixed outcomes" since at the follow-up point, only 50% of the patients were abstinent (the intended goal of the program) but there was a 70% reduction in frequency of drinking and a 50% reduction in medical and psychiatric symptoms. Meanwhile, an economist or health policy analyst might have used Medicaid data tapes to compare the health services utilization rates of a sample of discharged patients, two years prior to their treatment admission and two years following their discharge. The conclusion here might be that "treatment had very poor outcome" since there had been no decrease in health care utilization from the pre- to the posttreatment period, hence no "cost-offset" to the public.

This example illustrates two points. First, that these three common perspectives on outcome have different purposes for their evaluations and different expectations regarding treatment, they measure different elements of the treatment process and the patient population, and at different points in time. Following from the first point, these different measures of outcome are not well related to each other; and it has been the case that clinical research has often focused upon a rather narrow set of outcomes (e.g., abstinence from alcohol or drugs) to evaluate treatments while interventions delivered at community treatment organizations are being evaluated on a different and often broader set of outcomes (e.g., reduction of crime, reincarceration, reduction of family violence, reduction of Medicaid claims, etc.). If research is to be able to inform clinical practice, there should be efforts made to agree upon and adopt common expectations and measures.

REFERENCES

Alterman AI, O'Brien CP, McLellan AT, August DS, Snider EC, Droba M, Cornish JC, Hall CP, Raphaelson AH, Schrade FX. 1994. Effectiveness and costs of inpatient versus day hospital cocaine rehabilitation. *Journal of Nervous and Mental Disesase* 182(3):157–163.

Anglin MD, Speckart GR, Booth MW, Ryan TM. 1989. Consequences and costs of shutting off methadone. *Addictive Behaviors* 14:307–326.

Anton RF. 1995. New directions in the pharmacotherapy of alcoholism. *Psychiatric Annals* 25:353–362.

Azrin NH, Sisson RW, Meyers RW, Godley M. 1982. Alcoholism treatment by disulfiram and community reinforcement therapy. *Journal of Behavior Therapy and Experimental Psychiatry* 13:105–112.

Babor TF, Dolinsky Z, Rounsaville BJ, Jaffe JH. 1988. Unitary versus multidimensional models of alcoholism treatment outcome: An empirical study. *Journal of Studies on Alcohol* 49(2):167–177.

Ball JC, Ross A. 1991. *The Effectiveness of Methadone Maintenance Treatment*. New York: Springer-Verlag.

Bickel WK, Amass L, Higgins ST, Badger GJ, Esch RA. 1997. Effects of adding behavioral treatment to opioid detoxification with buprenorphone. *Journal of Consulting and Clinical Psychology* 65(5):803–810.

Brown SA, Irwin M, Schuckit MA. 1991. Changes in anxiety among abstinent male alcoholics. *Journal of Studies on Alcohol* 52:55–61.

Carroll KM, Rounsaville BJ, Gawin FH. 1991. A comparative trial of psychotherapies for ambulatory cocaine abusers: Relapse prevention and interpersonal psychotherapy. *American Journal of Drug and Alcohol Abuse* 17:229–247.

Carroll KM, Power MD, Bryant K, Rounsaville BJ. 1993. One-year follow-up status of treatment-seeking cocaine abusers: Psychopathology and dependence severity as predictors of outcome. *Journal of Nervous and Mental Disease* 181:71–79.

Carroll KM, Rounsaville BJ, Gordon LT, Nich C, Jatlow P, Bisighini RM, Gawin FH. 1994a. Psychotherapy and pharmacotherapy for ambulatory cocaine abusers. *Archives of General Psychiatry* 51:177–187.

Carroll KM, Rounsaville BJ, Nich C, Gordon LT, Wirtz PW, Gawin F. 1994b. One-year follow-up of psychotherapy and pharmacotherapy for cocaine dependence: Delayed emergence of psychotherapy effects. *Archives of General Psychiatry* 51(12):989–997.

Carroll KM, Nich C, Rounsaville BJ. 1995. Differential symptom reduction in depressed cocaine abusers treated with psychotherapy and pharmacotherapy. *Journal of Nervous and Mental Disease* 183:251–259.

Childress AR, McLellan AT, O'Brien CP. 1985. Assessment and extinction of conditioned opiate withdrawal-like responses. *NIDA Research Monograph* 55:202–210.

Childress AR, McLellan AT, O'Brien CP. 1986. Abstinent opiate abusers exhibit conditioned craving, conditioned withdrawal and reductions in both through extinction. *British Journal of the Addictions* 81:665–660.

Childress AR, Ehrman R, Rohsenow D, Robbins S, O'Brien CP. 1992. Classically conditioned factors in drug dependence. In: Lowinson J, Ruiz P, Millman RB, eds. *Substance Abuse: A Comprehensive Textbook*. Second Edition. Baltimore, MD: Williams and Wilkins. Pp. 56–69.

Cornelius JR, Salloum IM, Ehler JG, Jarrett PJ, Cornelius MD, Perel JM, Thase JE, Black A. 1997. Fluoxetine in depressed alcoholics: A double-blind, placebo controlled trial. *Archives of General Psychiatry* 54:700–705.

Cornish JW, Metzger D, Woody GE, Wilson D, McLellan AT, Vandergrift B, O'Brien CP. 1997. Naltrexone pharmacotherapy for opioid dependent federal probationers. *Journal of Substance Abuse Treatment* 14(6):529–534.

D'Aunno T, Vaughn TE. 1992. Variations in methadone treatment practices: Results from a national study. *Journal of the American Medical Association* 267:253–258.

D'Aunno TJ, Vaughn T. 1995. An organizational analysis of service patterns in drug abuse treatment. *Journal of Substance Abuse* 16:123–131.

DATOS (Drug Abuse Treatment Outcome Study). 1992. Drug Abuse Treatment Outcome Study. *NIDA Research Monograph 237*. Rockville, MD: National Institute on Drug Abuse.

De Leon G. 1984. The Therapeutic Community: Study of Effectiveness Treatment Research Monograph 51. Rockville, MD: National Institute on Drug Abuse.

De Leon G. 1994. Therapeutic communities: Toward a general theory and model. In: Tims FM, De Leon G, Jainchill N, eds. *NIDA Research Monograph 144*. Rockville, MD: National Institute on Drug Abuse.

Dennis ML, Karuntzos GT, McDougal GL, French MT. 1993. Developing training and employment programs to meet the needs of methadone treatment clients. *Evaluation Program Planning* 16:73–86.

DiClemente CC, Prochaska JO, Fairhurst SK, Velicer WF, Velasquez MM, Rossi JS. 1991. The process of smoking cessation: An analysis of precontemplation, contemplation, and preparation stages of change. *Journal of Consulting and Clinical Psychology* 59:295–304.

Everingham S, Rydell C. 1994. *Controlling Cocaine*. Santa Monica, CA: RAND Corporation.

Fals-Stewart W, Birchler GR, O'Farrell TJ. 1996. Behavioral couples therapy for male substance abusing patients: Effects on relationship adjustment and drug-using behavior. *Journal of Consulting and Clinical Psychology* 64:959–972.

Finnegan LP. 1991. Treatment issues for opioid-dependent women during the perinatal period. *Journal of Psychoactive Drugs* 23:191–199.

Finney JW, Moos RH. 1992. The long-term course of treated alcoholism: II. Predictors and correlates of 10-year functioning and mortality. *Journal of Studies on Alcohol* 53:142–153.

Finney JW, Hahn AC, Moos RH. 1996. The effectiveness of inpatient and outpatient treatment of substance abuse: The need to focus on mediators and moderators of setting effects. *Addiction* 91:1773–1796.

Fiore M, Bailey WC, Cohen SJ et al. 1996. *Smoking Cessation Guidelines from the Agency for Health Care Policy Research*. AHCPR Pub. No. 96-0692. Washington, DC: U.S. Department of Health and Human Services.

Fiorentine R, Anglin MD. 1997. Does increasing the opportunity for counseling increase the effectiveness of outpatient drug treatment? *American Journal of Drug and Alcohol Abuse* 23(3):369–382.

Fleming MF, Barry KL, eds. 1992. *Addictive Disorders*. St. Louis: Mosby Yearbook Primary Care Series.

Fox BS. 1997. Development of a therapeutic vaccine for the treatment of cocaine addiction. *Drug and Alcohol Dependence* 48:153–158.

French MT, Dennis ML, McDougal GL, Karuntzos GT, Hubbard RL. 1992. Training and employment programs in methadone treatment: Client needs and desires. *Journal of Substance Abuse Treatment* 9:293–303.

Fuller RK, Branchey L, Brightwell DR, Derman RM, Emrick CD, Iber FL, James KE, Lacoursiere RB, Lee KK, Lowenstram I et al. 1986. Disulfiram treatment of alcoholism: A Veterans Administration cooperative study. *Journal of the American Medical Association* 256:1449–1489.

Gastfriend D, McLellan AT. 1997. Treatment matching: Theoretical basis and practical implications. In: Samet J, Stein M, eds. *Medical Clinics of North America.* New York: W.B. Saunders.

Gerstein DR, Johnson RA, Harwood HJ, Fountain D, Suter N, Malloy K. 1994. *Evaluating recovery services: The California Drug and Alcohol Treatment Assessment (CALDATA).* Contract No. 92-001100. Sacramento, CA: State of California Department of Alcohol and Drug Programs. April.

Gomberg ESL, Nirenberg TD, eds. 1993. *Women and Substance Abuse.* Norwood, NJ: Ablex Publishing Corporation.

Greenstein R, O'Brien CP, Woody G, McLellan AT. 1981. Naltrexone: A short-term treatment alternative for opiate dependence. *American Journal of Alcohol and Drug Abuse* 8(1):291–296.

Hagan TA, Finnegan LP, Nelson L. 1994. Impediments to comprehensive drug treatment models for substance abusing women: Treatment and research questions. *Journal of Psychoactive Drugs* 26:163–171.

Hall SM, Loeb P, LeVois P, Cooper J. 1981. Increasing employment in ex-heroin addicts II: Methadone maintenance sample. *Behavioral Medicine* 12:453–460.

Havassy BE, Hall SM, Wasserman DA. 1991. Social support and relapse: Commonalities among alcoholics, opiate users, and cigarette smokers. *Addictive Behaviors* 16(5):235–246.

Heather N, Rollnick S, Bell A. 1993. Predictive validity of the Readiness to Change Questionnaire. *Addiction* 88:1667–1677.

Higgins ST, Delaney DD, Budney AJ, Bickel WK, Hughes JR, Foerg F, Fenwick JW. 1991. A behavioral approach to achieving initial cocaine abstinence. *American Journal of Psychiatry* 148:1218–1224.

Higgins ST, Budney AJ, Bickel WK, Hughes JR, Foeg FE, Badger GJ. 1993. Achieving cocaine abstinence with a behavioral approach. *American Journal of Psychiatry* 150:763–769.

Higgins ST, Budney AJ, Bickel WK, Foerg FE, Donham R, Badger GJ. 1994. Incentives improve outcome in outpatient behavioral treatment of cocaine dependence. *Archives of General Psychiatry* 51:568–576.

Higgins ST, Budney AJ, Bickel WK, Badger GJ, Foerg FE, Ogden D. 1995. Outpatient behavioral treatment for cocaine dependence: One-year outcome. *Experimental and Clinical Psychopharmacology* 3:205–212.

Holder HD, Longabaugh R, Miller WR, Rubonis A. 1991. The cost-effectiveness of treatment for alcohol problems: A first approximation. *Journal of Studies on Alcohol* 52:517–540.

Hubbard RL, Marsden ME. 1986. Relapse to use of heroin, cocaine and other drugs in the first year after treatment. In: National Institute on Drug Abuse. *Relapse and Recovery in Drug Abuse.* NIDA Research Monograph 72. Rockville, MD: National Institute on Drug Abuse.

Hubbard RL, Marsden ME, Rachal JV, Harwood HJ, Cavanaugh ER, Ginzburg HM. 1989. *Drug Abuse Treatment: A National Study of Effectiveness.* Chapel Hill, NC: University of North Carolina Press.

Hubbard RL, Craddock G, Flynn PM, Anderson J, Etheridge R. 1997. Overview of 1-year follow-up outcomes in the Drug Abuse Treatment Outcome Study (DATOS). *Psychology of Addictive Behavior* 11(4):261–278.

Inciardi JA. 1988. Some considerations on the clinical efficacy of compulsory treatment: Reviewing the New York experience. In: Leukefeld GC, Tims FM, eds. *Compulsory Treatment of Drug Abuse: Research and Clinical Practice.* NIDA Research Monograph 86. Rockville, MD: National Institute on Drug Abuse.

IOM (Institute of Medicine). 1989. *Prevention and Treatment of Alcohol Problems: An Agenda for Research.* Washington, DC: National Academy Press.

IOM. 1990a. *Broadening the Base of Treatment for Alcohol Problems.* Washington, DC: National Academy Press.

IOM. 1990b. *Treating Drug Problems.* Vol. 1. Washington, DC: National Academy Press.

IOM. 1995. Development of Medications for the Treatment of Opiate and Cocaine Addictions: Issues for the Government and Private Sector. Washington, DC: National Academy Press.

Kadden RM, Cooney NL, Getter H, Litt MD. 1990. Matching alcoholics to coping skills or interactional therapies: posttreatment results. *Journal of Consulting and Clinical Psychology* 57:698–704.

Kang SY, Kleinman PH, Woody GE, Millman RB, Todd TC, Kemp J, Lipton DS. 1991. Outcomes for cocaine abusers after once-a-week psychosocial therapy. *American Journal of Psychiatry* 148:630–635.

Kosten TR, Rounsaville BJ, Kleber HD. 1987. Multidimensionality and prediction and treatment outcome in opioid addicts: 2.5-year follow-up. *Comprehensive Psychiatry* 28:3–13.

Kranzler HR, Burleson JA, Del Boca FK, Babor TF, Korner P, Brown J, Bohn MJ. 1994. Buspirone treatment of anxious alcoholics: A placebo-controlled trial. *Archives of General Psychiatry* 51:720–731.

Ladewig D, Knecht T, Leher P, Fendl A. 1993. Acamprosate—A stabilizing factor in long-term withdrawal of alcoholic patients. *Therapeutische Umschau* 50(3):182–188.

Lawental E, McLellan AT, Grissom G, Brill P, O'Brien CP. 1996. Coerced treatment for substance abuse problems detected through workplace urine surveillance: Is it effective? *Journal of Substance Abuse* 8(1):115–128.

Lhuintre JP, Moore N, Tran G, Steru L, Langrenon S, Daoust M, Parot P, Ladure P, Libert C, Boismare F et al. 1990. Acamprosate appears to decrease alcohol intake in weaned alcoholics. *Alcohol and Alcoholism* 25:613–622.

Ling W, Charuvastra C, Kaim SC, Klett J. 1976. Methadyl acetate and methadone as maintenance treatments for heroin addicts. *Archives of General Psychiatry* 33:709–720.

Longabaugh R, Beattie M, Noel N, Stout R, Malloy P. 1993. The effect of social investment on treatment outcome. *Journal of Studies on Alcohol* 54:465–478.

Longabaugh R, Wirtz PW, Beattie MC, Noel N, Stout R. 1995. Matching treatment focus to patient social investment and support: 18 month follow-up results. *Journal of Consulting and Clinical Psychology* 63:296–307.

Luborsky L, McLellan AT, Woody GE, O'Brien CP. 1985. Therapist success and its determinants. *Archives of General Psychiatry* 42:602–611.

Marlatt GA. 1988. Matching clients to treatment: Treatment models and stages of change. In: Donovan DM, Marlatt A, eds. *Assessment of Addictive Behaviors.* New York: Guilford Press. Pp. 474–483.

Mason BJ, Kocsis JH, Ritvo EC, Cutler RB. 1996. A double-blind, placebo-controlled trial of desipramine for primary alcohol dependence stratified on the presence or absence of major depression. *Journal of the American Medical Association* 275:761–767.

Mattson ME, Allen JP, Longabaugh R, Nickless CJ, Connors GJ, Kadden RM. 1994. A chronological review of empirical studies matching alcoholics to treatment. *Journal of Studies on Alcohol* Suppl. 12:16–29.

McCaul M, Svikis D. 1991. Improving client compliance in outpatient treatment: Counselor-targeted interventions. *National Institute on Drug Abuse Research Monograph* 106:204–217.

McCrady BS, Miller WR, eds. 1993. *Research on Alcoholics Anonymous: Opportunities and Alternatives.* New Brunswick, NJ: Rutgers Center of Alcohol Studies.

McCrady BS, Noel NE, Abrams DB, Stout RL, Nelson HF, Hay WM. 1986. Comparative effectiveness of three types of spouse involvement in outpatient behavioral alcoholism treatment. *Journal of Studies on Alcohol* 47:459–467.

McGrath PJ, Nunes EV, Stewart JW, Goldman D, Agosti V, Ocepek-Welikson K, Quitkin FM. 1996. Imipramine treatment of alcoholics with primary depression: A placebo-controlled clinical trial. *Archives of General Psychiatry* 53:232–240.

McKay JR, McLellan AT, Alterman AI. 1992. An evaluation of the Cleveland Criteria for Inpatient Treatment of Substance Abuse. *American Journal of Psychiatry* 149:1212–1218.

McKay JR, Alterman AI, McLellan AT, Snider EC. 1994. Treatment goals, continuity of care, and outcome in a day hospital substance abuse rehabilitation program. *American Journal of Psychiatry* 151:254–259.

McKay JR, Alterman AI, McLellan AT, Snider EC, O'Brien CP. 1995. The effect of random versus nonrandom assignment in a comparison of inpatient and day hospital rehabilitation for male alcoholics. *Journal of Consulting and Clinical Psychology* 63:70–78.

McKay JR, Alterman AI, Cacciola JS, Rutherford MR, O'Brien CP, Koppenhaver J. 1997a. Group counseling vs. individualized relapse prevention aftercare following intensive outpatient treatment for cocaine dependence: Initial results. *Journal of Consulting and Clinical Psychology* 65:778–788.

McKay JR, Cacciola J, McLellan AT, Alterman AI, Wirtz PW. 1997b. An initial evaluation of the psychosocial dimensions of the ASAM criteria for inpatient and day hospital substance abuse rehabilitation. *Journal of Studies on Alcohol* 58:239–252.

McKay JR, McLellan AT, Alterman AI, Cacciola JS, Rutherford MJ, O'Brien CP. 1998. Predictors of participation in aftercare sessions and self-help groups following completion of intensive outpatient treatment for substance abuse. *Journal of Studies on Alcohol* 59(2):152–162.

McLatchie BH, Lomp KG. 1988. Alcoholics Anonymous affiliation and treatment outcome among a clinical sample of problem drinkers. *American Journal of Drug and Alcohol Abuse* 14:309–324.

McLellan AT, Weisner C. 1996. Achieving the public health potential of substance abuse treatment: Implications for patient referral, treatment "matching" and outcome evaluation. In: Bickel W, DeGrandpre R, eds. *Drug Policy and Human Nature.* Philadelphia: Williams and Wilkins.

McLellan AT, Luborsky L, O'Brien CP, Woody GE. 1980. An improved diagnostic instrument for substance abuse patients: The Addiction Severity Index. *Journal of Nervous and Mental Diseases* 168:26–33.

McLellan AT, Ball JC, Rosen L, O'Brien CP. 1981a. Pretreatment source of income and response to methadone maintenance: A follow-up study. *American Journal of Psychiatry* 138(6):785–789.

McLellan AT, O'Brien CP, Luborsky L, Woody GE, Kron R. 1981b. Are the addiction-related problems of substance abusers really related? *Journal of Nervous and Mental Diseases* 169(4):232–239.

McLellan AT, Luborsky L, Woody GE, Druley KA, O'Brien CP. 1983a. Predicting response to alcohol and drug abuse treatments: Role of psychiatric severity. *Archives of General Psychiatry* 40:620–625.

McLellan AT, Luborsky L, Woody GE, O'Brien CP, Druley KA. 1983b. Increased effectiveness of substance abuse treatment: A prospective study of patient-treatment "matching." *Journal of Nervous and Mental Diseases* 171(10):597–605.

McLellan AT, Griffith J, Childress AR, Woody GE. 1984. The psychiatrically severe drug abuse patient: Methadone maintenance or therapeutic community. *American Journal of Drug and Alcohol Abuse* 10(1):77–95.

McLellan AT, Woody GE, Luborsky L, Goehl L. 1988. Is the counselor an "active ingredient" in substance abuse rehabilitation? *Journal of Nervous and Mental Disease* 176:423–430.

McLellan AT, Alterman AI, Woody GE, Metzger D. 1992a. A quantitative measure of substance abuse treatments: The Treatment Services Review. *Journal of Nervous and Mental Disease* 180:100–109.

McLellan AT, Cacciola J, Kushner H, Peters R, Smith I, Pettinati H. 1992b. The Fifth Edition of the Addiction Severity Index: Cautions, additions and normative data. *Journal of Substance Abuse Treatment* 9(5):461–480.

McLellan AT, Grissom G, Durell J, Alterman AI, Brill P, O'Brien CP. 1993a. Substance abuse treatment in the private setting: Are some programs more effective than others? *Journal of Substance Abuse Treatment* 10:243–254.

McLellan AT, Arndt IO, Woody GE, Metzger D. 1993b. Psychosocial services in substance abuse treatment. *Journal of the American Medical Association* 269(15):1953–1959.

McLellan AT, Alterman AI, Metzger DS, Grissom G, Woody GE, Luborsky L, O'Brien CP. 1994. Similarity of Outcome Predictors Across Opiate, Cocaine and Alcohol Treatments: Role of Treatment Services. *Journal of Clinical and Consulting Psychology* 62 (6):1141–1158.

McLellan AT, Meyers K, Hagan T, Durell J. 1996a. Local data supports national trend in decline of substance abuse treatment system. *Connections* 4–8.

McLellan AT, Woody GE, Metzger D, McKay J, Durrell J, Alterman AI, O'Brien CP. 1996b. Evaluating the effectiveness of addiction treatments: Reasonable expectations, appropriate comparisons. *The Milbank Quarterly* 74(1):51–85.

McLellan AT, Woody GE, Metzger D, McKay J, Alterman AI, O'Brien CP. 1997a. Evaluating the effectiveness of treatments for substance use disorders: Reasonable expectations, appropriate comparisons. In: Egertson JA, Fox DM, Leshner AI, eds. *Treating Drug Abusers Effectively*. Malden, MA: Blackwell.

McLellan AT, Grissom G, Zanis D, Brill P. 1997b. Problem—Service "matching" in addiction treatment: A prospective study in four programs. *Archives of General Psychiatry* 54:730–735.

Merrill J. 1993. *The Cost of Substance Abuse to America's Health Care System, Report 1: Medicaid Hospital Hospital Costs*. New York: Center on Addiction and Substance Abuse, Columbia University.

Meyers RJ, Smith JE. 1995. *Clinical Guide to Alcohol Treatment: The Community Reinforcement Approach*. New York: Guilford.

Miller WR, Hester RK. 1986. Inpatient alcoholism treatment: Who benefits? *American Psychologist* 41:794–805.

Miller WR, Taylor CA, West JC. 1980. Focused versus broad-spectrum behavior therapy for problem drinkers. *Journal of Consulting and Clinical Psychology* 48:590–601.

Miller WR, Benefeld RG, Tonigan JS. 1993. Enhancing motivation for change in problem drinking: A controlled comparison of two therapist styles. *Journal of Consulting and Clinical Psychology* 61:455–461.

Moitto K, McKann MJ, Rawson RA, Frosch D, Ling W. 1997. Overdose, suicide attempts, and death among a cohort of naltrexone-treated opoid addicts. *Drug and Alcohol Dependence* 45(1–2):131–134.

Moos RH. 1974. *Evaluating Treatment Environments*. New York: Wiley.

Moos RH, Moos B. 1984. The process of recovery from alcoholism III: Comparing family functioning in alcoholic and matched control families. *Journal of Studies on Alcohol* 45:111–118.

Moos RH, Finney JW, Cronkite RC. 1990. *Alcoholism Treatment: Context, Process, and Outcome*. New York: Oxford University Press.

Morgenstern J, Labouvie E, McCrady BS, Kahler CW, Frey RM. 1997. Affiliation with Alcoholics Anonymous following treatment: A study of its therapeutic effects and mechanisms of action. *Journal of Consulting and Clinical Psychology* 65(5):768–777.

NIDA (National Institute on Drug Abuse). 1991. *See How Drug Abuse Takes the Profit Out of Business*. Rockville, MD: National Institute on Drug Abuse.

Najavits LM, Weiss RD. 1994. Variations in therapist effectiveness in the treatment of patients with substance use disorders: An empirical review. *Addiction* 89(6):679–688.

Nowinski J, Baker S. 1992. *The Twelve-Step Facilitation Handbook: A Systematic Approach to Early Recovery from Alcoholism and Addiction*. Lexington, MA: Lexington Books.

O'Brien CP. 1996. Recent developments in the pharmacotherapy of substance abuse. *Journal of Consulting and Clinical Psychology* 64:677–686.

O'Brien CP, McKay JR. In press. Psychopharmacological treatments of substance use disorders. In: Nathan PE, Gorman JM, eds. *Effective Treatments for DSM-IV Disorders*. Oxford University Press.

O'Brien CP, Childress AR, McLellan AT, Ternes J, Ehrman R. 1984. Use of naltrexone to extinguish opioid conditioned responses. *Journal of Clinical Psychiatry* 45(9):53–56.

O'Brien CP, Childress AR, Ehrman RA. 1991. A learning model of addiction. In: O'Brien CP, Jaffe J, eds. *Advances in Understanding the Addictive States*. New York: Raven. Pp. 157–177.

O'Farrell TJ, Choquette KA, Cutter HSG. In press. Couples relapse prevention sessions after behavioral marital therapy for male alcoholics: Outcomes during the three years after starting treatment. *Journal of Studies on Alcohol*.

O'Malley SS, Jaffe AJ, Chang G, Schottenfeld RS. 1992. Naltrexone and coping skills therapy for alcohol dependence: A controlled study. *Archives of General Psychiatry* 49:881–887.

OTA (Office of Technology Assessment). 1983. *The Effectiveness and Costs of Alcoholism Treatment*. Health Technology Case Study 22. Washington, DC: U.S. Government Printing Office.

Pettinati HM, Belden PP, Evans BD, Ruetsch CR, Meyers K, Jensen JM. 1998. The natural history of outpatient alcohol and drug abuse treatment in a private health care setting. *Alcoholism: Clinical and Experimental Research* 55(10):53–56.

Platt JJ. 1995. Vocational rehabilitation of drug abusers. *Psychological Bulletin* 117:416–435.

Powell BJ, Pennick EC, Othemer E, Bingham SF, Rice AS. 1982. Prevalence of additional psychiatric syndromes among male alcoholics. *Journal of Clinical Psychiatry* 43:404–407.

Prochaska JO, DiClemente CC. 1984. *The Transtheoretical Approach: Crossing Traditional Boundaries of Therapy*. Homewood, IL: Dow Jones, Irwin.

Prochaska JO, DiClemente CC, Norcross JC. 1992. In search of how people change: Applications to addictive behaviors. *American Psychologist* 47(9):1102–1114.

Project MATCH Research Group. 1997. Matching alcoholism treatments to client heterogeneity: Project MATCH posttreatment drinking outcomes. *Journal of Studies on Alcohol* 58:7–29.

Roman P. 1988. Growth and transformation in workplace alcoholism programming. In: Galanter M, ed. *Recent Developments in Alcoholism*. Vol. 11. New York: Plenum. Pp. 131–158.

Rounsaville BJ, Glazer W, Wilber CH, Weissman MM, Kleber H. 1983. Short-term interpersonal psychotherapy in methadone-maintained opiate addicts. *Archives of General Psychiatry* 40:630–636.

Rounsaville BJ, Dolinsky ZS, Babor TF, Meyer RE. 1987. Psychopathology as a predictor of treatment outcome in alcoholics. *Archives of General Psychiatry* 44:505–513.

Satel SL, Price LH, Palumbo JM, McDougle CJ, Krystal JH, Gawin F, Charney DS, Heninger GR, Kleber HD. 1991. Clinical phenomenology and neurobiology of cocaine abstinence: A prospective inpatient study. *American Journal of Psychiatry* 148:1712–1716.

Schmidt L, Weisner C. 1995. The emergence of problem-drinking women as a special population in need of treatment. In: Galanter M, ed. *Alcoholism and Women*. New York: Plenum Press. Pp. 309–334.

Schuckit MA, Monteiro MG. 1988. Alcoholism, anxiety and depression. *British Journal of Addiction* 83:1373–1380.

Schuckit MA, Irwin M, Brown SA. 1990. History of anxiety symptoms among 171 primary alcoholics. *Journal of Studies on Alcohol* 51:34–41.

Silverman K, Higgins HT, Brooner RK, Montonya ID, Cone EJ, Schuster CR, Preston KL. 1996. Sustained cocaine abstinence in methadone maintenance patients through voucher-based reinforcement therapy. *Archives of General Psychiatry* 53:409–415.

Simpson DD. 1981. Treatment for drug abuse: Follow-up outcomes and length of time spent. *Archives of General Psychiatry* 38:875–880.

Simpson DD. 1997. Effectiveness of drug abuse treatment: Review of research from field settings. In: Egertson JA, Fox DM, Leshner AI, eds. *Treating Drug Abusers Effectively*. Malden, MA: Blackwell.

Simpson DD, Savage L. 1980. Drug abuse treatment readmissions and outcomes. *Archives of General Psychiatry* 37:896–901.

Simpson DD, Joe GW, Broome KM, Hiller ML, Knight K, Rowan-Szal GA. 1997a Program diversity and treatment retention rates in the Drug Abuse Treatment Outcome Study (DATOS). *Psychology of Addictive Behaviors* 11(4):279–293.

Simpson DD, Joe GW, Brown BS. 1997b Treatment retention and follow-up outcomes in the Drug Abuse Treatment Outcome Study (DATOS). *Psychology of Addictive Behaviors* 11(4):294–301.

Stanton MD. 1979. The client as family member. In: Brown BS, ed. *Addicts and Aftercare*. New York: Sage Publications.

Stanton MD, Todd T. 1982. *The Family Therapy of Drug Abuse and Addiction*. New York: Guilford Press.

State of Oregon, Department of Substance Abuse Services. 1996. *Evaluation of Alcohol and Drug Abuse Treatments In The State of Oregon*. Portland, OR: Oregon Office of Publications.

Stewart RG, Ware LG. 1989. *The Medical Outcomes Study*. Santa Monica, CA: The Rand Corporation Press.

Strain EC, Stitzer IA, Liebson IA, Bigelow GE. 1993. Dose-response effects of methadone in the treatment of opiod dependence. *Annals of Internal Medicine* 119:23–27.

Strain EC, Bigelow GE, Liebson IA, Stitzer ML. 1996. Moderate versus high dose methadone in the treatment of opioid dependence. Poster session presented at the annual meeting of the College on Problems of Drug Dependence. San Juan, Puerto Rico. June.

Timko C, Moos RH, Finney JW, Moos BS. 1994. Outcome of treatment for alcohol abuse and involvement in Alcoholics Anonymous among previously untreated problem drinkers. *Journal of Mental Health Administration* 21:145–160.

Tonigan JS, Toscova R, Miller WR. 1996. Meta-analysis of the literature on Alcoholics Anonymous: Sample and study characteristics moderate findings. *Journal of Studies on Alcohol* 57:65–72.

Valle S. 1981. Interpersonal functioning of alcoholism counselors and treatment outcome. *Journal of Studies on Alcohol* 42:783–790.

Volpicelli JR, Alterman AI, Hayashida M, O'Brien CP. 1992. Naltrexone in the treatment of alcohol dependence. *Archives of General Psychiatry* 49:876–880.

Walsh DC, Hingson RW, Merrigan DM, Levenson SM, Cupples LA, Heeren T, Coffman GA,Becker CA,Barker TA, Hamilton SK et al. 1991. A randomized trial of treatment options for alcohol-abusing workers. *New England Journal of Medicine* 325:775–782.

Weddington WW. 1992. Cocaine abstinence: "Withdrawal" or residua of chronic intoxication? *American Journal of Psychiatry* 149:1761–1762.

Widman M, Platt JJ, Marlowe D, Lidz V, Mathis DA, Metzger DS. 1997. Patterns of service use and treatment involvement of methadone maintenance patients. *Journal of Substance Abuse Treatment* 14(1):29–35.

Weisner C, Schmidt L. 1992. Gender disparities in treatment for alcohol problems. *Journal of the American Medical Association* 268:1872–1876.

Wilsnack SC, Wilsnack RW. 1993. Epidemiological research on women's drinking: Recent progress and directions for the 1990s. In: Gomberg ESL, Nirenberg TD, eds. *Women and Substance Abuse*. Norwood, NJ: Ablex Publishing Corporation. Pp. 62–99.

Woody GE, Luborsky L, McLellan AT, O'Brien CP, Beck AT, Blaine J, Herman I, Hole A. 1983. Psychotherapy for opiate addicts: Does it help? *Archives of General Psychiatry* 40:639–645.

Woody GE, McLellan AT, Luborsky L. 1984. Psychiatric severity as a predictor of benefits from psychotherapy. *American Journal of Psychiatry* 141(10):1171–1177.

Woody GE, McLellan AT, Luborsky L, O'Brien CP. 1987. Twelve-month follow-up of psychotherapy for opiate dependence. *American Journal of Psychiatry* 144:590–596.

Woody GE, McLellan AT, Luborsky L, O'Brien CP. 1995. Psychotherapy in community methadone programs: A validation study. *American Journal of Psychiatry* 152(9):1302–1308.

E

The Substance Abuse Treatment System: What Does It Look Like and Whom Does It Serve?

Preliminary Findings from the Alcohol and Drug Services Study

Constance M. Horgan and Helen J. Levine
Institute for Health Policy, Heller Graduate School,
Brandeis University

INTRODUCTION

The substance abuse treatment system is a complex mixture of different types of providers, serving a diverse array of clients with varying treatment needs. The system continues to evolve in response to changes in the external environment, including the financing of treatment with its increasing emphasis on managed care, and the multiple needs of its clients which are frequently nonmedical in nature. Despite these changes, the substance abuse treatment system remains one that is essentially community based with substantial funding from the public sector. It is in the context of this diversity of providers and clients that one examines the interface between research and community-based treatment.

The purpose of this paper is to describe what the substance abuse treatment system looked like in late 1996 as background for the IOM report on the effective transfer of information between research and community-based drug treatment. The paper is structured by answering a series

The Alcohol and Drug Services Study is supported by the Office of Applied Studies (OAS), Substance Abuse and Mental Health Administration (SAMHSA), U.S. Department of Health and Human Services. It is being conducted under contract by Brandeis University in collaboration with Westat, Inc. We thank Grant Ritter and Paula Wolk for their programming assistance, Margaret Lee and Sharon Reif for their research assistance, and Lisa Andersen for manuscript preparation. We are also grateful for comments received from other colleagues, including Daniel Ames, Sara Lamb, Carla Maffeo, Mary Ellen Marsden, and Dennis McCarty and the advice we received from SAMHSA/OAS in the preparation of the paper.

of questions about the organization and financing of alcohol and drug treatment facilities, and the characteristics of the clients that these facilities serve. This paper relies on data from the 1997 Alcohol and Drug Services Study (ADSS), which includes as one of its components a nationally representative sample survey of all types of alcohol and drug abuse treatment facilities in the United States. The Substance Abuse and Mental Health Services Administration (SAMHSA) contracted with Brandeis University to direct and analyze ADSS. The subcontractor for conducting the field data collection was Westat, Inc.

METHODOLOGY

ADSS encompasses a three-phase research design and is based on a complex national sample of alcohol and drug abuse treatment facilities in the United States. Phase I consisted of a mail questionnaire collected by telephone interview of a stratified random sample of 2,400 noncorrectional alcohol and drug treatment facilities. Phase II consists of two components: (1) an administrator interview which collects more detailed cost information and other facility level data from a subset of approximately 300 facilities, and (2) record abstraction of over 6,000 clients. Phase III consists of up to six in-person follow-up interviews with Phase II clients, accompanied by urine testing to be conducted at six-month intervals. Data are being collected on treatment history, characteristics at admission to the index treatment, characteristics at follow-up including alcohol and drug use, employment, mental and physical health status indicators, illegal activities, and readmission to treatment. Facility level data collected in Phases I and II, combined with client level data collected in Phases II and III will allow for cost-effectiveness analyses, as well as other measures of treatment outcome.

This paper relies entirely on preliminary data from Phase I. The sampling frame was SAMHSA's 1995 National Master Facility Inventory augmented to encompass the universe of substance abuse treatment facilities. Phase I was conducted during early 1997 with data collected for the point-prevalence date of October 1, 1996 and for the most recent twelve-month reporting period of the facility. Data were collected which described facility characteristics as well as aggregate information on clients in the sampled facilities. Facility directors or administrators completed the questionnaire. The Phase I response rate was 92 percent.

The Phase I sampling design incorporates a stratified random probability sample that allows for estimates of parameters at the national level. The strata were selected to reflect the different modalities of care within the substance abuse treatment system. Since ADSS is based on sample data, weights have been developed to produce national estimates of facilities and characteristics of clients in treatment. The sampling weights adjust for facility nonresponse, as well as differential response rates within strata. The data presented in this report are weighted, but do not contain imputation for any missing values. Sampling errors are calculated using WESVAR, a procedure for complex survey data employing replicated estimates of variance, developed by Westat, Inc. Calculations for these sampling errors are available from the authors upon request. The data in this paper should be considered preliminary until final weights for Phase I are produced after adjustments are made based on Phase II data.

HOW IS THE SYSTEM ORGANIZED?

Each facility in the survey answered a series of questions about its ownership and location (Table E-1). The majority of substance abuse treatment facilities (63 percent) are owned by private not-for-profit entities and another 14 percent are publicly owned by either federal, state, or local governments. Almost one-quarter of facilities are organized as private for-profit entities (23 percent). This is reflective of the increasing shift to for-profit ownership in health care more generally.

These sampled facilities reflect the fact that substance abuse treatment takes place in many types of treatment settings. A sizable minority of facilities reported that they were located in hospitals (10 percent in general hospitals and 4 percent in psychiatric or other specialized hospitals). Almost one in five reported being in some type of free-standing residential setting. Only seven percent of all facilities are therapeutic communities and 6 percent are half-way houses. Many facilities reported a link to the mental health system and described themselves as being located in a community mental health center (19 percent). More than two-fifths were in other types of outpatient treatment settings.

Other organizational questions were asked, including the types of care offered, the facility's relationship with other entities, and other services provided (Table E-2). The majority of sampled substance abuse treatment facilities provide some type of outpatient treatment. Over 61 percent of facilities offered only outpatient nonmethadone services and another 5 percent delivered outpatient methadone treatment either alone or in combination with outpatient nonmethadone services. About 3 percent offered only inpatient treatment, 17 percent offered only residential, and 14 percent offered inpatient or residential care combined with outpatient treatment. Many treatment facilities were engaged in providing not only substance abuse services, but also mental health treatment (55 percent) and medical treatment (27 percent).

Most treatment facilities are connected to some other organization, with 62 percent reporting that they were legally part of another organization. About 56 percent of facilities that were part of another organization

TABLE E-1 Organizational Characteristics of Substance
Abuse Treatment Facilities, October 1, 1996: Percentage of
Facilities by Ownership and Treatment Setting

Ownership	
Private for-profit	23.4%
Private nonprofit	62.3%
Public	14.2%
Total[a]	100.0%
Treatment Setting[b]	
General hospital	10.3%
VA hospital	1.3%
Psychiatric or specialized hospital	4.1%
Nonhospital residential	19.2%
Therapeutic community	6.9%
Halfway house	5.6%
Community mental health center	18.7%
Solo practice	2.3%
Group practice	5.1%
School	1.4%
Outpatient, other than above	44.2%
Other	6.1%

SOURCE: 1997 Alcohol and Drug Services Study—Phase I—Preliminary Data. Office of Applied Studies, Substance Abuse and Mental
Health Services Administration.

[a]Does not total to 100% because of rounding.

[b]Does not total to 100% because facilities could respond to as many
categories as applied.

reported that this parent organization was an administrative office. The
parent organization for 30 percent of facilities was a substance abuse treatment facility and for 20 percent was a hospital.

ADSS does not have any direct measures of a facility's capacity to
conduct and/or participate in research. It does however have information
on the existence of an operational computerized information system. While
such systems serve administrative functions, sometimes data in these systems are used for research purposes. Table E-3 shows that the majority of
facilities have an operational computerized information system, but its existence varies along a number of dimensions. For example, using the point
prevalence client count as a measure of facility size, we see the existence of
a computerized system is directly related to size. Almost 80 percent of
facilities with a client census of greater than 100 active clients have comput-

TABLE E-2   Organizational Characteristics of Substance Abuse
Treatment Facilities, October 1, 1996: Percentage Distribution of
Facilities by Type of Care, and Percentage of Facilities by Relationship
with Other Organization, Mental Health, or Medical Treatment Provider

Type of Care	
Inpatient only	3.0%
Residential only	17.4%
Outpatient methadone[a]	5.0%
Outpatient nonmethadone only	61.1%
Combination inpatient and/or residential with outpatient nonmethadone	13.6%
Total[b]	100.0%
Legally Part of Other Organization	61.9%
Types of Other Organization[c,d]	
Administrative office	55.5%
Substance abuse treatment facility	29.8%
Hospital	19.7%
Government agency	11.9%
Other organization	27.0%
Provision of Other Services[a]	
Mental health treatment	54.3%
Medical treatment	27.0%

SOURCE: 1997 Alcohol and Drug Services Study—Phase I—Preliminary Data.
Office of Applied Studies, Substance Abuse and Mental Health Services Administration.

[a]Twenty-six percent of outpatient methadone treatment facilities also provide
outpatient nonmethadone treatment.

[b]Does not total to 100% because of rounding.

[c]Does not total to 100% because facilities could respond to as many categories
as applied.

[d]Distribution is for facilities indicating that they are legally part of another
organization.

erized systems compared with about 60% for small facilities. Residential
programs are the least likely to use a computerized information system with
54 percent having a computerized system. Interestingly, facilities that rely
more heavily on public dollars are more likely to report having a computerized system. Whether this is related to the mandated reporting requirements
for facilities receiving public dollars, or other factors, is unknown.

TABLE E-3   Characteristics of Facilities with an Operational
Computerized Information System: Percentage of Facilities with System
by Organizational and Financial Characteristics

Facility Characteristics	Percentage with a Computerized Information System
Type of Care	
Inpatient only	72.4%
Residential only	54.3%
Outpatient methadone*	77.4%
Outpatient nonmethadone only	69.2%
Combination inpatient and/or residential with outpatient nonmethadone	70.3%
Size	
Small (≤16)	58.9%
Medium (17–40)	64.0%
Large (41–100)	68.9%
Extra large (>100)	78.1%
Ownership	
Private for-profit	61.1%
Private nonprofit	67.1%
Public	77.0%
Percentage of Revenue from Public Sources	
0–50%	64.3%
50–90%	67.1%
90–100%	71.0%

SOURCE: 1997 Alcohol and Drug Services Study—Phase I—Preliminary Data.
Office of Applied Studies, Substance Abuse and Mental Health Services Administration.
    *Twenty-six percent of outpatient methadone treatment facilities also provide
outpatient nonmethadone treatment.

Table E-4 demonstrates the substantial role played by others in getting
clients into treatment. Of all clients in treatment on October 1, 1996, only
21 percent were classified by facilities as being self-referred. The criminal
justice system was the largest source of referrals, accounting for over one-
third of referrals. Other substance abuse treatment facilities referred 12
percent and health or mental health providers accounted for 9 percent of
referrals. Over 7 percent were referred by welfare or other social service

TABLE E-4   Referral to Substance Abuse Treatment Facilities, October 1, 1996: Percentage Distribution of Clients by Referral Sources

Percentage of Clients from:	
Criminal justice system	34.0%
Self-referred/voluntary	21.3%
Other treatment facility	11.6%
Health or mental health provider	9.1%
Welfare or social service agency	7.2%
Family	5.1%
Employer	4.5%
Friend	2.3%
Other	4.8%
Total*	100.0%

SOURCE: 1997 Alcohol and Drug Services Study—Phase I—Preliminary Data. Office of Applied Studies, Substance Abuse and Mental Health Services Administration.

*Does not total to 100% because of rounding.

agencies. Family and employers each accounted for about 5 percent of the referrals.

The vast majority of clients in treatment on October 1, 1996 were being treated on an outpatient basis (89 percent) as shown in Table E-5, with most clients being served in outpatient nonmethadone programs (75 percent) and the remainder in outpatient methadone programs (14 percent). Almost one in ten clients were receiving treatment in a residential setting, with 8 percent in residential rehabilitation and 2 percent in residential detoxification programs. The numbers of patients served in hospital inpatient settings continues to dwindle, accounting for just over 1 percent of all clients in treatment on the ADSS point prevalence date.

The mean number of clients per facility in treatment on October 1, 1996 varied by type of setting. Outpatient methadone programs were the largest with 216 mean number of active clients in treatment, followed by other outpatient programs with a mean number of 82 active clients. The mean number of active clients in treatment was 27 in both residential rehabilitation and residential detoxification programs. The mean number of clients in hospital inpatient settings was 12.

WHO ARE THE CLIENTS?

A typical client treated in the substance abuse treatment system is a white, young adult male whose primary drug of abuse is alcohol. The

TABLE E-5 Type of Care of Active Clients in Substance Abuse Treatment Facilities, October 1, 1996: Percentage Distribution and Mean Number of Clients in Treatment

	Percentage Distribution	Mean Number of Clients in Treatment
Total Hospital Inpatient	1.4%	
Hospital detoxification	0.7%	7.0
Hospital rehabilitation	0.7%	11.3
Total Residential	**9.4%**	
Residential detoxification	1.8%	26.9
Residential rehabilitation	7.6%	27.3
Total Outpatient	**89.2%**	
Outpatient methadone	13.9%	215.6
Outpatient nonmethadone	75.3%	82.2
Total	**100.0%**	**82.8**

SOURCE: 1997 Alcohol and Drug Services Study—Phase I—Preliminary Data. Office of Applied Studies, Substance Abuse and Mental Health Services Administration.

diversity of clients is shown in Table E-6 which summarizes selected demographic characteristics of clients in treatment on October 1, 1996. Over two-thirds of those in treatment were male (68 percent). The majority of clients were white of non-Hispanic origin (57 percent); however, a substantial number of clients were of minority origin (24 percent black, non-Hispanic; 12 percent Hispanic, and 3 percent Native American).

The age distribution of clients in treatment shows a distinctly youthful population. More than one in five clients are less than 25 years old. Well over one-half of clients are less than 35 and 80 percent of clients are under 45 years of age. Alcohol remains the primary drug of abuse for the largest number of clients in treatment (43 percent). As expected, the use of heroin, cocaine, and marijuana, as primary drugs of abuse, is significant. The number of heroin clients has been increasing relative to other illicit drugs, consistent with trends of drug abuse in this country.

WHAT SERVICES ARE OFFERED?

A variety of services are offered in conjunction with substance abuse treatment reflecting the diverse needs of the treatment population. Table E-

TABLE E-6   Aggregate Client Characteristics of Substance Abuse
Treatment Facilities, October 1, 1996: Percentage Distribution of Active
Clients by Selected Demographic Characteristics

Gender	
Male	68.1%
Female	30.4%
Unknown	1.6%
Total*	100.0%
Race/Ethnicity	
White, not Hispanic	57.1%
Black, not Hispanic	23.7%
Hispanic	11.8%
Asian or Pacific Islander	0.8%
American Indian/Alaskan Native	3.0%
Unknown	3.7%
Total*	100.0%
Age at Admission	
Under 18	8.4%
18–24	13.0%
25–34	30.8%
35–44	27.5%
≥45	14.3%
Unknown	6.1%
Total*	100.0%
Primary Drug of Use	
Alcohol	43.4%
Heroin/other opiates	17.6%
Cocaine	15.1%
Marijuana	9.7%
Amphetamines	2.9%
Benzodiazepines	1.0%
PCP/LSD	0.8%
Barbiturates	0.5%
Other (not alcohol)	3.1%
Unknown	5.8%
Total*	100.0%

SOURCE: 1997 Alcohol and Drug Services Study—Phase I—Preliminary Data.
Office of Applied Studies, Substance Abuse and Mental Health Services Administration.
    *Does not total to 100% because of rounding.

7 summarizes the types of services offered in treatment facilities during the course of their most recent 12-month reporting period. It should be noted that ADSS determined only if the services were offered at the facility during the twelve-month reporting period. The data do not indicate how frequently the services were available and whether they were available to all clients, targeted subpopulations, or on an ad hoc basis. Well over 90 percent of facilities offered comprehensive assessment and diagnosis, individual therapy, and group therapy. More than 75 percent provided family counseling, HIV/AIDS counseling, relapse prevention, and aftercare (after the cessation of routine treatment) services. Far fewer facilities were likely to offer services of a nonmedical nature. Employment counseling/training was offered in 41 percent of facilities; academic education/GED classes in 17 percent; and child care in 13 percent.

TABLE E-7 Percentage of Facilities Offering Selected Services in Substance Abuse Treatment Facilities (over 12-month reporting period)

Facilities Offering:*	
Individual therapy	96.6%
Comprehensive assessment/diagnosis	93.7%
Group therapy (not including relapse prevention)	91.7%
Family counseling	85.6%
Aftercare	82.3%
Relapse prevention groups	78.4%
HIV/AIDS counseling	75.5%
Self-help or mutual-help groups	71.3%
Outcome follow-up	66.8%
Combined substance abuse and mental health	66.5%
Transportation	48.6%
TB screening	42.1%
Employment counseling/training	40.7%
Detoxification	25.6%
Smoking cessation	24.4%
Academic education/GED classes	17.2%
Child care	12.9%
Prenatal care	11.7%
Acupuncture	4.7%

SOURCE: 1997 Alcohol and Drug Services Study—Phase I—Preliminary Data. Office of Applied Studies, Substance Abuse and Mental Health Services Administration.

*Does not total to 100% because facilities indicated as many services as they offered.

WHO PAYS FOR TREATMENT?

The substance abuse treatment system in this country has always been largely publicly supported and continues to be so as shown in Table E-8, albeit to a diminishing extent. The majority of funding (65 percent) comes from public sources, with nearly half coming from public noninsurance mechanisms such as the federal, state, and local grants and contracts (47 percent). The remaining private revenue sources (30 percent) are divided between client fees (17 percent) and private insurance (13 percent). This differs substantially from the rest of the health care system where private and public insurance accounts for the majority of revenue.

The relative importance of public funding in facilities varies depending on facility ownership. As expected, private for-profit facilities do not rely heavily on public dollars, with only 22 percent of revenues coming from public sources. Publicly owned facilities are heavily but not completely reliant on public dollars (84 percent). The majority of treatment facilities are private nonprofit organizations, and they too rely heavily on public sources with over 71 percent of funding coming from the public sector.

CONCLUSION

In summary, although the substance abuse treatment system is generally publicly funded and serves patients largely on an outpatient basis, there is still considerable diversity along a number of dimensions. It is unknown the degree to which substance abuse treatment facilities participate either actively or passively in research studies, or how quickly research findings disseminate into the delivery of services. The data suggest that given such a diverse substance abuse treatment system, there will be varying abilities and willingness to engage and benefit from research, particularly in a system that many view as underfunded.

TABLE E-8 Revenue Type of Substance Abuse Treatment Facilities (over 12-month reporting period): Percentage Distribution by Sources of Revenue and Mean Percentage of Public Revenue by Ownership

Sources of Revenue	
Private	**30.3%**
Client fees	16.9%
Private insurance, fee for service	6.8%
Private insurance, managed care	6.6%
Public	**64.9%**
Medicaid, unspecified	10.7%
Medicaid, managed care	1.8%
Medicare	2.3%
Other federal funds (VA, CHAMPUS)	3.1%
Other public funds (federal, state, and local block grants, contracts)	47.1%
Other	**4.7%**
Other (philanthropy, in-kind)	3.6%
Unknown	1.1%
Total*	**100.0%**

	Mean Percentage of Revenue from Public Sources
Ownership	
Private for-profit	21.7%
Private nonprofit	71.4%
Public	83.7%
Total	62.5%

SOURCE: 1997 Alcohol and Drug Services Study—Phase I—Preliminary Data. Office of Applied Studies, Substance Abuse and Mental Health Services Administration.

*Does not total to 100% because of rounding.

F
National Institutes of Health Consensus Development Statement on Effective Medical Treatment of Heroin Addiction

NIH Consensus Statements are prepared by a nonadvocate, non-Federal panel of experts, based on (1) presentations by investigators working in areas relevant to the consensus questions during a 2-day public session; (2) questions and statements from conference attendees during open discussion periods that are part of the public session; and (3) closed deliberations by the panel during the remainder of the second day and morning of the third. This statement is an independent report of the consensus panel and is not a policy statement of the NIH or the Federal Government.

ABSTRACT

Objective. To provide health care providers, patients, and the general public with a responsible assessment of the effective approaches for treating opiate dependence.

SOURCE: National Institutes of Health. 1997. NIH Consensus Development Statement: Effective Medical Treatment of Heroin Addiction. November 17–19, 1997 [WWW Document]. URL http://odp.od.nih.gov/consensus/statements/cdc/108/108_stmt.html (Accessed March 27, 1998).

This statement will be published as: Effective Medical Treatment of Opiate Addiction. NIH Consensus Statement 1997 November 17–19;15(6): in press. For making bibliographic reference to consensus statement No. 108 in the electronic form displayed here, it is recommended that the following format be used: NIH Consensus Statement Online 1997 November 17–19 [cited year, month, day]; 15(6): in press.

Participants. A non-Federal, nonadvocate, 12-member panel representing the fields of psychology, psychiatry, behavioral medicine, family medicine, drug abuse, epidemiology, and the public. In addition, 25 experts from these same fields presented data to the panel and a conference audience of 600.

Evidence. The literature was searched through Medline and an extensive bibliography of references was provided to the panel and the conference audience. Experts prepared abstracts with relevant citations from the literature. Scientific evidence was given precedence over clinical anecdotal experience.

Consensus Process. The panel, answering predefined questions, developed their conclusions based on the scientific evidence presented in open forum and the scientific literature. The panel composed a draft statement that was read in its entirety and circulated to the experts and the audience for comment. Thereafter, the panel resolved conflicting recommendations and released a revised statement at the end of the conference. The panel finalized the revisions within a few weeks after the conference. The draft statement was made available on the World Wide Web immediately following its release at the conference and was updated with the panel's final revisions.

Conclusions. Opiate dependence is a brain-related medical disorder that can be effectively treated with significant benefits for the patient and society, and society must make a commitment to offer effective treatment for opiate dependence to all who need it. All opiate-dependent persons under legal supervision should have access to methadone maintenance therapy, and the U.S. Office of National Drug Control Policy and the U.S. Department of Justice should take the necessary steps to implement this recommendation. There is a need for improved training for physicians and other health care professionals and in medical schools in the diagnosis and treatment of opiate dependence. The unnecessary regulations of methadone maintenance therapy and other long-acting opiate agonist treatment programs should be reduced, and coverage for these programs should be a required benefit in public and private insurance programs.

INTRODUCTION

In the United States, prior to 1914, it was relatively common for private physicians to treat opiate-dependent patients in their practices by prescribing narcotic medications. While the passage of the Harrison Act did not prohibit the prescribing of a narcotic by a physician to treat an addicted patient, this practice was viewed as problematic by Treasury officials charged with enforcing the law. Physicians who continued to prescribe were indicted and prosecuted. Because of withdrawal of treatment by physicians, various local governments and communities established formal morphine clinics for treating opiate addiction. These clinics were eventually closed when the AMA, in 1920, stated that there was unanimity that prescribing opiates to addicts for self-administration (ambulatory treatment) was not an acceptable medical practice. For the next 50 years, opiate addiction was basically managed in this country by the criminal justice system and the two Federal Public Health Hospitals in Lexington, Kentucky, and Fort Worth, Texas. The relapse rate for opiate use from this approach was close to 100 percent. During the 1960s opiate use reached epidemic proportions in the United States, spawning significant increases in crime and in deaths from opiate overdose. The increasing number of younger people entering an addiction lifestyle indicated that a major societal problem was emerging. This stimulated a search for innovative and more effective methods to treat the growing number of individuals dependent upon opiates. This search resulted in the emergence of drug-free therapeutic communities and the use of the opiate agonist, methadone, to maintain those with opiate dependence. Furthermore, a multimodality treatment strategy was designed to meet the needs of the individual addict patient. These three approaches remain the main treatment strategies being used to treat opiate dependence in the United States today.

Opiate dependence has long been associated with increased criminal activity. For example, in 1993 more than one-quarter of the inmates in State and Federal prisons were incarcerated for drug offenses (234,600), and prisoners serving drug sentences were the largest single group (60 percent) in Federal prisons.

In the past 10 years, there has been a dramatic increase in the prevalence of human immunodeficiency virus (HIV), hepatitis B and C viruses, and tuberculosis among intravenous opiate users. From 1991 to 1995, in major metropolitan areas, the annual number of opiate related emergency room visits has increased from 36,000 to 76,000, and the annual number of opiate-related deaths has increased from 2,300 to 4,000. This associated morbidity and mortality further underscore the human, economic, and societal costs of opiate dependence.

During the last two decades, evidence has accumulated on the neurobiology of opiate dependence. Whatever conditions that may lead to opiate exposure, opiate dependence is a brain-related disorder, with the requisite characteristics of a medical illness. Thus, opiate dependence as a medical illness will have varying causative mechanisms. There is a need to identify discrete subgroups of opiate-dependent people and the most relevant and effective treatments for each subgroup. The safety and efficacy of narcotic agonist (methadone) maintenance treatment has been unequivocally established. Although there are other medications (e.g., *levo*-alpha-acetyl-methadol [LAAM] and naltrexone, an opiate antagonist, etc.) that are safe and effective in the treatment of opiate addicts, the focus of this consensus development conference was primarily on methadone maintenance treatment (MMT). MMT is effective in reducing illicit opiate drug use, in crime reduction, in enhancing social productivity, and in reducing the spread of viral diseases such as AIDS and hepatitis.

Approximately 115,000 of the estimated 600,000 opiate-dependent persons in the United States are in MMT. Science has not yet overcome the stigma of addiction and the negative public perception about MMT. Some leaders in the Federal Government, public health officials, members of the medical community, and the public-at-large frequently conceive of opiate dependence as a self-inflicted disease of the will or a moral flaw. They also regard MMT as an ineffective narcotic substitution and believe that a drug-free state is the only valid treatment goal. Other obstacles to MMT include Federal and State government regulations that restrict the number of treatment providers and patient access. Some of these Federal and State regulations are driven by disproportionate concerns about methadone diversion, concern about premature (e.g., in 12-year-olds) initiation of maintenance treatment, and concern about provision of methadone without any other psychosocial services.

Although a drug-free state represents an optimal treatment goal, research has demonstrated that this goal cannot be achieved or sustained by the majority of opiate-dependent people. However, other laudable treatment goals including decreased drug use, reduced crime, and gainful employment can be achieved in most MMT patients.

To address the most important issues surrounding effective medical treatment of opiate dependence, the NIH organized this 2 1/2-day conference to present data on opiate agonist treatment for opiate dependence. The conference brought together national and international experts in the fields of the basic and clinical medical sciences, epidemiology, natural history, prevention and treatment of opiate dependence, and broad representation from the public.

After 1-1/2 days of presentations and audience discussion, an independent, non-Federal consensus panel chaired by Lewis L. Judd, M.D., Mary Gilman Marston Professor, Chair of the Department of Psychiatry, University of California, San Diego School of Medicine, weighed the scientific evidence and wrote a draft statement that was presented to the audience on the third day. The consensus statement addressed the following key questions:

- What is the scientific evidence to support conceptualization of opiate addiction as a medical disorder including natural history, genetics and risk factors, pathophysiology, and how is diagnosis established?
- What are the consequences of untreated opiate addiction to individuals, families and society?
- What is the efficacy of current treatment modalities in the management of opiate addiction including detoxification alone, nonpharmacological/psychosocial treatment, treatment with opiate antagonists, and treatment with opiate agonists (short-term and long-term)? And, what is the scientific evidence for the most effective use of opiate agonists in the treatment of opiate addiction?
- What are the important barriers to effective use of opiate agonists in the treatment of opiate addiction in the U.S. including perceptions and adverse consequences of opiate agonist use, legal, regulatory, financial and programmatic barriers?
- What are the future research areas and recommendations for improving opiate agonist treatment and improving access?

The primary sponsors of this meeting were the National Institute on Drug Abuse and the NIH Office of Medical Applications of Research. The conference was cosponsored by the NIH Office of Research on Women's Health.

1. What Is the Scientific Evidence to Support a Conceptualization of Opiate Dependence as a Medical Disorder Including Natural History, Genetics and Risk Factors, and Pathophysiology, and How Is Diagnosis Established?

The Natural History of Opiate Dependence

Individuals addicted to opiates often become dependent on these drugs by their early twenties and remain intermittently dependent for decades. Biological, psychological, sociological, and economic factors determine when an individual will start taking opiates. However, it is clear that when use begins, it often escalates to abuse (repeated use with adverse consequences) and then to dependence (opioid tolerance, withdrawal symptoms, compulsive drug taking). Once dependence is established there are usually repeated cycles of cessation and relapse extending over decades. This "addiction career" is often accompanied by periods of imprisonment.

Treatment can alter the natural history of opiate dependence, most commonly, by prolonging periods of abstinence from illicit opiate abuse. Of the various treatments available, MMT, combined with attention to medical, psychiatric, and socioeconomic issues, as well as drug counseling, has the highest probability of being effective.

Addiction-related deaths, including accidental overdose, drug-related accidents, and many illnesses directly attributable to chronic drug dependence explain one-fourth to one-third of the mortality in an opiate-addicted population. As a population of opiate addicts age, there is a decrease in the percentage who are still addicted.

There is clearly a natural history of opiate dependence, but causative factors are poorly understood. It is especially unclear for a given individual whether repeated use begins as a medical disorder, (e.g., a genetic predisposition) or whether socioeconomic and psychological factors lead an individual to try and then later compulsively use opiates. However, there is no question that once the individual is dependent on opiates, such dependence constitutes a medical disorder.

Molecular Neurobiology and Pathogenesis of Opiate Dependence: Genetic and Other Risk Factors for Opiate Dependence

Twin, family, and adoption studies show that vulnerability to drug abuse may be a partially inherited condition with strong influences from environmental factors. Cross-fostering adoption studies have demonstrated that both inherited and environmental factors operate in the etiology of drug abuse. These cross-fostering adoption studies identified two distinct genetic pathways to drug abuse/dependence. The first is a direct effect of substance abuse in a biologic parent. The second pathway is an indirect effect from antisocial personality disorder in a biologic parent, leading to both antisocial personality disorder and drug abuse/dependence in the adoptee. Family studies report significantly increased relative risk for substance abuse (6.7-fold increased risk), alcoholism (3.5), antisocial personality (7.6), and unipolar depression (5.1) among the first-degree relatives of opiate-dependent patients compared with relatives of controls. The siblings of opiate-dependent patients have very high susceptibility to abuse and dependence after initial use of illicit opioids. Twin studies indicate substantial heritability for substance abuse and dependence, with half the risk attributable to additive genetic factors.

Neurobiological Substrates of Opiate Dependence

Dopaminergic pathways from the ventral tegmentum (VT) to the nucleus accumbens (NA) and medial frontal cortex (MFC) are activated during rewarding behaviors. Opiates exert their rewarding properties by binding to the "mu" opioid receptor (OPRM) at several distinct anatomical locations in the brain, including the VT, NA, MFC, and possibly the locus coeruleus (LC). Opiate agonist administration causes inhibition of the LC. Chronic administration of opioid agonists causes adaptation to the LC inhibition. Rapid discontinuation of opioid agonists (or administration of antagonists) results in excessive LC neuronal excitation and the appearance of withdrawal symptoms. Abnormal LC excitation is thought to underlie many of the physical symptoms of withdrawal, and this hypothesis is consistent with the ability of clonidine, an alpha 2 noradrenergic agonist, to ameliorate opiate withdrawal.

Regional Cerebral Glucose Metabolism in Opiate Abusers

Two independent human studies (using positron emission tomography) suggest that opiates reduce cerebral glucose metabolism in a global manner, with no regions showing increased glucose utilization. A third study demonstrates decreased D2 receptor availability in opiate-dependent patients compared with controls. Opiate antagonist administration produced an intense withdrawal experience but did not change D2 receptor availability.

Diagnosis of Opioid Dependence

Opioid dependence (addiction) is defined as a cluster of cognitive, behavioral, and physiological symptoms in which the individual continues use of opiates despite significant opiate-induced problems. Opioid dependence is characterized by repeated self-administration that usually results in opioid tolerance, withdrawal symptoms, and compulsive drug-taking. Dependence may occur with or without the physiological symptoms of tolerance and withdrawal. Usually, there is a long history of opioid self-administration, typically via intravenous injection in the arms or legs, although recently, the intranasal route or smoking also is used. Often there is a history of drug-related crimes, drug overdoses, and family, psychological, and employment problems. There may be a history of physical problems including skin infections, hepatitis, HIV infection, or irritation of the nasal and pulmonary mucosa. Physical examination usually reveals puncture marks along veins in the arms and legs and "tracks" secondary to sclerosis of veins. If the patient has not taken opiates recently, he/she may also demonstrate symptoms of withdrawal, including anxiety, restlessness, runny nose, tearing, nausea, and vomiting. Tests for opioids in saliva and urine can help support a diagnosis of dependence. However, by itself, neither a positive nor a negative test can rule dependence in or out. Further evidence for opioid dependence can be obtained by a naloxone (Narcan) challenge test to induce withdrawal symptoms.

Evidence That Opioid Dependence Is a Medical Disorder

For decades, opioid dependence was viewed as a problem of motivation, willpower, or strength of character. Through careful study of its natural history and through research at the genetic, molecular, neuronal, and epidemiological levels, it has been proven that opiate addiction is a medical disorder characterized by predictable signs and symptoms. Other arguments for classifying opioid dependence as a medical disorder include:

• Despite varying cultural, ethnic, and socioeconomic backgrounds, there is clear consistency in the medical history, signs, and symptoms exhibited by individuals who are opiate-dependent.
• There is a strong tendency to relapse after long periods of abstinence.
• The opioid-dependent person's craving for opiates induces continual self-administration even when there is an expressed and demonstrated strong motivation and powerful social consequences to stop.
• Continuous exposure to opioids induces pathophysiologic changes in brain.

2. What Are the Consequences of Untreated Opiate Dependence to Individuals, Families, and Society?

Of the estimated total opiate-dependent population of 600,000, only 115,000 are known to be in methadone maintenance treatment (MMT) programs. Research surveys indicate that the untreated population of opiate-addicted people are younger than those in treatment. They are typically in their late teens and early to mid-twenties, during their formative, early occupational, and reproductive years. The financial costs of untreated opiate dependence to the individual, the family, and society are estimated to be approximately $20 billion per year. The costs in human suffering are incalculable.

What is currently known about the consequences of untreated opiate dependence to individuals, families, and society?

Mortality

Prior to the introduction of MMT, annual death rates reported in four American studies of opiate dependence varied from 13 per 1,000 to 44 per 1,000, with a median of 21 per 1,000. Although it cannot be causally attributed, it is interesting that after the introduction of MMT, the death rates of opiate-dependent persons in four American studies had a narrower range, from 11 per 1,000 to 15 per 1,000, and a median of 13 per 1,000.

The most striking evidence of the effectiveness of MMT on death rates are studies directly comparing these rates in opiate-dependent persons, on and off methadone. Every study showed that death rates were lower in opiate-dependent persons maintained on methadone compared with those who are not. The median death rate for opiate-dependent persons in MMT was 30 percent of the death rate of those not in treatment. A clear consequence of not treating opiate dependence, therefore, is a death rate that is more than three times greater than that experienced by those engaged in MMT.

Illicit Drug Use

Multiple studies conducted over several decades and in different countries demonstrate clearly that MMT results in a marked decrease in illicit opiate use. In addition, there is also a significant and consistent reduction in the use of other illicit drugs including cocaine and marijuana, and in the abuse of alcohol, benzodiazepines, barbiturates, and amphetamines.

Criminal Activity

Opiate dependence in the United States is unequivocally associated with high rates of criminal behavior. More than 95 percent of opiate-dependent persons report committing crimes during an 11-year at-risk interval. These crimes range in severity from homicides to other crimes against people and property. Stealing in order to purchase drugs is the most common criminal offense. Over the past two decades, clear and convincing evidence has been collected from multiple studies that effective treatment of opiate dependence markedly reduces the rates of criminal activity. Therefore, it is clear that significant amounts of crime perpetrated by opiate-dependent persons is a direct consequence of untreated opiate dependence.

Health Care Costs

Although the general health status of people with opiate dependence is substantially worse than that of their contemporaries, they do not routinely use medical services. Typically, they seek medical care in hospital emergency rooms only after their medical conditions are seriously advanced. The consequences of untreated opiate dependence include much higher incidence of bacterial infections, including endocarditis, thrombophlebitis, and skin and soft tissue infections; tuberculosis; hepatitis B and C; AIDS and sexually transmitted diseases; and alcohol abuse. Because those who are opiate-dependent present for medical care late in their diseases, medical care is generally more expensive. Health care costs related to opiate dependence have been estimated to be $1.2 billion per year.

Joblessness

Opiate dependence prevents many users from maintaining steady employment. Much of their time each day is spent in drug-seeking and drug-taking behavior. Therefore, many seek public assistance because they are unable to generate the income needed to support themselves and their families. Long-term outcome data show that opiate-dependent persons in MMT earn more than twice as much money annually as those not in treatment.

Outcomes of Pregnancy

A substantial number of pregnant women dependent upon opiates also have HIV/AIDS. Based on preliminary data, women who receive MMT are more likely to be treated with zidovudine. It has been well established that administration of zidovudine to HIV-positive pregnant women reduces by two-thirds the rate of HIV transmission to their babies. Comprehensive MMT, along with sound prenatal care, has been shown to decrease obstetrical and fetal complications as well.

3. What Is the Efficacy of Current Treatment Modalities in the Management of Opiate Dependence Including Detoxification Alone, Nonpharmacological/Psychosocial Treatment, Treatment with Opiate Antagonists, and Treatment with Opiate Agonists (Short Term and Long Term). And, What Is the Scientific Evidence for the Most Effective Use of Opiate Agonists in the Treatment of Opiate Dependence?

The Pharmacology of Commonly Prescribed Opiate Agonists and Antagonists

The most frequently used agent in medically supervised opiate withdrawal and maintenance treatment is methadone. Methadone's half-life is approximately 24 hours and leads to a long duration of action and once-a-day dosing. This feature, coupled with its slow onset of action, blunts its euphoric effect, making it unattractive as a principal drug of abuse. LAAM, a presently less commonly used opiate agonist, has a longer half-life and may prevent withdrawal symptoms for up to 96 hours. An emerging treatment option, buprenorphine, a partial opioid agonist, appears also to be effective for detoxification and maintenance.

Naltrexone is a nonaddicting specific "mu" antagonist with a long half-life permitting once-a-day administration. It effectively blocks the cognitive and behavioral effects of opioids, and its prescription does not require special registration. The opioid-dependent person considering treatment should be informed of the availability of naltrexone maintenance treatment. However, in actively using opiate addicts, it produces immediate withdrawal symptoms with potentially serious effects.

Medically Supervised Withdrawal

Methadone can also be used for detoxification. This can be accomplished over several weeks after a period of illicit opiate use or methadone maintenance. If methadone withdrawal is too rapid, abstinence symptoms are likely. They may lead the opiate-dependent person to illicit drug use and relapse into another cycle of abuse. Buprenorphine holds promise as an option for medically supervised withdrawal, because its prolonged occupation of "mu" receptors attenuates withdrawal symptoms.

More rapid detoxification options include use of opiate antagonists alone; the alpha-2 agonist clonidine alone; or clonidine followed by naltrexone. Clonidine reduces many of the autonomic signs and symptoms of opioid withdrawal. These strategies may be used in both inpatient and outpatient settings and allow medically supervised withdrawal from opioids in as little as 3 days. Most patients successfully complete detoxification using these strategies, but information concerning relapse rates is not available.

The Role of Psychosocial Treatments

Nonpharmacologic supportive services are pivotal to successful MMT. The immediate introduction of these services as the opiate-dependent patient applies for MMT leads to significantly higher retention and more comprehensive and effective treatment. Comorbid psychiatric disorders require treatment. Other behavioral strategies have been successfully used in substance abuse treatment. Ongoing substance abuse counseling and other psychosocial therapies enhance program retention and positive outcome. Stable employment is an excellent predictor of clinical outcome. Therefore, vocational rehabilitation is a useful adjunct.

Efficacy of Opiate Agonists

It is now generally agreed that opiate dependence is a medical disorder and that pharmacologic agents are effective in its treatment. Evidence presented to the panel indicates that availability of these agents is severely limited and that large numbers of patients with this disorder have no access to treatment.

The greatest experience with such agents has been with the opiate agonist methadone. Prolonged oral treatment with this medication diminishes and often eliminates opiate use, reduces transmission of many infections, including HIV and hepatitis B and C, and reduces criminal activity. Evidence is now accumulating that suggests the effectiveness in such patients of LAAM and buprenorphine. For more than 30 years, the daily oral administration of methadone has been used to treat tens of thousands of individuals dependent upon opiates in the United States and abroad. The effectiveness of MMT is dependent on many factors, including adequate dosage, duration plus continuity of treatment, and accompanying psychosocial services. A dose of 60 mg given once daily may achieve the desired treatment goal: abstinence from opiates. But higher doses are often required by many patients. Continuity of treatment is crucial—patients who are treated for less than 3 months generally show little or no improvement, and most, if not all, patients require continuous treatment over a period of years, and perhaps for life. Therefore, the program has come to be termed methadone "maintenance" treatment (MMT). Patient attributes that have sometimes been linked to better outcomes include older age, later age of dependence onset, lesser abuse of other substances including cocaine and alcohol, and lesser criminal activity. Recently, it has been reported that high motivation for change has been associated with positive outcomes.

The effectiveness of MMT is often dependent on the involvement of a knowledgeable and empathetic staff and the availability of psychotherapy and other counseling services. The latter are especially important since individuals with opiate dependence are often afflicted with comorbid mental and personality disorders.

Because methadone-treated patients generally are exposed to much less or no intravenous opiates, they are much less likely to transmit and contract HIV and hepatitis. This is especially important since recent data have shown that up to 75 percent of new instances of HIV infection are attributable to intravenous drug use. Since for many patients a major source of financing the opiate habit is criminal behavior, MMT generally leads to much less crime.

Although methadone is the primary opioid agonist used, other full and partial opioid agonists have been developed for treatment of opiate dependence. An analog of methadone, levo-alpha acetyl-methadol (LAAM) has a longer half-life than methadone and so can be administered less frequently. A single dose of LAAM can prevent withdrawal symptoms and drug craving for 2 to 4 days. Buprenorphine, a recently developed partial opiate agonist, has the advantage over methadone that its discontinuation leads to much less severe withdrawal symptoms. The use of these medications is at an early stage, and it may be some time before their usefulness has been adequately evaluated.

4. What Are the Important Barriers to Effective Use of Opiate Agonists in the Treatment of Opiate Dependence in the United States, Including Perceptions and the Adverse Consequences of Opiate Agonist Use and Legal, Regulatory, Financial, and Programmatic Barriers?

Misperceptions and Stigmas

Many of the barriers to effective use of MMT in the treatment of opiate dependence stem from misperceptions and stigmas attached to opiate dependence, the people who are addicted, the people who treat them, and the settings in which services are provided. Opiate-dependent persons are often perceived not as individuals with a disease, but as "other" or "different." Factors such as racism play a large role here but so does the popular image of dependence itself. Many people believe that dependence is self-induced or a failure of willpower and also believe that efforts to treat it will inevitably fail. Vigorous and effective leadership is needed to inform the public that dependence is a medical disorder that can be effectively treated with significant benefits for the patient and society.

Increasing Availability of Effective Services

Unfortunately, MMT programs are not readily available to all who could and wish to benefit from them. We as a society must make a commitment to offer effective treatment for opiate dependence to all who need it. Accomplishing that goal will require:

• Making treatment as cost-effective as possible without sacrificing quality.
• Increasing the availability and variety of treatment services.
• Including and ensuring wider participation by physicians trained in substance abuse who will oversee the medical care.
• Providing additional funding for opiate dependence treatments and coordinating these services with other necessary social services and medical care.

Training Physicians and Other Health Care Professionals

One barrier to availability of MMT is the shortage of physicians and other health care professionals prepared to care for opiate dependence. All primary care medical specialties (including general practice, internal medicine, family practice, obstetrics and gynecology, geriatrics, pediatrics, and adolescent medicine) should be taught the principles of diagnosing and treating patients with opiate dependence. Nurses, social workers, psychologists, physician assistants, and other health care professionals should also be trained in these areas. The greater the number of trained physicians and other health care professionals, the greater the supply not only of professionals who can competently treat the opiate dependent but also of members of the community who are equipped to provide leadership and public education on these issues.

Reducing Unnecessary Regulation

Of critical importance in improving MMT of opiate dependence is the recognition that, as in every other area of medicine, treatment must be tailored to the needs of the individual patient. Current Federal regulations make this difficult if not impossible. By prescribing MMT procedures in minute detail, FDA's regulations limit the flexibility and responsiveness of the programs, require unproductive paperwork, and impose administrative and oversight costs greater than what are necessary for many patients. Yet these regulations seem to have little if any effect on quality of MMT care. We know of no other area where the Federal government intrudes so deeply and coercively into the practice of medicine. For example, although providing a therapeutic dose is central to effective treatment and the therapeutic dose is now known to be higher than had previously been understood, FDA's regulations discourage such higher doses. However well-intended the FDA's treatment regulations were when written in 1972, they are no longer helpful. We recommend that these regulations be eliminated. Alternative means, such as accreditation, for improving quality of MMT programs should be instituted. The U.S. Department of Health and Human Services can more effectively, less coercively, and much more inexpensively discharge its statutory obligation to provide treatment guidance to MMT programs, physicians, and staff by means of publications, seminars, Web sites, continuing medical education, and the like.

We also believe current laws and regulations should be revised to eliminate the extra level of regulation on methadone compared with other Schedule II narcotics. Currently, methadone can be dispensed only from facilities that obtain an extra license and comply with extensive extra regulatory requirements. These extra requirements are unnecessary for a medication that is not often diverted for recreational or casual use but rather to individuals with opiate dependence who lack access to MMT programs.

If extra levels of regulation were eliminated, many more physicians and pharmacies could prescribe and dispense methadone, making treatment available in many more locations than is now the case. Not every physician will choose to treat opiate-dependent persons, and not every methadone-treated person will prefer to receive services from an individual physician rather than receive MMT in a clinic setting. But if some additional physicians and groups treat a few patients each, aggregate access to MMT would be expanded.

We also believe that State and local regulations and enforcement efforts should be coordinated. We see little purpose to having separate State and Federal inspections of MMT programs. State and Federal regulators should coordinate their efforts, agree which programs each will inspect to avoid duplication, and target "poor performers" for the most intensive scrutiny while reducing scrutiny for MMT programs that consistently perform well. The States should address the problem of slow approval (at the State level) of FDA-approved medications. LAAM, for example, has not yet been approved by many States. States should harmonize their requirements with those of the Federal Government.

We would expect these changes in the current regulatory system to reduce unnecessary costs both to MMT programs and to enforcement agencies at all levels. The savings could be used to treat more patients.

In the end, an infusion of additional funding will be needed—funding sufficient to provide access to treatment for all who require treatment. We strongly recommend that legislators and regulators recognize that providing MMT is both cost-effective and compassionate and that it constitutes a health benefit that should be a component of public and private health care.

5. What Are the Future Research Areas and Recommendations for Improving Opiate Agonist Treatment and Improving Access?

- What initiates opiate use?
  - Define genetic predispositions
  - Do some individuals take opiates to treat a preexisting disorder?
  - Which of the multiple psychological, sociological, and economic factors believed to predispose individuals to try opiates are most important as causative factors?
- If the above are known, can one prevent opiate dependence?
- What are the changes in the human brain that result in dependence when individuals repeatedly use opiates?
- What are the underlying anatomical and neurophysiological substrates of craving?
- What are the differences between individuals who can successfully terminate opiate dependence and those who cannot?
- A scientifically credible national epidemiological study of the prevalence of opiate dependence in the United States is strongly recommended.
- Rigorous study of the economic costs of opiate dependence in the

United States and the cost-effectiveness of methadone maintenance therapy is also needed.

- Longer term followup studies of patients who complete rapid detoxification is necessary.
- The feasibility of alternative routes of administration for agonist and antagonist therapy should be explored.
- Systematic pharmacokinetic studies of methadone during MMT maintenance therapy are essential.
- Physiologic factors that may influence adequate methadone dose in pregnant women need to be defined.
- The effects of reduction of entitlement programs for those patients on MMT must be assessed.
- The effects of the early and systematic introduction of rehabilitation services in MMT should be evaluated.
- Variables that determine barriers must be defined.
- Research on changing attitudes of the public, of health professionals, and of legislators is needed.
- Research on improving educational methods for health professionals should be performed.
- Research on prevention methods is necessary.
- Research on efficacy of other opiate agonists/antagonists should be compared to methadone.

CONCLUSIONS AND RECOMMENDATIONS

- Vigorous and effective leadership is needed within the Office of National Drug Control Policy (ONDCP) (and related Federal and State agencies) to inform the public that dependence is a medical disorder that can be effectively treated with significant benefits for the patient and society.
- Society must make a commitment to offer effective treatment for opiate dependence to all who need it.
- The panel calls attention to the need for opiate-dependent persons under legal supervision to have access to MMT. The ONDCP and the U.S. Department of Justice should implement this recommendation.
- The panel recommends improved training of physicians and other health care professionals in diagnosis and treatment of opiate dependence. For example, we encourage the National Institute on Drug Abuse and other agencies to provide funds to improve training for diagnosis and treatment of opiate dependence in medical schools.
- The panel recommends that unnecessary regulation of MMT and all long-acting agonist treatment programs be reduced.
- Funding for MMT should be increased.

• We advocate MMT as a benefit in public and private insurance programs, with parity of coverage for all medical and mental disorders.

• We recommend targeting opiate-dependent pregnant women for MMT.

• MMT must be culturally sensitive to enhance a favorable outcome for participating African American and Hispanic persons.

• Patients, underrepresented minorities, and consumers should be included in bodies charged with policy development guiding opiate dependence treatment.

• We recommend expanding the availability of opiate agonist treatment in those States and programs where this treatment option is currently unavailable.

CONSENSUS DEVELOPMENT PANEL

Lewis L. Judd, M.D.
Conference and Panel Chair
Mary Gilman Marston Professor
    Chair
Department of Psychiatry
School of Medicine
University of California, San Diego
La Jolla, California

Clifford Attkisson, Ph.D.
Dean of Graduate Studies
Associate Vice Chancellor for
    Student Academic Affairs
Professor of Medical Psychology
University of California, San
    Francisco
San Francisco, California

Wade Berrettini, M.D., Ph.D.
Professor of Psychiatry and
    Director
Center for Neurobiology and
    Behavior
Department of Psychiatry
School of Medicine
University of Pennsylvania
Philadelphia, Pennsylvania

Nancy L. Buc, Esq.
Buc & Beardsley
Washington, DC

Benjamin S. Bunney, M.D.
Charles B.G. Murphy Professor
    and Chairman
Professor of Pharmacology
Department of Psychiatry
Yale University School of Medicine
New Haven, Connecticut

Roberto A. Dominguez, M.D.
Professor and Director of Adult
    Outpatient Clinic
Department of Psychiatry
University of Miami School of
    Medicine
Miami, Florida

Robert O. Friedel, M.D.
Heman E. Drummond Professor
    and Chairman
Department of Psychiatry and
    Behavioral Neurobiology
The University of Alabama at
    Birmingham
Birmingham, Alabama

John S. Gustafson
Executive Director
National Association of State
    Alcohol and Drug Abuse
    Directors, Inc.
Washington, DC

Donald Hedeker, Ph.D.
Associate Professor of Biostatistics
Division of Epidemiology and
    Biostatistics
School of Public Health
University of Illinois, Chicago
Chicago, Illinois

Howard H. Hiatt, M.D.
Professor of Medicine
Harvard Medical School
Senior Physician
Division of General Medicine
Brigham and Women's Hospital
Boston, Massachusetts

Radman Mostaghim, M.D., Ph.D.
Greenbelt, Maryland

Robert G. Petersdorf, M.D.
Distinguished Professor of
    Medicine
University of Washington
Seattle, Washington

SPEAKERS

M. Douglas Anglin, Ph.D.
"The Natural History of Opiate
    Addiction"
Director
UCLA Drug Abuse Research
    Center
Los Angeles, California

Donald C. Des Jarlais, Ph.D.
"Transmission of Bloodborne
    Viruses Among Heroin
    Injectors"
Director of Research
Chemical Dependency Institute
Beth Israel Medical Center and
    National Development and
    Research Institutes
New York, New York

David P. Desmond, M.S.W.
"Deaths Among Heroin Users In
    and Out of Methadone
    Maintenance"
Instructor
Department of Psychiatry
University of Texas Health Science
    Center
San Antonio, Texas

Rose Etheridge, Ph.D.
"Factors Related to Retention and
    Posttreatment Outcomes in
    Methadone Treatment:
    Replicated Findings Across
    Two Eras of Treatment"
Senior Research Psychologist
National Development and
    Research Institutes, Inc.
    (NDRI, Inc.)
Raleigh, North Carolina

Igor I. Galynker, M.D., Ph.D.
"Methadone Maintenance and
   Regional Cerebral Glucose
   Metabolism in Opiate Abusers:
   A Positron Emission
   Tomographic Study"
Physician-in-Charge
Division of Psychiatric Functional
   Brain Imaging
Department of Psychiatry
Beth Israel Medical Center
New York, New York

G. Thomas Gitchel
"Diversion of Methadone:
   Expanding Access While
   Reducing Abuse"
Chief
Liaison and Policy Section
Office of Diversion Control
U.S. Drug Enforcement
   Administration
Washington, DC

Michael Gossop, Ph.D.
"Methadone Substitution
   Treatment in the United
   Kingdom: Outcome Among
   Patients Treated in Drug
   Clinics and General Practice
   Settings"
Head of Research, National
   Addiction Centre
Institute of Psychiatry
Maudsley Hospital
London, United Kingdom

John Grabowski, Ph.D.
"Behavioral Therapies: A
   Treatment Element for Opiate
   Dependence"
Director
Substance Abuse Research Center
Professor
Department of Psychiatry
Health Science Center
University of Texas, Houston
Houston, Texas

Henrick J. Harwood
"Societal Costs of Heroin
   Addiction"
Senior Manager
The Lewin Group
Fairfax, Virginia

Jerome H. Jaffe, M.D.
"The History and Current Status
   of Opiate Agonist Treatment"
Director
Office for Scientific Analysis and
   Evaluation
Center for Substance Abuse
   Treatment
Substance Abuse and Mental
   Health Services Administration
Rockville, Maryland

Herbert D. Kleber, M.D.
"Detoxification with or without
   Opiate Agonist Treatment"
Professor of Psychiatry
Division of Substance Abuse
Department of Psychiatry
Columbia University College of
   Physicians and Surgeons
New York, New York

Mary Jeanne Kreek, M.D.
"Opiate Agonist Treatment,
   Molecular Pharmacology, and
   Physiology"
Professor and Head
Senior Physician
Laboratory of the Biology of
   Addictive Diseases
Rockefeller University
New York, New York

David C. Lewis, M.D.
"Access to Narcotic Addiction
   Treatment and Medical Care"
Director, Center for Alcohol and
   Addiction Studies
Brown University
Providence, Rhode Island

Dennis McCarty, Ph.D.
"Narcotic Agonist Treatment as a
   Benefit Under Managed Care"
Human Services Research
   Professor
Institute for Health Policy
Heller Graduate School
Brandeis University
Waltham, Massachusetts

A. Thomas McLellan, Ph.D.
"Problem-Service Matching in
   Methadone Maintenance
   Treatment: Policy Suggestions
   From Two Prospective
   Studies"
Scientific Director
DeltaMetrics in Association with
   Treatment Research Institute
Philadelphia, Pennsylvania

Jeffrey Merrill, Ph.D.
"Impact of Methadone
   Maintenance on HIV
   Seroconversion and Related
   Costs"
Director
Economic and Policy Research
Treatment Research Institute
University of Pennsylvania
Philadelphia, Pennsylvania

Eric J. Nestler, M.D., Ph.D.
"Neurobiological Substrates for
   Opiate Addiction"
Elizabeth Mears and House
   Jameson Professor of
   Psychiatry and Pharmacology
Department of Psychiatry
Connecticut Mental Health Center
Yale University School of Medicine
New Haven, Connecticut

David N. Nurco, D.S.W.
"Narcotic Drugs and Crime:
   Addict Behavior While
   Addicted Versus Nonaddicted"
Research Professor
Department of Psychiatry
University of Maryland School of
   Medicine
Baltimore, Maryland

Mark W. Parrino, M.P.A.
"Legal, Regulatory, and Funding
   Barriers to Good Practice and
   Associated Consequences"
President
American Methadone Treatment
   Association, Inc.
New York, New York

J. Thomas Payte, M.D.
"Methadone Dose and Outcome"
Medical Director
Drug Dependence Associates
San Antonio, Texas

Roy W. Pickens, Ph.D.
"Genetic and Other Risk Factors in
    Opiate Addiction"
Senior Scientist
Division of Intramural Research
Addiction Research Center
National Institute on Drug Abuse
National Institutes of Health
Baltimore, Maryland

D. Dwayne Simpson, Ph.D.
"Patient Engagement and Duration
    of Treatment"
Director and S.B. Sells Professor of
    Psychology
Institute of Behavioral Research
Texas Christian University
Fort Worth, Texas

Barbara J. Turner, M.D.
"Prenatal Care and Antiretroviral
    Use Associated with
    Methadone Treatment of HIV-
    Infected Pregnant Women"
Professor of Medicine
Director of Research in Health
    Care
Thomas Jefferson University
The Center for Research in
    Medical Education and Health
    Care
Philadelphia, Pennsylvania

George E. Woody, M.D.
"Establishing a Diagnosis of
    Heroin Abuse and Addiction"
Chief, Substance Abuse Treatment
    Unit
Veterans Affairs Medical Center
Clinical Professor
Department of Psychiatry
University of Pennsylvania
Philadelphia, Pennsylvania

Joan E. Zweben, Ph.D.
"Community, Staff, and Patient
    Perceptions and Attitudes"
Executive Director
14th Street Clinic and East Bay
    Community Recovery Project
Clinical Professor of Psychiatry
University of California, San
    Francisco
Berkeley, California

PLANNING COMMITTEE

James R. Cooper, M.D.
Planning Committee Chair
Associate Director for Medical
    Affairs
Division of Clinical and Services
    Research
National Institute on Drug Abuse
National Institutes of Health
Rockville, Maryland

Elsa A. Bray
Program Analyst
Office of Medical Applications of
    Research
National Institutes of Health
Bethesda, Maryland

Mona Brown
Press Officer
National Institute on Drug Abuse
National Institutes of Health
Rockville, Maryland

Kendall Bryant, Ph.D.
Coordinator
AIDS Behavioral Research
National Institute on Alcohol
    Abuse and Alcoholism
National Institutes of Health
Rockville, Maryland

Jerry Cott, Ph.D.
Chief
Pharmacologic Treatment Research
    Program
National Institute of Mental
    Health
National Institutes of Health
Rockville, Maryland

Donald C. Des Jarlais, Ph.D.
Director of Research
Chemical Dependency Institute
Beth Israel Medical Center and
    National Development and
    Research Institutes
New York, New York

John H. Ferguson, M.D.
Director
Office of Medical Applications of
    Research
National Institutes of Health
Bethesda, Maryland

Bennett Fletcher, Ph.D.
Acting Chief
Services Research Branch
Division of Clinical and Services
    Research
National Institute on Drug Abuse
National Institutes of Health
Rockville, Maryland

Joseph Frascella, Ph.D.
Chief
Etiology and Clinical Neurobiology
    Branch
Division of Clinical and Services
    Research
National Institute on Drug Abuse
National Institutes of Health
Rockville, Maryland

G. Thomas Gitchel
Chief, Liaison and Policy Section
Office of Diversion Control
U.S. Drug Enforcement Agency
Washington, DC

William H. Hall
Director of Communications
Office of Medical Applications of
    Research
National Institutes of Health
Bethesda, Maryland

Jerome H. Jaffe, M.D.
Director, Office for Scientific
    Analysis and Evaluation
Center for Substance Abuse
    Treatment
Substance Abuse and Mental
    Health Services Administration
Rockville, Maryland

Lewis L. Judd, M.D.
Panel and Conference Chair
Mary Gilman Marston Professor
Chair, Department of Psychiatry
School of Medicine
University of California, San Diego
La Jolla, California

Herbert D. Kleber, M.D.
Professor of Psychiatry
Division of Substance Abuse
Department of Psychiatry
Columbia University College of
    Physicians and Surgeons
New York, New York

Mitchell B. Max, M.D.
Chief, Clinical Trials Unit
Neurobiology and Anesthesiology
    Branch
National Institute of Dental
    Research
National Institutes of Health
Bethesda, Maryland

A. Thomas McLellan, Ph.D.
Scientific Director
DeltaMetrics in Association with
    Treatment Research Institute
Philadelphia, Pennsylvania

Eric J. Nestler, M.D., Ph.D.
Elizabeth Mears and House
    Jameson Professor of
    Psychiatry and Pharmacology
Department of Psychiatry
Connecticut Mental Health Center
Yale University School of Medicine
New Haven, Connecticut

Stuart Nightingale, M.D.
Associate Commissioner for Health
    Affairs
U.S. Food and Drug
    Administration
Rockville, Maryland

Roy W. Pickens, Ph.D.
Senior Scientist, Division of
    Intramural Research
Addiction Research Center
National Institute on Drug Abuse
National Institutes of Health
Baltimore, Maryland

Nick Reuter, M.P.H.
Associate Director for Domestic
    and International Drug
    Control
U.S. Food and Drug
    Administration
Rockville, Maryland

Charles R. Sherman, Ph.D.
Deputy Director
Office of Medical Applications of
   Research
National Institutes of Health
Bethesda, Maryland

Alan Trachtenberg, M.D., M.P.H.
Medical Officer
Office of Science Policy and
   Communications
National Institute on Drug Abuse
National Institutes of Health
Rockville, Maryland

Frank Vocci, Ph.D.
Acting Director
Medications Development Division
National Institute on Drug Abuse
National Institutes of Health
Rockville, Maryland

Anne Willoughby, M.D., M.P.H.
Chief
Pediatric, Adolescent and Maternal
   AIDS Branch
Center for Research for Mothers
   and Children
National Institute of Child Health
   and Human Development
National Institutes of Health
Rockville, Maryland

Stephen R. Zukin, M.D.
Director
Division of Clinical and Services
   Research
National Institute on Drug Abuse
National Institutes of Health
Rockville, Maryland

CONFERENCE SPONSORS

Office of Medical Applications of
   Research, NIH
John H. Ferguson, M.D., Director

National Institute on Drug Abuse
Alan I. Leshner, Ph.D.

CONFERENCE COSPONSORS

Office of Research on Women's
   Health, NIH
Vivian W. Pinn, M.D., Director

BIBLIOGRAPHY

The speakers listed above identified the following key references in developing their presentations for the consensus conference. A more complete bibliography prepared by the National Library of Medicine at NIH, along with the references below, were provided to the consensus panel for their consideration. The full NLM bibliography is available at the following Web site: http://www.nlm.nih.gov/pubs/cbm/heroin_addiction.html.

Institute of Medicine. Managing managed care: quality improvement in behavioral health. Washington: National Academy Press; 1997.

National evaluations of drug abuse treatment outcomes. Psych Addict Behav [Special Issue]. In press.

Anglin MD, Speckart GR, Booth MW, Ryan TM. Consequences and costs of shutting off methadone. Addict Behav 1989;14:307–26.

Anglin MD, Hser Y. Treatment of drug abuse. In: Tonry M, Wilson JQ, editors. Drugs and crime. Chicago: University of Chicago Press; 1990. Pp. 393–58.

Ball JC, Ross A. The effectiveness of methadone maintenance treatment. New York: Springer Verlag; 1991.

Barrett DH, Luk AJ, Parrish RG, Jones TS. An investigation of medical examiner cases in which methadone was detected, Harris County, Texas, 1987–1992. J Forensic Sci 1996 May;41(3):442–8.

Cadoret RJ, Troughton E, O'Gorman TW, Heywood E. An adoption study of genetic and environmental factors in drug abuse. Arch Gen Psychiatry 1986;43:1131–6.

Capelhorn JR, Hartel DM, Irwig L. Measuring and comparing the attitudes and beliefs of staff working in New York methadone maintenance clinics. Subst Use Misuse 1997;32(4)1:399–413.

Caplehorn JR, Dalton MS, Haldar F, Petrenas AM, Nisbet JG. Methadone maintenance and addicts' risk of fatal heroin overdose. Subst Use Misuse 1996; 31(2):177–96.

Cooper JR. Methadone treatment and acquired immunodeficiency syndrome. JAMA 1989;252:1664–8.

Cooper JR. Establishing a methadone quality assurance system: rationale and objectives. In: Improving drug abuse treatment. National Institute on Drug Abuse Research Monograph Series #106. Washington: DHHS; 1991. Pp. 358–64.

Cooper JR. Including narcotic addiction treatment in an office-based practice. JAMA 1995a;273:1619–20.

Courtwright DT. A century of American narcotic policy. In: Gerstein DR, Harwood HJ, editors. Treating drug problems. Vol. 2. Institute of Medicine. Washington: National Academy Press; 1992.

Des Jarlais DC. Research design, drug use, and deaths: cross study comparisons. In: Serban G, editor. The social and medical aspects of drug abuse. Jamaica (NY): Spectrum Publications; 1984. Pp. 229–35.

Dole VP. Implications of methadone maintenance for theories of narcotic addiction. JAMA 1988;260(20):3025–9.

Dole VP. On federal regulation of methadone treatment. Conn Med 1996;60:428–9.

Dole, VP. Hazards of process regulations: the example of methadone maintenance. JAMA 1992;267:2234–5.

Edwards G, Gross MM. Alcohol dependence: previsional description of a clinical syndrome. Br Med 1996;1:1058–61.

Elk R, Grabowski J, Rhoades HM, McLellan AT. A substance abuse research-treatment clinic. Substance Abuse Treatment. 1993;10(5):459–71.

Etheridge RM, Craddock SG, Dunteman GH, Hubbard RL. Treatment services in two national studies of community-based drug abuse treatment programs. J Subst Abuse Treat 1995;7:9–26.

Frances A, Pincus HA, First MB, editors. Substance related disorders. In: Diagnostic and statistical manual of mental disorders. Fourth Edition. (DSM-IV). Washington: American Psychiatric Association Press; 1994. Pp. 175–272.

Gerstein DR, Harwood HJ, editors. Treating drug problems. Vol. 1. Institute of Medicine. Washington: National Academy Press; 1990.

Goldstein A. Heroin addiction: neurobiology, pharmacology, and policy. J Psychoactive Drugs 1991;23:(2)123–33.

Gossop M, Griffiths P, Bradley B, Strang J. Opiate withdrawal symptoms in response to 10-day and 21-day methadone withdrawal programmes. Br J Psychiatry 1989;154:360–3.

Gronbladh L., Ohlund LS, Gunne LM. Mortality in heroin addiction: impact of methadone treatment. Acta Psychiatr Scand 1990;82(3):223–7.

Grudzinskas CV, Woosley RL, Payte JT, Collins J, Moody DE, Tyndale RF, et al. The documented role of pharmacogenetics in the identification and administration of new medications for treatment drug abuse. Problems of drug dependence 1995: Proceedings of the 57th Annual Scientific Meeting. NIDA research monograph; 1995. Pp. 60–3.

Hser Y, Anglin MD, Powers K. A 24-year follow-up of California narcotics addicts. Arch Gen Psychiatry 1993;50:577–84.

Hser Y, Anglin MD, Grell, C, Longshore D, Prendergast M. Drug treatment careers: a conceptual framework and existing research findings. J Subst Abuse 1997;14(3):1–16.

Hser Y, Yamaguchi K, Anglin MD, Chen J. Effects of interventions on relapse to narcotics addiction. Eval Rev 1995;19:123–40.

Hubbard RL, Marsden ME, Rachal JV, Harwood HJ, Cavanaugh ER, Ginzburg HM. Drug abuse treatment: a national study of effectiveness. Chapel Hill: The University of North Carolina Press; 1995.

Hubbard RL, Craddock SG, Flynn PM, Anderson J, Etheridge RM. Overview of one-year followup outcomes in DATOS. Psychol Addictive Behav 1997;11(4).

Joe GW, Simpson DD, Sells SB. Treatment process and relapse to opioid use during methadone maintenance. Am J Drug Alcohol Abuse 1994;20(2):173–97.

Kleber HD. Outpatient detoxification from opiates. Primary Psychiatry 1996;1:42–52.

Kosten TR, Morgan C, Kleber HD. Treatment of heroin addicts using buprenorphine. Am J Drug Alcohol Abuse 1991;7(1):119–28.

Krystal JH, Woods SW, Kosten TR, Rosen MI, Seibyl JP. Opiate dependence and withdrawal: preliminary assessment using single photon emission computerized tomography (SPECT). Am J Drug Alcohol Abuse 1995;21(1):47–63.

Lewis D, Gear C, Laubli Loud M, Langenick-Cartwright D, English edition editors. The medical prescription of narcotics, Rihs-Middel M, editor. Toronto: Hogrefe & Huber Publishers; 1997.

Loimer N, Schmid R, Grünberger J, Jagsch R, Linzmayer L, Presslich O. Psychophysiological reactions in methadone maintenance patients do not correlate with methadone plasma levels. Psychopharmacology 1991;103:538–40.

London ED, Broussolle EP, Links JM, Wong DF, Cascella NG, Dannals RF, et al. Morphine-induced metabolic changes in human brain. Studies with positron emission tomography and [fluorine 18]fluorodeoxyglucose. Arch Gen Psychiatry 1990;47(1):73–81.

McLellan AT, Woody GE, Luborsky L, O'Brien CP. Is the counselor an "active ingredient" in substance abuse treatment? J Nerv Ment Dis 1988;176(7):423–30.

McLellan AT, Arndt IO, Alterman AI, Woody GE, Metzger D. Psychosocial services in substance abuse treatment: a dose-ranging study of psychosocial services. JAMA 1993.

McLellan AT, Alterman AI, Metzger DS, Grissom G, Woody GE, Luborsky L, et al. Similarity of outcome predictors across opiate, cocaine and alcohol treatments: role of treatment services. J Consult Clin Psychol 1994;62:1141–58.

Mechanic D, Schlesinger M, McAlpine DD. Management of mental health and substance abuse services: state of the art and early results. Milbank Q 1995;73:19–55.

Merikangas KR, Rounsaville BJ, Prusoff BA. Familial factors in vulnerability to substance abuse. In: Glantz M, Pickens R, editors. Vulnerability to drug abuse. Washington: American Psychological Association; 1992. Pp. 75–97.

Molinari SP, Cooper JR, Czechowicz DJ. Federal regulation of clinical practice in narcotic addiction treatment: purpose, status, and alternatives. J Law Med Ethics 1994; 22(3)231–9.

Murphy S, Irwin J. "Living with the dirty secret": Problems of disclosure for methadone maintenance clients. J Psychoactive Drugs 1992;24(3):257–64.

Musto DF. The American disease. Origins of narcotic control. Expanded edition. New York: Oxford University Press; 1987.

Nestler EJ. Under seige: the brain on opiates. Neuron 1996;16:897–900.

Novick M, Joseph H, Salsitz EA, Kalin MF, Keefe JB, Miller EL, et al. Outcomes of treatment of socially rehabilitated methadone maintenance patients in physicians' offices (medical maintenance): follow-up at three and a half to nine and a fourth years. J Gen Intern Med 1994;9:127–30.

Nurco DN, Hanlon TE, Balter MB, Kinlock TW, Slaght E. A classification of narcotic addicts based on type, amount, and severity of crime. J Drug Issues 1991;21:429–48.

Nurco DN, Cisin IH, Balter MB. Addicts career II: the first ten years. Addict 1981; 8: 1327–56.

Nurco DN, Ball JC, Shaffer JW, Hanlon TE. The criminality of narcotic addicts. J Nerv Ment Dis 1985;173:94–102.

Nurco DN, Shaffer JW, Ball JC, Kinlock TW. Trends in the commission of crime among narcotic addicts over successive periods of addiction and nonaddiction. Am J Drug Alcohol Abuse 1984;10:481–9.

Pickens RW, Svikis DS, McGue M, Lykken DT, Heston LL, Clayton PJ. Heterogeneity in the inheritance of alcoholism. A study of male and female twins. Arch Gen Psychiatry 1991;48:19–28.

Rettig RA, Yarmolinsky A, editors. Federal regulation of methadone treatment. Institute of Medicine. Washington: National Academy Press; 1995.

Rhoades H, Creson D, Elk R, Schmitz J, Grabowski J. Retention, HIV risk, and illicit drug use during treatment: methadone dose and visit frequency. Am J Public Health 1997;88:34–9.

Rogowski JA. Insurance coverage for drug abuse. Health Aff 1992;11(3):137–48.

Scott JE, Greenberg D, Pizzaro J. A survey of state insurance mandates covering alcohol and other drug treatment. J Ment Health Adm 1992;19(1):96–118.

Senay EC, Barthwell AG, Marks R, Boros P, Gillman D, White G. Medical maintenance: a pilot study. J Addict Dis 1993;12(4):59–76

Simpson DD. Effectiveness of drug-abuse treatment: a review of research from field settings. In: Egertson JA, Fox DM, Leshner AI, editors. Treating drug abusers effectively. Cambridge, MA: Blackwell Publishers of North America; 1997. Pp. 42–73.

Simpson DD, Joe GW, Dansereau DF, Chatham LR. Strategies for improving methadone treatment process and outcomes. J Drug Issues 1997;27(2):239–60.

Tennant FS, Rawson RA, Cohen A, Tarver A, Clabout C. Methadone plasma levels and persistent drug abuse in high dose maintenance patients. Subst Alcohol Actions Misuse 1983;4:369–74.

Tsuang MT , Lyons MJ, Eisen SA, Goldberg J, True W, Lin N, et al. Genetic influences on DSM-III-R drug abuse and dependence: a study of 3,372 twin pairs. Am J Med Genet 1996;67:473–7.

Vining E, Kosten TR, Kleber HD. Clinical utility of rapid clonidine-naltrexone detoxification for opioid abuse. Br J Addict 1988;83:567–75.

Walsh SL, Gilson SF, Jasinski DR, Stapleton JM, Phillips RL, Dannals RF, et al. Buprenorphine reduces cerebral glucose metabolism in polydrug abusers. Neuropsychopharmacology 1994;10(3):157–70.

Yancovitz SR, Des Jarlais DC, Peyser NP, Drew E, Friedmann P, Trigg HL, et al. Am J Public Health 1991;81(9):1185–91.

Zweben JE, Payte JT. Methadone maintenance in the treatment of opioid dependence: a current perspective. West J Med 1990;152(5):588–99.

G

Useful Internet Resources—Examples

SELECTED ALCOHOL AND DRUG ABUSE WEBSITES

Government

Agency for Health Care Policy Research (AHCPR)
http://www.ahcpr.gov/
Instant Fax: 301-594-2800 or 301-594-2801

Center for Substance Abuse Treatment (CSAT)
http://www.samhsa.gov/csat/csat.htm/
CSAT by Fax: 301-403-8329 (voice)

National Clearinghouse for Alcohol and Drug Information
http://www.health.org/
Information: 1-800-SAY-NO-TO

National Criminal Justice Reference Service (NCJRS)
http://www.ncjrs.org/

National Institute on Drug Abuse (NIDA)
http://www.nida.nih.gov/
NIDA InfoFax: 1-888-NIH-NIDA

National Institute on Alcohol Abuse and Alcoholism (NIAAA)
http://www.niaaa.nih.gov/

NIH Consensus Development Program
http://consensus.nih.gov/

Office of National Drug Control Policy (ONDCP)
http://www.whitehousedrugpolicy.gov/

Treatment Improvement Exchange (TIE)
http://www.treatment.org/

Providers

CAB Health and Recovery Services
http://www.cabhrs.org/

Haight-Asbury Free Clinics, Inc.
http://www.hafci.org/hafci/

Hazelden
http://www.hazelden.org/

Step One
http://www.stepone.org/

Walden House
http://www.waldenhouse.org/

Associations/Advocacy

Association for Health Services Research (AHSR)
http://www.ahsr.org/

Join Together
http://www.jointogether.org/

National Alliance of Methadone Advocates
http://www.methadone.org/

National Association of Alcohol and Drug Abuse Counselors (NAADAC)
http://www.naadac.org/

National Association of Drug Court Professionals (NADCP)
http://www.drugcourt.org/

National Association of State Alcohol and Drug Abuse Directors (NASADAD)
http://www.nasadad.org/

Research and Education

Addiction Research Foundation
http://www.arf.org/

Center for Alcohol and Addiction Studies (CAAS)
http://center.butler.brown.edu/

Center for Education and Drug Abuse (CEDAR)
http://www.pitt.edu/~mmv/cedar.html

Center for Substance Abuse Research (CESAR)
http://www.bsos.umd.edu/cesar/cesar.html

Emory University Health Sciences Center Library MEDWEB—Substance Dependence
http://www.gen.emory.edu/MEDWEB/keyword/substance_dependence.html

National Center on Addiction and Substance Abuse (CASA)
http://www.casacolumbia.org/

UCLA Drug Abuse Research Center
http://www.medsch.ucla.edu/som/npi/DARC/

NIDA CAPSULE: METHAMPHETAMINE ABUSE

Methamphetamine Abuse

Methamphetamine is a drug that strongly activates certain systems in the brain. Methamphetamine is closely related chemically to amphetamine, but the central nervous system effects of methamphetamine are greater. Both drugs have some medical uses, primarily in the treatment of obesity, but their therapeutic use is limited.

Methamphetamine is made in illegal laboratories and has a high potential for abuse and dependence. Street methamphetamine is referred to by many names, such as "speed," "meth," and "chalk." Methamphetamine hydrochloride, clear chunky crystals resembling ice, which can be inhaled by smoking, is referred to as "ice," "crystal," and "glass."

Extent of Abuse

The Monitoring the Future Study assesses the extent of drug use among adolescents (8th-, 10th-, and 12th-graders) and young adults across the country. Recent data from the survey:

- In 1996, 4.4 percent of high school seniors had used crystal methamphetamine at least once in their lifetimes, an increase from 2.7 percent in 1990.
- Data show that 2.8 percent of seniors had used crystal methamphetamine in 1996, more than doubling the 1.3 percent reported in 1990.

Methods of Abuse

Methamphetamine is taken orally or intranasally (snorting the powder), by intravenous injection, and by smoking. Immediately after inhalation or intravenous injection, the methamphetamine user experiences an intense sensation, called a "rush" or "flash," that lasts only a few minutes and is described as extremely pleasurable. Oral or intranasal use produces euphoria—a high, but not a rush.

Because methamphetamine elevates mood, people who experiment with it tend to use it with increasing frequency and in increasing doses, although this was not their original intent.

Health Effects and Hazards

The central nervous system (CNS) actions that result from taking even small amounts of methamphetamine include increased wakefulness, increased physical activity, decreased appetite, increased respiration, hyper-thermia, and euphoria. Other CNS effects include irritability, insomnia, confusion, tremors, convulsions, anxiety, paranoia, and aggressiveness. Hyperthermia and convulsions can result in death. Cardiovascular side effects, which include chest pain and hypertension, also can result in cardio-vascular collapse and death. In addition, methamphetamine causes increased heart rate and blood pressure and can cause irreversible damage to blood vessels in the brain, producing strokes. Other effects of methamphetamine include respiratory problems, irregular heartbeat, and extreme anorexia.

Supply

Methamphetamine is a Schedule II drug under Federal regulations, meaning it has a high potential for abuse with severe liability to cause dependence. During World War II, methamphetamine was used by soldiers as an aid to fight fatigue and enhance performance. In Japan, intravenous methamphetamine abuse reached epidemic proportions immediately after World War II, when supplies stored for military use became available to the public.

In the United States in the 1950s, legally manufactured tablets of meth-amphetamine were used nonmedically by college students, truck drivers, and athletes, who usually did not become severely addicted. This pattern changed drastically in the 1960s with the increased availability of injectable methamphetamine. The 1970 Controlled Substances Act severely restricted the legal production of injectable methamphetamine, causing its use to decrease greatly.

According to the Drug Enforcement Administration, methamphetamine has been the most prevalent clandestinely produced controlled substance in the United States since 1979. The clandestine manufacture of methamphet-amine was based primarily in the West and Southwest. Since the 1980s, ice has been smuggled from Taiwan and South Korea into Hawaii. However, it was not until the summer of 1988 that its use became relatively widespread in that State. By 1990, distribution of ice had spread to the U.S. mainland, although distribution remained limited.

Part of the NIDA Capsule Series—(C-89-06) [Revised September, 1997]

SOURCE: National Institute on Drug Abuse. 1997. NIDA Capsule Meth-amphetamine Abuse [WWW Document]. URL http://www.nida.nih.gov/NIDACapsules/NCMethamphetamine.html (Accessed December 19, 1997).

CSAT BY FAX:
WHAT MAKES AN EFFECTIVE ADDICTIONS COUNSELOR?

CSAT by Fax
May 7, 1997
Vol. 2, Issue 8

A Special Edition of CESAR *FAX* ➤

A Collaborative Effort of the Center for Substance Abuse Treatment (CSAT) and the Center for Substance Abuse Research (CESAR)/University of Maryland at College Park

What Makes an Effective Addictions Counselor?

In April 1995, a CSAT-appointed task force met to discuss the characteristics of addictions counselors who work successfully with clients. The Task Force on the Characteristics of Effective Addictions Counselors included experts with experience in clinical practice, training, and research. Participants were asked to enumerate what characteristics they thought would help them predict a counselor's effectiveness in working toward positive client outcomes. Using their intuition and the results of the limited research done on this question, the task force reached consensus on the importance of the following counselor characteristics:

- the mental health and personal adjustment of the individual counselor;

- therapeutic optimism;

- organizational ability;

- the ability to recognize and maintain appropriate boundaries and balance client and counselor needs;

- positive experience and convictions about recovery;

- investment in personal and professional growth;

- appropriate ethics and values; and

- sense of humor.

The task force suggested that future research focus on identifying the most important counselor characteristics, and on investigating whether these characteristics can be taught.

SOURCE: Center for Substance Abuse Treatment, *Task Force on the Characteristics of Effective Addictions Counselors Progress Review*, April 1995. For more information, contact Sue Rohrer at 301-443-8521.

National Methamphetamine Consensus Meeting Report Now Available

Proceedings of the National Consensus Meeting on the Use, Abuse and Sequelae of Abuse of Methamphetamine with Implications for Prevention, Treatment and Research is now available from the National Clearinghouse for Alcohol and Drug Information at 800-729-6686 or 301-468-6433. Please ask for publication number BKD219.

CSAT by Fax is supported by funding from CSAT, Substance Abuse and Mental Health Services Administration, and may be copied without permission with appropriate citation. For mailing list modifications contact CESAR at
•• 301-403-8329 (voice) •• 301-403-8342 (fax) •• CESAR@cesar.umd.edu (e-mail) ••

SOURCE: Center for Substance Abuse Research. 1998. GIF Image, 592 × 768 Pixels [WWW Document]. URL http://www.bsos.umd.edu/cesar/csat2/CSAT2-8.GIF (Accessed January 28, 1998).

SUBSTANCE ABUSE AND MENTAL HEALTH DATA ARCHIVE SUMMARY OF SAMHSA'S TREATMENT EPISODE DATA SET AND NIDA'S MONITORING THE FUTURE STUDY

Treatment Episode Data Set (1992–1995)

The Treatment Episode Data Set (TEDS) is an administrative data system providing descriptive information about the national flow of admissions to specialty providers of substance abuse treatment. TEDS is designed to supply annual data on the number and characteristics of persons admitted to public and private nonprofit substance abuse treatment programs in all 50 states, DC, and Puerto Rico. The unit of analysis is treatment admissions to substance abuse treatment units receiving public funding. TEDS includes both a Minimum Data Set (required reporting) and a Supplemental Data Set (optional reporting). The data include demographics, services, substance(s) of abuse, number of prior treatments, referral source, employment status, frequency of use, age at first use, veteran and pregnancy status, insurance type, and income.

TEDS is sponsored by the Office of Applied Studies at the Substance Abuse and Mental Health Services Administration.

SOURCE: Substance Abuse and Mental Health Data Archive (SAMHDA). 1998. TEDS [WWW Document]. URL http://www.icpsr.umich.edu/ SAMHDA/teds.html (Accessed February 1, 1998).

Monitoring the Future (1976–1995)

MTF explores changes in values, behaviors, and lifestyle of American youth. Provides an annual systematic and accurate description of the youth population and quantifies the direction and rate of change occurring over time. Respondents are nationally representative of high school seniors in the U.S. and respond to about 100 drug-use and demographic questions as well as to about 200 questions on subjects such as attitudes toward government, social institutions, race relations, changing roles for women, educational aspirations, occupational aims, and marital and family plans.

MTF is sponsored by the National Institute on Drug Abuse.

SOURCE: SAMHDA. 1998. MTF [WWW Document]. URL http://www. icpsr.umich.edu/ SAMHDA/mtf.html (Accesssed February 1, 1998).

H

List of Currently Available CSAT Treatment Improvement Protocols (TIPs)

TIP 1   State Methadone Treatment Guidelines

TIP 2   Pregnant, Substance-Abusing Women

TIP 3   Screening and Assessment of Alcohol- and Other Drug-Abusing Adolescents

TIP 4   Guidelines for the Treatment of Alcohol- and Other Drug-Abusing Adolescents

TIP 5   Improving Treatment for Drug-Exposed Infants

TIP 6   Screening for Infectious Diseases Among Substance Abusers

TIP 7   Screening and Assessment for Alcohol and Other Drug Abuse Among Adults in the Criminal Justice System

TIP 8   Intensive Outpatient Treatment for Alcohol and Other Drug Abuse

TIP 9   Assessment and Treatment of Patients with Coexisting Mental Illness and Alcohol and Other Drug Abuse

TIP 10   Assessment and Treatment of Cocaine-Abusing Methadone-Maintained Patients

TIP 11   Simple Screening Instruments for Outreach for Alcohol and Other Drug Abuse and Infectious Diseases

TIP 12   Combining Substance Abuse Treatment with Intermediate Sanctions for Adults in the Criminal Justice System

TIP 13   The Role and Current Status of Patient Placement Criteria in the Treatment of Substance Use Disorders

TIP 14   Developing State Outcomes Monitoring Systems for Alcohol and Other Drug Abuse Treatment

TIP 15   Treatment for HIV-Infected Alcohol and Other Drug Abusers

TIP 16   Alcohol and Other Drug Screening of Hospitalized Trauma
         Patients
TIP 17   Planning for Alcohol and Other Drug Abuse Treatment for Adults
         in the Criminal Justice System
TIP 18   The Tuberculosis Epidemic: Legal and Ethical Issues for Alcohol
         and Other Drug Treatment Providers
TIP 19   Detoxification from Alcohol and Other Drugs
TIP 20   Matching Treatment to Patient Needs in Opioid Substitution
         Therapy
TIP 21   Combining Alcohol and Other Drug Abuse Treatment with
         Diversion for Juveniles in the Justice System
TIP 22   LAAM in the Treatment of Opiate Addiction
TIP 23   Treatment Drug Courts: Integrating Substance Abuse Treatment
         with Legal Case Processing
TIP 24   A Guide to Substance Abuse Services for Primary Care Physicians
TIP 25   Substance Abuse Treatment and Domestic Violence

I

Opportunities for Collaboration

Joseph Westermeyer
University of Minnesota and
Minneapolis VA Medical Center

Many clinical areas will benefit from empirical scrutiny and investigations where clinicians collaborate with research teams to articulate research questions, design research protocols, collect and analyze data, and interpret results. The descriptions of opportunities for collaboration presented in this appendix are examples of a few such areas. They may also serve as a model for writing up a "one pager" to begin the discussion of a collaborative research project.

Table I-1 identifies some of the major gaps between what is known from treatment research and what is actually practiced in the outpatient drug abuse treatment system. It suggests questions that could be addressed with more services research and collaboration with treatment providers.

In the same volume, an assessment of drug abuse treatment research completed in field settings concluded that studies of phases of treatment have been uneven and will benefit from additional attention in at least six areas: (1) identification and recruitment of individuals in need of treatment, (2) motivation and readiness for treatment, (3) treatment induction processes, (4) matching services to client needs, (5) engaging and retaining individuals in care, and (6) understanding postdischarge improvements (Simpson, 1997).

A separate analysis of factors that affect access to care observed that changes in health care financing may alter access to care and the types of services available to clients (Horgan, 1997). Studies of the effects of managed care on the organization and financing of drug abuse treatment require substantial cooperation from the community-based programs that

TABLE I-1   Drug Abuse Treatment—What We Know and
Current Practice

Treatment Processes and Inputs	What We Know and Current Practice
Treatment Process	**Review Findings**
Assessment	Advances in assessment methods recently achieved
	Physical health not routinely assessed in drug-free outpatient treatment
	Mental health assessed, formal diagnosis less frequently
	Prevalence of addiction severity assessment unknown
	HIV assessment infrequent but growing
Treatment planning	Research on patient-treatment matching increasing
	Prevalence of individualized treatment planning unknown
	Current treatment goals are abstinence, physical health, relationship improvement, not "responsible use"
Core treatment mechanisms	Expert opinion identifies acceptance of responsibility, relapse prevention, denial reduction as core mechanisms of effective treatment
	Current practice involves individual and group therapy and addiction education
	High-dose methadone treatment is effective but many programs restrict dosage levels and client participation in treatment planning
Supportive treatment services	Supportive legal, family, job, and medical services are important for effective treatment
	Less than half of treatment settings provide supportive services
	AIDS prevention and counseling infrequent
Aftercare	New relapse prevention treatment and education available
	Follow-up and aftercare is critical to effective treatment
	Less than three-quarters of outpatient and half of methadone units have formal written follow-up plans

TABLE I-1 Continued

Treatment Processes and Inputs	What We Know and Current Practice
Treatment Process	**Review Findings**
	Less than two-thirds of outpatient services collect any follow-up information at all
Treatment Inputs	
Staffing	Majority of staff are BA and MA level
	Only half have special training or certification in substance-abuse treatment
	Work experience and special training seen as important hiring qualifications
	Recovering addict status not seen as special qualification. Effectiveness unclear
	Understaffing and poor client-staff ratios produce poorer outcomes
Client characteristics	Women substance abuse clients have special service needs associated with pregnancy, sexual abuse, child care, and homelessness
	Less than half of outpatient services have special services for women, one-fifth have special services for pregnant women
	Minority clients need culturally sensitive supportive services to improve recruitment and reduce dropout
	New services for minority clients are not being developed rapidly
Organization	Staffing, client assessment, client characteristics vary in methadone vs. outpatient drug-free programs
	Hospital and mental health settings utilize more professionals in treatment
	Public programs provided better access than private-for-profit programs
	Private-for-profit programs may achieve lower cost by reducing individual treatment intensity

SOURCE: Price RH. 1997. What we know and what we actually do: Best practices and their prevalence. In: Egertson JA, Fox DM, Leshner AI, eds. *Treating Drug Problems Effectively.* Bodmin, Cornwall: Blackwell Publishers. Pp. 125–155. Reprinted by permission of Blackwell Publishers. Copyright 1997. All rights reserved.

provide treatment services. Similarly, investigations of staffing patterns and the characteristics of the drug abuse treatment workforce can not be completed without the direct participation of treatment agencies (Brown, 1997; Price, 1997). There is also insufficient information on the characteristics of individuals seeking care and the interventions that best meet the unique needs of women, minorities, and adolescents (Price, 1997).

Case management has been widely adopted and promoted for the care of men and women with serious mental illness but has not been well developed for the treatment of chronic alcohol and drug dependence (Willenbring, 1995; Willenbring et al., 1991). Managed care organizations, however, often promote case management as an essential tool. While investigations of case management for drug abuse treatment demonstrate that case managed clients receive more services, evidence that outcomes improve has emerged less clearly (Orwin et al., 1993) and more slowly (Shwartz et al., 1997). Thus, there is much opportunity for treatment providers with effective mature models of case management to collaborate with researchers and examine the factors that contribute to more beneficial outcomes.

The committee heard many additional areas highlighted in testimony from both researchers and practitioners. The list of areas where collaboration between researchers and treatment programs will improve theory and enhance practice may be nearly infinite.

REFERENCES

Brown BS. 1997. Staffing patterns and services for the war on drugs. In: Fox DM, Egertson J, Leshner AI eds. *Treating Drug Abusers Effectively*. Malden, MA: Blackwell Publishers. Pp. 99–124.

Horgan CM. 1997. Need and access to drug-abuse treatment. In: Egertson JA, Fox DM, Leshner AI eds. *Treating Drug Abusers Effectively*. Malden, MA: Blackwell Publishers.

Orwin RG, Goldman HH, Sonnefeld LJ, Smith NG, Ridgely MS, Garrison-Morgren R, O'Neill E, Luchese J, Sherman A, O'Connell ME. 1993. *Community Demonstration Grant Projects for Alcohol and Drug Abuse Treatment of Homeless Individuals: Final Evaluation Report*. NIH Pub. No. 92-3541. Rockville, MD: National Institute on Alcohol Abuse and Alcoholism.

Price RH. 1997. What we know and what we actually do: Best practices and their prevalence. In: Egertson JA, Fox DM, Leshner A eds. *Treating Drug Abusers Effectively*. Malden, MA: Blackwell Publishers. Pp. 125–155.

Shwartz M, Baker G, Mulvey KP, Plough A. 1997. Improving publicly funded substance abuse treatment. *American Journal of Public Health* 87:1659–1664.

Simpson DD. 1997. Effectiveness of drug-abuse treatment: A review of research from field settings. In: Egertson JA, Fox DM, Leshner AI eds. *Treating Drug Abusers Effectively*. Malden, MA: Blackwell Publishers.

Willenbring ML. 1995. Case management application in substance use disorders. *Journal of Case Management* 3:150–157.

Willenbring ML, Ridgely MS, Stinchfield R, Rose M. 1991. *Application of Case Management in Alcohol and Drug Dependence: Matching Techniques and Populations.* DHHS Pub. No. ADM 91-1766. Rockville, MD: National Institute on Alcohol Abuse and Alcoholism.

OPPORTUNITIES FOR COLLABORATION:
ADOLESCENT OUTREACH AND EARLY INTERVENTION

Studies of substance use among youth go back a half-century in the United States (Glad, 1947). Four decades ago an official at the World Health Organization first identified a worldwide pandemic of substance abuse among youth (Cameron, 1968). Since that time, investigators have identified the association of substance abuse with numerous social and behavior problems among youth, including:

- delinquency (Farrow and French, 1986);
- risk of physical and sexual abuse (Dembo et al., 1987);
- suicide, at least in some subgroups of adolescents (Berlin, 1987; Bechtold, 1988; Dizmang et al., 1974; Grossman et al., 1991);
- driving while intoxicated (Harwood and Leonard, 1989);
- illegitimate pregnancy (Gilchrist et al., 1990); and
- running away, especially among females (Fors and Rojek, 1991).

Considerable information exists regarding the epidemiology and clinical characteristics of adolescent substance abuse (Johnson and Marcos, 1988). Young substance abusers are more apt to abuse alcohol, cannabis, inhalants (Beauvais et al., 1985; Padilla et al., 1979; Schwartz, 1988; Westermeyer et al., 1994) and less apt to abuse cocaine and heroin. Antisocial behavior is especially apt to accompany substance abuse in adolescents (Osuna and Luna, 1988) although many cases do not involve such behavior. High rates of several comorbid psychiatric disorders accompany early-onset substance abuse in adolescents (Burke et al., 1994; Deykin et al., 1992; King et al., 1993; Myers et al., 1990; Westermeyer et al., 1994). Institutionalized youth are at particular risk to substance abuse (Cockerham, 1975), as are particular ethnic and socioeconomic groups (Cockerham et al., 1976).

Prevention services for adolescents have been developed and well studied (Perry, 1986). However, much of these data indicate a delay in substance use rather than prevention of eventual substance abuse. Most data on adolescent treatment focuses on description of services, anecdotal reports, or uncontrolled studies (Tarter, 1990). Data on outreach, early intervention, treatment outcome, and cost efficacy for adolescent substance abusers is remarkably sparse. Special treatment alternatives for adolescents (e.g., school-based adult-led self-help groups, switching schools, relocation of families with affected adolescents to a new neighborhood) remain essentially unstudied, although they often undertaken and sometimes even recommended by clinicians. Some interesting models for working with adolescents in groups have been developed, but not well researched (Red Horse, 1982). Local mass media may be a useful means for reaching adolescents in particular (Skirrow, 1987). In order to conduct quantitative research among adolescents, adolescent-specific instruments are needed (Mayer and Filstead, 1979). Issues regarding validity of data obtained from adolescents differ in certain respects from adults (Winters et al., 1991).

REFERENCES

Beauvais F, Oetting ER, Edward RW. 1985. Trends in the use of inhalants among American Indian adolescents. *White Cloud Journal* 3:3.

Bechtold DW. 1988. Cluster suicide in American Indian adolescents. *American Indian and Alaska Native Mental Health Research* 1(3):26–35.

Berlin IN. 1987. Suicide among American Indian adolescents: An overview. *Suicide and Life-Threatening Behavior* 17(3):218–232.

Burke JD, Burke KC, Rae DS. 1994. Increased rates of drug abuse and dependence after onset of mood or anxiety disorders in adolescence. *Hospital Community Psychiatry* 45(5):451–455.

Cameron DC. 1968. Youth and drugs: A world view. *Journal of the American Medical Association* 206:1267–1271.

Cockerham WC. 1975. Patterns of drinking behavior among institutionalized and non-institutionalized Wyoming youth. *Journal of Studies on Alcohol* 36:993–995.

Cockerham WC, Forslund MA, Roboin RM. 1976. Drug use among White and American Indian high school youth. *International Journal of Addiction* 11(2):209–220.

Dembo R, Derthke M, LaVoie L, Borders S, Washburn M. 1987. Physical abuse, sexual victimization and illicit drug use: A structural analysis among high risk. *Journal of Adolescence* 10(1):10–34.

Deykin EY, Buka SL, Zeena TH. 1992. Depressive illness among chemically dependent adolescents. *American Journal of Psychiatry* 149(10):1341–1347.

Dizmang LH, Watson J, May PA, Bopp J. 1974. Adolescent suicide at an Indian reservation. *American Journal of Orthopsychiatry* 44(1):43–49.

Farrow JA, French J. 1986. The drug abuse-delinquency connection revisited. *Adolescence* 21:951–960.

Fors SW, Rojek DG. 1991. A comparison of drug involvement between runaways and school youths. *Journal of Drug Education* 21(1):13–25.

Gilchrist LD, Gillmore MR, Lohr MJ. 1990. Drug use among pregnant adolescents. *Journal of Consulting and Clinical Psychology* 58(4):402–407.

Glad DD. 1947. Attitudes and experiences of American-Jewish and American-Irish male youth as related to differences in adult rates of inebriety. *Quarterly Journal of Studies of Alcohol* 8:406–472.

Grossman DC, Milligan BC, Deyo RA. 1991. Risk factors for suicide attempts among Navajo adolescents. *American Journal of Public Health* 81(7):870–874.

Harwood MK, Leonard KE. 1989. Family history of alcoholism, youthful antisocial behavior and problem drinking among DWI offenders. *Journal of Studies on Alcohol* 50(3):210–216.

Johnson RE, Marcos AC. 1988. Correlates of adolescent drug use by gender and geographic location. *American Journal of Drug and Alcohol Abuse* 14(1):51–63.

King CA, Naylor MW, Hill EM, Shain BN, Greden JF. 1993. Dysthymia characteristics of heavy alcohol use in depressed adolescents. *Biological Psychiatry* 33(3):210–212.

Mayer J, Filstead WJ. 1979. The Adolescent Alcohol Involvement Scale: An instrument for measuring adolescents' use and misuse of alcohol. *Journal of Studies on Alcohol* 40(3):291–300.

Myers WC, Burket RC, Lyles WB, Stone L, Kemph JP. 1990. DSM-III diagnoses and offenses in committed female juvenile delinquents. *Bulletin of the American Academy of Psychiatry and the Law* 18(1):47–54.

Osuna E, Luna A. 1988. Adolescent drug use and antisocial behavior. *Medicine and Law* 7(4):365–330.

Padilla ER, Padilla AM, Morales A. 1979. Inhalant, marijuana and alcohol abuse among barrio children and adolescents. *International Journal of the Addictions* 14:945–964.

Perry CI. 1986. Results of prevention programs with adolescents. *Drug and Alcohol Dependence* 20:13–19.

Red Horse Y. 1982. A cultural network model: Perspectives for adolescent services and paraprofessional training. In: Manson S ed. *New Directions in Prevention Among American Indian and Alaska Native Communities*. Portland, OR: University of Oregon.

Schwartz RH. 1988. Deliberate inhalation of isobutyl nitrate during adolescence: A descriptive study. *NIDA Research Monograph* 83:81–85.

Skirrow J. 1987. II. Influencing the adolescent life style: The role of mass media. *Drug and Alcohol Dependence* 20:21–26.

Tarter RE. 1990. Evaluation and treatment of adolescent substance abuse: A decision tree method. *American Journal of Drug and Alcohol Abuse* 16(1–2):1–46.

Westermeyer J, Specker S, Neider J, Lingenfelter MA. 1994. Substance abuse and associated psychiatric disorder among 100 adolescents. *Journal of Addictive Diseases* 13(1):67–83.

Winters KC, Stinchfield RD, Henly GA, Schwartz R. 1991. Validity of adolescent self-report of substance involvement. *International Journal of the Addictions* 25:1379–1395.

OPPORTUNITIES FOR COLLABORATION:
COMMUNITY REINFORCEMENT

Formal research on Community Reinforcement began 25 years ago, with the work of Hunt, Azrin and coworkers (Azrin, 1976; Hunt and Azrin, 1973). Despite the utility of their early work and the time that has elapsed since then, relatively few studies have been undertaken regarding community reinforcement. Those few that have been undertaken have demonstrated the cost efficacy of this approach. They include the following:

- the role of the community in motivating drug abusers to seek treatment, organizing groups of addicts to seek treatment concurrently, and in providing family/household support for the addict in treatment (Westermeyer and Bourne, 1978);

- the adjunctive role of disulfiram in the Community Reinforcement treatment of alcoholism (Azrin et al., 1982);
- the effectiveness of a work program for young drug abusers in the community (Stead et al., 1990);
- the application of these principles to the chronic public inebriate (Willenbring et al., 1990); and
- the utility of the Community Reinforcement treatment in the care of substance abusers and addicts, as well as in rural settings and among ethnic minority groups (Miller et al., 1992).

Although these investigators have demonstrated the effectiveness, and even the cost efficacy of these methods, they have not been widely applied. This is probably due to the complexity of the approach, the need for community and treatment resources to cooperate, the requirement for an overarching plan with "reinforcement" of the respective positive as well as negative consequences. In order to work effectively, the reinforcements must be consistently and fairly applied over lengthy periods of time. Political support and diverse funding streams add to the further difficulty of establishing and maintaining Community Reinforcement programs.

REFERENCES

Azrin NH. 1976. Improvements in the community-reinforcement approach to alcoholism. *Behavior Research Therapy* 14:339–348.

Azrin NH, Sisson RW, Meyers R, Godley M. 1982. Alcoholism treatment by disulfiram and community reinforcement therapy. *Journal of Behavior Therapy and Experimental Psychiatry* 13:105–112.

Hunt GM, Azrin NH. 1973. A community-reinforcement approach to alcoholism. *Behavior Research Therapy* 11:91–104.

Miller WR, Meyers RF, Tonigan JS, Hester RK. 1992. *Effectiveness of the Community Reinforcement Approach*. Albuquerque, NM: Center on Alcoholism, Substance Abuse, and Addictions.

Stead P, Rozynko V, Berman S. 1990. The SHARP carwash: A community-oriented work program for substance abuse patients. *Social Work* 35(1):79–80.

Westermeyer J, Bourne P. 1978. Treatment outcome and the role of the community in narcotic addiction. *Journal of Nervous Mental Disorders* 166:51–58.

Willenbring ML, Whelan JA, Dahlquist JS, O'Neal MW. 1990. Community treatment of the chronic public inebriate: I. Implementation. *Alcoholism Treatment Quarterly* 7(1):79–98.

OPPORTUNITIES FOR COLLABORATION: OUTREACH STRATEGIES FOR EARLY INTERVENTION AND TREATMENT FOLLOW-UP

Outreach activities can be used for two purposes: to intervene early in the course of addiction and bring substance abusers to treatment before their resources diminish and their problems exacerbate. However, there are several difficulties associated with outreach, as follows:

- expense for personnel, material, and other resources;
- deciding how to target endeavors in the most cost-effective manner;
- the need to collaborate closely with social institutions with which addiction treatment facilities have limited experience (e.g., churches, schools, police, private associations);
- risk to violence, especially in certain lower socioeconomic neighborhoods or in groups that might be threatened by early intervention activities (e.g., gangs, certain clubs or bars); and
- many clinicians and researchers have little experience in outreach activities, or virtually any intervention activities outside of the clinic or laboratory.

Despite the obstacles, outreach efforts have been successful in several settings. These include:

- outpatient clinics (Lowe and Alston, 1973);
- seeking community cohorts of addicts to enter treatment concurrently or at least within months of one another (Westermeyer and Bourne, 1978);
- schools (Red Horse, 1982);
- community programs for mentally retarded persons (Westermeyer et al., 1988); and
- building a community consensus about modal or acceptable use versus unacceptable use (Beauvais, 1992).

Outreach has not been studied in a variety settings in which results might be fruitful. One of these involves individuals who have been injured and/or involved in vehicular crashes (*Morbidity and Mortality Weekly Report*, 1989). Cost efficacy of various outreach strategies are not available.

REFERENCES

Beauvais F. 1992. The need for community consensus as a condition of policy implementation in the reduction of alcohol abuse on Indian reservations. *American Indian and Alaska Native Mental Health Research* 4(3):77–81.

Lowe GD, Alston JP. 1973. An analysis of racial differences in services to alcoholics in a southern clinic. *Hospital Community Psychiatry* 24:547–551.

Morbidity and Mortality Weekly Report. 1989. Motor vehicle crashes and injuries in an Indian community-Arizona. *Morbidity and Mortality Weekly Report* 38:589–591.

Red Horse Y. 1982. A cultural network model: Perspectives for adolescent services and para-professional training. In: Manson S ed. *New Directions in Prevention Among American Indian and Alaska Native Communities*. Portland, OR: University of Oregon.

Westermeyer J, Bourne P. 1978. Treatment outcome and the role of the community in narcotic addiction. *Journal of Nervous Mental Disorders* 166:51–58.

Westermeyer J, Phaobtong T, Neider J. 1988. Substance use and abuse among mentally retarded persons: A comparison of patients and a survey population. *American Journal of Drug and Alcohol Abuse* 14(1):109–123.

OPPORTUNITIES FOR COLLABORATION: RESEARCHING SPIRITUAL, "FOLK," AND OTHER NONTRADITIONAL INTERVENTIONS

Large numbers of substance abusers seek relief in a variety of spiritual, religious, ethnic, and nontraditional treatments and programs. Acupuncture, one example of this category, has been addressed elsewhere in this report. Students of addiction, such as Galanter, have described the potent influence of religious influence on the lives of those affiliating with religious groups (Galanter and Westermeyer, 1980). Of interest, active substance abuse and religious practice tend to be inversely related (Westermeyer and Walzer, 1975). Certain modern treatments for addiction, such as the "anonymous" self-help groups, have their bases in religious movements (Johnson and Westermeyer, 1997).

So far, most studies in this area have focused on descriptions (Jilek, 1976; Westermeyer, 1988). Several qualitative and anecdotal reports have documented religious affiliation as a successful means of recovering from substance abuse (Kearny, 1970). A few studies have shown the feasibility of studying addiction treatment in religious settings (Westermeyer, 1980). In one quasi-experimental comparison of a religion-based program versus a medically based program for opiate addicts in Asia, the religion-based program had a higher mortality during opiate withdrawal; but follow-up failed to show differences between abstinence rates between the two therapies (Westermeyer and Bourne, 1978). In the latter study, community factors (e.g., community cohort treatment, a clinician or mentor committed to the addict's sobriety) were potent correlates of abstinence in both groups. More such studies are needed in a variety of settings in order to establish those dimensions of such interventions that may be efficacious in abating drug misuse, abuse, and dependence.

REFERENCES

Galanter M, Westermeyer J. 1980. Charismatic religious experience and large-group psychology. *American Journal of Psychiatry* 137(12):1550–1552.

Jilek WG. 1976. "Brainwashing" as a therapeutic technique in contemporary Canadian Indian spirit dancing: A case in theory building. *Anthropology and Mental Health* 201–213.

Johnson DR, Westermeyer J. 1997. Psychiatric therapies influenced by religious movements. In: Boehnlein J ed. *Textbook on Religion and Psychiatry.* Washington, DC: American Psychiatric Press.

Kearny M. 1970. Drunkenness and religious conversion in a Mexican village. *Quarterly Journal of Studies on Alcohol* 31:248–249.

Westermeyer J. 1980. Treatment for narcotic addiction in a Buddhist monastary. *Journal of Drug Issues* 10:221–228.

Westermeyer J. 1988. Folk medicine in Laos: A comparison between two ethnic groups. *SocialScience and Medicine* 27(8):769–778.

Westermeyer J, Bourne P. 1978. Treatment outcome and the role of the community in narcotic addiction. *Journal of Nervous Mental Disorders* 166:51–58.

Westermeyer J, Walzer V. 1975. Drug usage: An alternative to religion? *Diseases of the Nervous System* 36(9):492–495.

J

Summary of Interviews with Minnesota State Alcoholism-Addiction Leaders

Cindy Turnure, Ph.D.
Single State Agency Chief

Patricia Harrison, Ph.D.
Chief of Alcoholism/Addictions Research/Evaluation

POSITIVE STRATEGIES AND CONTRIBUTIONS OF RESEARCH TO COMMUNITY PROGRAMS

1. Research studies (especially treatment outcome studies) have produced *a few major findings*, discernible largely through meta-analyses, that do guide state-level planners (although may not yet affect community programs and private health organizations). These are as follows:

- virtually any kind of *treatment helps* (message: look for the low cost treatment);
- *brief but frequent contacts* with patients work better than intensive but short-term contacts; and
- treatment should be for the *long term*, with the expectation that many patients will surface repeatedly in treatment over a lifetime.

2. Nationwide data on addiction have not been particularly helpful. States and communities vary too greatly. More specific *data on similar states and communities* have been helpful.

NONPRODUCTIVE STRATEGIES AND PROBLEMS OF RESEARCH IN RELATION TO COMMUNITY PROGRAMS

1. They discern a growing *"research gap"* that is, the field has more and *more findings* that are less and *less used* in community settings.

246

2. *Dissemination of research results* to practitioners in the community:

• *expensive* to get information to community practitioners; they do not read the newsletters often produced by research centers or federal agencies;
• application of some research results requires additional staff *training*; there are no funds to pay for this;
• some research findings would require considerably *increased staff time* and/or staff *credentials* to bring these findings to the patient; these cannot be implemented in a time of declining state and private budgets for addiction services;
• some research findings require *sophisticated resources, additional financing*, etc., to apply; such findings have low-to-nil utility in the community (e.g., much "matching" research).

3. The highly selective criteria for many research protocols bias the research towards *atypical* rather than typical *patient-subjects*. For example, most research appears to involve "proactive" patients, urban patients, patients who have transportation to a center where research is conducted, can get referred into a research program, or come across the "right" gate keepers. These traits do not apply to most patients in community settings.
4. Much of the research appears to be based on models or concepts that clearly have not worked in this field. Examples, include research strategies that have approached patients as though addiction were an "acute care" disorder, rather than a chronic relapsing disorder in which recovery (even if it does occur) continues over years rather than weeks. Another flawed approach has been the search for a psychosocial or biomedical "silver bullet," in which one acute or subacute treatment method will "cure" addiction.

RECOMMENDATIONS FOR FUTURE RESEARCH FUNDING

1. More *clinicians* (or at least clinicians who are active applied researchers) should be *appointed to committees* charged with funding research.
2. Research goals should have as a *criterion* the *applicability* of any anticipated research findings to patients in community settings.
3. Research *models* should *reflect the realities* of addictive disorders (e.g., chronic, often recurrent disorders; associated psychosocial and biomedical problems; requiring years for recovery-maintenance-management).
4. Is there a way that *public policy* (on state as well as national levels)

can be tied to research findings? Currently, research findings do not seem to influence public policy.

5. Is there a way that research findings can inform *public perceptions* and opinions? Currently, public opinion leaders (e.g., mass media, heads of managed health care organizations, elected officials, health professionals, educational system, etc.) hold opinions counter to research findings (e.g., treatment for addiction does not work, treatment is more expensive than "supply reduction").

6. State planners would like to have research findings that address the following issues facing community programs:

• *How "brief"* can brief contacts be and still be effective? One hour, half hour, fifteen minutes, five minutes?

• How much do interventions *cost* in terms of assessment, total costs (including training, consultation, administrative costs, cost efficacy, cost offsets)?

• *Where* should treatment be best provided? Medical center? Home? Workplace? What about telephone contacts?

1. Any research findings, to be utilized at a community level, must be *simple* to apply (KISS principle). Interventions requiring special interviews (e.g., ASI), or costly psychological evaluation, or special assessments of staff members (e.g., personality types) are not used.

2. More *research* should be conducted *in community settings*. Much research now is conducted in large university or VA medical centers.

3. Community personnel, programs, and planners need *algorithms* to help in guiding patients through treatment. Examples include patients who are failing in treatment, special demographic groups, those with associated biomedical or psychosocial problems.

4. Managed care has become an integral part of health care. How can *managed care methods* be brought to the service of addicted patients? What are reasonable criteria for the involvement of managed care organizations and personnel in the care of addicted patients?

5. The *distinction* between *private and public* patients is fading fast in the addiction field. Previously "private" programs are taking public patients, as private programs no longer pay for addiction services. In addition, employed addicted persons either cannot get health insurance nowadays or lose private insurance coverage more readily than in the past. How can these "mixed" patients be best managed in the same system? What kind of case manager (or what kind of case management) should apply to either or both systems? How much does such case management cost? Case managers currently seem to add to treatment costs, rather than decrease costs. In addition, the cost efficacy of case management is far from obvious.

6. The *model of paying for addiction services* varies from community to community. Research might address whether "carve in" administration/funding is better than, worse than, or the same as "carve out" administration/funding. There are many theoretical advantages and disadvantages to both, or to perhaps some combination of both. Research is needed to assess the influence of these different approaches on addiction treatment.

7. The *distinction* between *prevention* (especially early intervention at the point of heavy use or early prediagnostic problematic use) *and treatment* are less relevant in the addictions than they may be in infectious disease, cardiovascular disease, cancer, etc. Currently, the "prevention" people receive different funding streams and do not address "early case" or "precase" finding. Likewise, clinicians do encounter early cases and heavy users, but cannot be funded to provide care if the person does not meet diagnostic severity or if their social impairment is still minimal. This is especially apropros of adolescents, who often do not meet diagnostic criteria, but are vulnerable to an addictive career. Can research address the special dimensions of prevention in the addiction field?

8. Research regarding *addiction services under welfare reform* is urgently needed. These reforms are cutting off payments to addicted persons. Most people at the community level believe that this may have serious social effects, but are not agreed on what is apt to occur. States and communities would like information about the consequences of welfare reform on addicted persons, along with how best to manage this.

9. More *quasi-experimental designs* would be appreciated, since these seem to provide more practical information than highly controlled (but also highly biased and nonapplicable controlled, random assignment studies). For example, the results from policies and strategies employed in the fifty different states should be informative. Could such data be collected, compared, and analyzed?

10. *Long term* studies and *longitudinal studies* (over at least one year, and sometimes several years or a few decades) are needed. Community agencies provide services for years and even decades in many, perhaps most cases.

11. *Cocaine* abusers are going to prison in large numbers, relative to alcohol, cannabis, opiate, etc. abusers. Overlapping this is the fact that *Afro-American patients* are using cocaine more and going to prison more often. Community people would like to find ways of keeping cocaine patients and Afro-American patients in treatment rather than in prison. Can research help address this issue? Understanding of the complexities involved might also help (e.g., organic brain damage from cocaine, reversible vs. irreversible effects, ethnic differences in the acceptance of cocaine, community approaches to getting cocaine out of the community).

12. Can research tell us how best to detect and treat patients with

comorbid psychiatric disorders in community settings? What is the best way to provide combined addiction and mental health services in the community, especially in a time of dwindling resources?

13. At a community level, much resources continue to be devoted to patients whose benefit or outcomes from treatment are poor or nil. How can we identify when to reduce services to *such patients*? How should treatment of chronic, relapsing patients be managed? Should they have special assessments to ascertain whether a treatable condition exists? How much would this cost. Who would do this and where should it be done? What ethical, legal, and socially acceptable alternatives can be brought to bear (e.g., case management, asylum, methods of managing their money, or other resources)?

14. The *research "turn around time"* needs to be faster. Much research now being published was conceived several years or a decade ago, when a much different system was in place. Research funding should support more exploratory, quasi-experimental, clinically relevant studies. Secondary analyses and meta-analyses of state agency data might reveal useful trends or information.

15. Federal *"on-site" visits/reviews* and *technical assistance* to states and communities should be expanded. Perhaps these could include researchers who have conducted community-applicable research. Those who have a national or cross-state perspective can tell community, state, and regional people what is being tried and what has been successful in similar settings. Community and state program leaders and planners have found these contacts helpful.

16. Providing care to addicted persons *in rural areas* is a growing problem. More drug use now occurs in rural areas; it is no longer "contained" in urban settings. All aspects of care are multiplied: access to care; support over time back in the community; special help for people with special needs (e.g., solo mothers, adolescents, elderly). We need new models of care such as more use of primary care, telemedicine, and mobile treatment teams.

Conducted by Joseph Westermeyer
July 1997

Index

A

Academic programs and research, 3, 12, 15, 20
  attitudes toward, 79
  collaborative research with CBOs, 12-13, 76, 79, 87, 96, 98-99, 102-103, 140, 141, 144
  information linkages with CBOs, 12-13, 20, 35, 68, 111-112, 119, 135, 137
  preventive interventions, 102-103
  primary care services, 35
  state funding, 8
  see also Medical education; Professional education
Acupuncture, 37-38, 150, 175, 195, 244
ADAMHA Reorganization Act of 1992, 95-96
Addiction Severity Index, 103, 155-156, 172
Administrators and managers, 211, 248
  associations of, opinions, 65, 95-97
  CBOs, 5, 10, 27-29, 35, 41-42, 47-51, 59-60, 64, 66, 68, 76, 77, 90, 93, 94, 99, 100, 112, 117, 123, 135, 187, 189, 190, 232, 247, 249
  state agency, 31, 35
  see also Case management; Management information systems
Adolescents, 34, 74, 87, 148, 194, 238, 239-240
Advocacy groups, 11-13, 31, 46-47, 51, 118-120 *passim*, 198, 227
  Internet sites, 227-228
African Americans, 139, 140, 143, 159, 160, 193, 194, 214, 249
Aftercare, *see* Followup treatment
Age factors, 152, 153, 193, 194, 209
  see also Adolescents; Children
Agency for Health Care Policy Research, 10, 14, 63-64, 226
Agricultural Extension Service, 69
AHCPR, *see* Agency for Health Care Policy Research
AIDS, *see* Human immunodeficiency virus
Alcohol abuse, 27-28, 49, 50, 61, 73, 95
  adolescents, 239
  Alcohol and Drug Services Survey, 192, 193, 194
  cocaine abuse and, 38-39
  Community Reinforcement Approach, 169
  driving while under the influence, 19, 239
  naltrexrone, 33, 167

NIH heroin addiction treatment guidelines, 209
outcome monitoring, 153-160 *passim*, 167, 168, 169
pregnant women, 36
Alcohol and Drug Research Study, 37
Alcohol and Drug Services Survey, 187-197
Alcoholics Anonymous, 24, 27-29, 85, 138, 140, 160, 162-164, 169, 175
Aliviane, 77
American Cancer Society, 46
American Heart Association, 46
American Lung Association, 46
American Medical Association, 62, 200
American Psychiatric Association, 61
American Society of Addiction Medicine, 61, 100, 161
Amphetamines, *see* Methamphetamines
Antabuse (disulfiram), 167, 169, 242
Antidepressants, 170
Anxiolytic buspirone, 170
Arapaho House Comprehensive Substance Abuse Treatment Center, 73-75, 78, 79, 82
Arizona, 20
ASI, *see* Addiction Severity Index
Asians/Pacific Islanders, 139, 194, 244
Assessment methodology, *see* Evaluation methodology; Quality control
Attitudes, *vi*
AA members, 27-29
abuser motivation, 33, 50, 80, 156-157, 162, 163, 175, 235, 241-242, 247
contingency management, 34
methadone maintenance, 32, 49-50
researchers, 77, 98
research subjects, 98, 99
self-esteem, 80
stigma, 9, 11, 16, 17, 25, 32, 46-48, 49-50, 116, 153, 205, 210, 213
treatment facilities placement, local residents, 38, 46, 47, 49-50
trust building, *xv*, 3, 5, 56, 57, 66-70, 74, 98, 112

B

Barbiturates, 194
Behavioral interventions, 2, 6, 7, 18, 19, 20, 24, 59, 67, 74, 86, 150, 164-165, 170-171

NIH heroin addiction treatment guidelines, 202, 208, 209
see also Contingency management; Counseling and counselors; Group therapy
Benzodiazepines, 194
Biopsychological factors, *vii*, 6, 16, 17, 80
methamphetamine abuse, 229
opiate addiction, 200-201, 203-204, 212
outcome analysis, 152
recovering addicts, 149
see also Drugs to treat abusers; Genetic factors; Medical interventions; Mental illness; Withdrawal
Black persons, *see* African Americans
Block grants, 7, 17, 27, 42-43, 65, 114, 197
methadone, 31
Buprenorphine, 49, 151, 166, 207, 209

C

California, 20, 22, 35, 36
Cancer treatment, 11, 46, 68-69, 96, 100-102, 107
cost-effectiveness, 5, 101, 112
see also Community Clinical Oncology Program
Case management, 34, 74, 97, 173, 238, 248, 250
CASPAR, 102
CBOs, *see* Community-based drug treatment organizations
CCOP, *see* Community Clinical Oncology Program
Center for Mental Health Services, 95
Center for Substance Abuse Prevention, 94-95
Center for Substance Abuse Treatment, *v*, *vii*, 9, 17-18, 116, 124, 231
collaborative research support, 10, 13-15, 18, 74, 94, 100, 117-118, 120
definitional issues, 23
technology transfer, 58, 59-60, 115, 120, 136
treatment protocols, list of approved, 233-234
Center on Alcohol, Substance Abuse, and Addiction, 20, 96, 98-99, 108
Certification, *see* Licensing and certification
Chestnut Health Systems and Interventions, 99, 107

Children, 32, 34, 35, 36, 65, 153-154
    Alcohol and Drug Services Survey, 194,
        195
    school-based preventive interventions,
        73-74, 97, 102-103, 240
    see also Adolescents
Chinese Americans, 139
Clinical protocols, 6, 49, 96, 100, 161
    CSAT, list of approved, 233-234
Clinical trials, 32, 37, 38, 62, 68, 79, 86,
        90, 100-101, 106, 148, 152, 174
CME, see Continuing medical education
Cocaine, 20, 22, 30, 33, 40(n.1), 49
    adolescents, 239
    alcohol abuse and, 38-39
    Alcohol and Drug Services Survey, 193,
        194
    NIH heroin addiction treatment
        guidelines, 206, 209
    outcome monitoring, 153, 155, 159,
        160-161, 163, 164, 167-168, 171
    prison treatments, 249
    treatment guidelines, 61
Colleges and universities, see Academic
        programs and research
Colorado, 73-74
Community-based drug treatment
        organizations, 2, 5, 6, 17, 18, 42-
        43
    academic researchers, collaboration, 12-
        13, 76, 79, 87, 96, 98-99, 102-
        103, 140, 141, 144
    academic researchers, information
        linkages, 12-13, 20, 35, 68, 111-
        112, 119, 135, 137
    administrators and managers, 5, 10, 27-
        29, 35, 41-42, 47-51, 59-60, 64,
        66, 68, 76, 77, 90, 93, 94, 99,
        100, 112, 117, 123, 135, 187,
        189, 190, 232, 247, 249
    Agricultural Extension Service as model,
        69
    Alcohol and Drug Services Survey, 187-
        197
    cancer treatment as model, 5-6, 11, 46,
        68-69, 96, 100-102, 107-108,
        112-113, 118
    counselors in recovery, 24, 27, 41, 44,
        45, 75
    cultural factors, 20, 24, 98, 131

definitional issues, 2-3, 23-25, 135-141
    employment issues, staff, 12-13, 15, 41,
        43-46, 59, 76-68, 113
    training, 12-13, 15, 41, 43-46, 59, 76-
        68, 113
    historical perspectives, 21-23, 138, 141-
        143
    models, 5-6, 58-70, 83, 85, 101-102,
        107-108, 112-113
    multimodal treatments, 35
    research contributions of, 73-88, 96,
        111-114
    research recommendations, 7, 12-13
    site visit vignettes, 27, 28, 29, 31, 74,
        89-90
    small providers, 27, 29, 41, 59, 60, 84,
        85, 141, 190, 191
    structural factors, 40-42, 51-52, 59-60
    training of staff, 12-13, 15, 41, 43-46,
        59, 76-68, 113
    understudied approaches, 35-40
    underutilized research, 32-34, 116-117,
        135-136, 147-176
    woman-centered, 36
Community Clinical Oncology Program
        (NCI), 5-6, 68-69, 96, 100-102,
        107-108, 112-113
    infrastructure, 5, 101-102, 106, 112-
        113
Community-level factors, other, 87, 101
    adolescent outreach, 240
    definitional issues, 136-137
    education and training, 43-44
    treatment facilities placement, attitudes,
        38, 46, 47, 49-50
Community Reinforcement Approach, 169-
        170, 240-242
Connecticut, 22, 141
Consensus conferences, 63-64, 117, 199
Consumer participation, 2, 4, 6, 10, 31-32,
        84, 113, 118-119, 120, 214
    cost factors, 5, 11-12, 119
    cultural factors, 24(n.4)
    foreign language speakers, 20, 99
    HIV treatment, 11, 105, 108
    professional licensing, 8, 44, 115
    standards, 8, 12, 119
    training, 13, 113
    see also Advocacy groups; Public
        education; Stakeholders

Consumer scorecards, 11, 61-63, 118
Contingency management, 30-31, 33-34,
      43, 169-170, 175
Continuing care, *see* Followup treatment
Continuing medical education, 8, 12, 15, 48
      guidelines, 62-64
Cost and cost-effectiveness factors, *vi*, 1, 18,
      31, 35, 49, 93, 95, 247, 248
   adolescents, treatment, 239-240
   cancer treatment as model, 5, 101, 112
   consumer participation, 5, 11-12, 119
   drug addiction, national losses, 144,
      147, 206, 212-213
   drugs to treat abusers, 28, 33
   employer treatment programs, 147
   innovation, 60(n.2)
   institutional care, 25
   literature review parameters, 148
   NIDA/NIAAA efforts, 9, 116
   NIH heroin addiction treatment
      guidelines, 206, 209, 212-213
   outreach, 239-240, 243
   research design, 81, 101
   research/practice links, 4, 76-77, 111-
      112
   treatment/patient matching, multiple
      problems, 173
   see also Funding
Counseling and counselors, 20, 37, 41, 44,
      86, 231
   abusers as counselors, 24, 27, 41, 44,
      45, 75, 138; *see also* Group
      therapy
   mentors, 45, 48, 111, 244
   NIH heroin addiction treatment
      guidelines, 203
   outcome monitoring, 164-165, 170-172,
      175
   theoretical basis, 80
   therapy *vs*, 164-165, 170-171, 175
   training, 84
   see also Marital status and therapy; Peer
      support
Crime and criminal justice system, *vi*, 2, 3,
      20, 43, 96, 143, 144
   adolescents, 239
   Alcohol and Drug Services Survey, 191,
      192
   Department of Justice, 213
   driving while under the influence, 19
   heroin addiction and, 200, 206, 209

   historical perspectives, 22
   naltrexone use by probationers, 167
   outcome monitoring, 152, 160, 165,
      171, 176, 209
   outreach, 239, 243
   see also Prisons and jails
CSAT, *see* Center for Substance Abuse
      Treatment
Cultural factors
   addiction, 80, 139, 214
   community-based treatment, 20, 24, 98,
      131
   organizational, *vii*, 5, 27-29, 60, 85-86,
      108, 112, 136
   religious factors, 24, 85-86, 138, 140,
      244
   research collaboration, *vii*, 24, 77, 96
   see also Social factors; *specific groups*

D

Databases, 5, 87, 95, 189-190
   TEDIS, 232
Data collection, 4, 21, 81, 82, 87, 93, 96,
      99, 100, 101
   adolescents, 239-240
   Alcohol and Drug Services Survey, 187-
      188
   homeless persons, 103-104
   see also Management information
      systems; Research methodology
Demographic factors, 142-143
   Alcohol and Drug Services Survey, 193,
      194
   clinical factors and, 16
   NIH heroin addiction treatment
      guidelines, 205-206
   outcome analysis, 152-152
   types of research, 81
   see also Age factors; Children;
      Employment factors; Gender
      factors; Homeless persons;
      Minority groups; Rural areas;
      Socioeconomic status; Urban
      areas
Department of Health and Human Services,
      see specific agencies
Department of Justice, 213
Department of Veterans Affairs, 3, 67, 138,
      160, 166

Detoxification methods and centers, 22, 31, 73-74, 148-176
  Alcohol and Drug Services Survey, 192, 193, 195
  see also Drugs to treat abusers
Diagnosis, *see* Identification of abusers
Diagnostic and Statistical Manual of Mental Disorders, 100, 148
Directors, *see* Administrators and managers
Diseases, other than alcohol/substance abuse, 41, 46, 59, 147, 152, 204
  outcome analysis, 63-64
  see also Mental illness; *specific diseases*
District of Columbia, 20-21
Disulfiram, *see* Antabuse
Doctors, *see* Physicians
Driving while under the influence, 19, 239
Drug Abuse Treatment Outcome Study, 34
Drug Outcome Monitoring System, 99-100
Drugs of abuse, specific, *see specific drugs*
Drugs to treat abusers, 41, 49, 67, 80, 117, 149, 150, 166-168, 175, 202, 208, 214
  underutilized, 32-33
  see also Antabuse; Buprenorphine; Methadone; Naltrexone
DSM-IV, *see Diagnostic and Statistical Manual of Mental Disorders*
Duration of treatment, 35, 147, 149, 150, 151, 154, 181, 161-162, 166, 207, 209, 248

see also* Medical education; Professional education; Public education; Technology transfer
Employee assistance programs, 18
Employment factors, 47, 49, 139, 142
  Alcohol and Drug Services Survey, 187, 192, 195
  drug rehabilitation organizations, 59, 95, 237, 238
    CBO staff, 12-13, 15, 41, 43-46, 59, 76-68, 113
  job training/finding, 34, 80, 95, 169, 172, 195
  labor unions, 140, 143
  outcome monitoring, 157-158, 160, 165, 169, 171, 172, 173
  self-insured employers, 11-12, 119
  unemployment, 20, 47, 143, 152, 158, 165, 207
Etiology, 1, 16, 31, 150
  NIH heroin addiction treatment guidelines, 202-204
Evaluation methodology, 9, 39, 77, 117
  guidelines, 61-62, 236
  scorecards, 11, 61-63, 118
  state policy on service delivery, 9
  see also Cost and cost-effectiveness factors; Grant review processes; Outcome monitoring
Evidence-based treatments, 10-11, 14, 17, 56, 59-60, 63-64, 118

E

EAP, *see* Employee assistance programs
Economic factors, 16, 19-20, 51-52, 112
  health services research, 94
  knowledge development, 9
  see Cost and cost-effectiveness factors; Socioeconomic status
Educational attainment, 152, 153
Education and training, 2, 12-13, 15, 43-45, 47, 56, 97, 99, 111, 119-120
  addicts, 175, 195
  costs, 35
  counselors, 44, 113
  families, 13
  Internet sites, 228
  organizational learning, 6, 76, 79, 111-112, 113
  school-based preventive interventions, 73-74, 97, 102-103, 240

F

Faith, *see* Religious factors
Families, 8, 11, 84, 119, 152
  adolescents, 240
  Alcohol and Drug Services Survey, 192, 195
  NIH heroin addiction treatment guidelines, 203
  outcome monitoring, 158-159, 160, 167, 168, 173, 175, 176
  training, 13
  see also Parents
Federal government, *vii*, 2, 22, 29-30, 114, 117
  Internet sites, 226-227, 232
  see also Legislation; Regulatory issues; *specific departments and agencies*

Fluoxetine, 170
Followup treatment, 34, 87, 101, 150, 163,
    195, 235, 236
    see also Relapse and relapse prevention
Food and Drug Administration, 33, 152,
    166, 167, 211, 212
Foreign language speakers, 20, 99
For-profit organizations, 137, 138, 140,
    188, 189, 191, 196, 237
    see also Health insurance; Health
        maintenance organizations
Foundations, 18-19, 46, 141
Funding, vi, 7-8, 12, 14, 17, 21, 42, 49, 77,
    97, 98-99, 113-115, 120, 141,
    196
    advocacy, 46
    CBO site visit vignettes, 27-29, 31, 73-
        74, 89-90
    clinical involvement, 247
    historical perspectives, 22, 23, 25, 27
    homeless persons, treatment, 104
    ineffective treatments, 10
    managed care reimbursement, 27
    prevention programs, 102
    small research projects, 7, 76, 84, 114
    top-down, 64-66
    see also Block grants; Grant review
        processes; Incentives, financial

G

Gay Men's Health Crisis, 46-47
Gender factors, 7, 114, 152, 153, 194
    see also Men; Women
Genetic factors, 150, 202, 203, 205, 212
Global Appraisal of Individual Needs, 99-
    100
Government, see Federal government; Local
    government; State government
Grant review processes, 7, 28, 106-107
Group therapy, 22, 164, 175, 195
    see also Peer support

H

Halfway houses, 22, 27-28
Harrison Act, 199
Health insurance, 42, 196, 214
    consumer participation, 11-12
    Mathematica study, vi

Mental Health Parity Act, vi
    self-insured employers, 11-12, 119
    see also Medicaid; Medicare
Health maintenance organizations, 19, 101,
    135-136, 140, 141, 143
Health Plan Employer Data and
    Information Set, 63
Hepatitis, 25, 204, 206, 209
Heredity, see Genetic factors
Here's Looking at You, 102
Heroin, 22, 30, 138, 139, 167
    adolescents, 239
    Alcohol and Drug Services Survey, 193,
        194
    crime and, 200, 206, 209
    NIH treatment guidelines, 198-225
    outcome monitoring, 153, 158
    see also Methadone
Hispanic persons, 20, 77, 194, 214
Historical perspectives, 1, 21-23, 25, 27,
    73, 94, 136, 138, 141-143, 199-
    200
    collaborative research, 90-95
    community-based defined, 137, 138, 140
    demonstration initiatives, 102
    funding, 22, 23, 25, 27
    hospitals, 21-22, 25
    methamphetamine abuse, 230
    technology transfer, 48-49, 57, 58
HIV, see Human immunodeficiency virus
HMOs, see Health maintenance
    organizations
Homeless persons, 74, 102, 103-105, 108,
    237
Hospitals, 97, 100, 135, 137-141 passim,
    143, 237
    Alcohol and Drug Services Survey, 188,
        193
    historical perspectives, 21-22, 25
    outcome monitoring, 150, 159-161, 169
Human immunodeficiency virus, 7, 25, 34-
    35, 42, 49, 65, 114, 118, 142
    advocacy groups, 46
    Alcohol and Drug Services Survey, 195
    consumer participation in treatment, 11,
        105, 108
    demonstration projects, 105, 108
    NIH heroin addiction treatment
        guidelines, 200, 201, 204, 209
    outreach, 105, 114

I

Idaho, 30
Identification of abusers, 36, 235
  DSM-IV, 10, 148
  NIH heroin addiction treatment
      guidelines, 204
  saliva testing, 204
  urine testing, 33, 49, 151, 160, 164,
      166, 187, 204
  see also Outreach; Referral
Ideology, see Political and ideological
      factors
Illinois, 22, 96, 99-100, 141
Incentives, behavioral, see Behavioral
      interventions
Incentives, financial, 56, 115, 120, 127
  CBOs, 8, 14, 112, 115
  top-down models, 64-66
Information dissemination, 4, 6, 9-11, 18,
      19, 21, 45, 49, 58, 76, 84, 95,
      116-117, 124, 131, 247
  academic/CBO collaboration, 12-13, 20,
      35, 68, 111-112, 119, 135, 137
  bidirectional, general, 2, 3, 18, 23, 36,
      58-59, 66-67, 121, 123, 135-137,
      144, 186-197
  CBO administrators, 42, 84
  definitional issues, 58
  guidelines, 62-64
  lag time, 19, 29, 31, 250
  NIDA role, 12-15, 28, 48-49, 58, 116-
      118, 119-120, 136
  policymakers, 7-8, 9-11, 19, 31-32, 113
  see also Education and training;
      Management information
      systems; Technology transfer
Informed consent, 78, 99
Infrastructure, 19, 56, 69, 106
  CCOP strategy, 5, 101-102, 106, 112-
      113
  DHHS support, 65
  NIDA support, 6, 14
  state support, 97
Inhalants, 239
Innovation, 60, 61, 62
Inpatient treatment
  Alcohol and Drug Services Study, 188-
      193 passim
  block grants and, 42-43
  heroin addiction, NIH treatment
      statement, 208

  outcome monitoring, 149, 150-155
      passim, 158, 159-163, 170, 172
  see also Residential treatment
Institute of Medicine, v, viii-ix, 1, 4, 17-18,
      23, 48, 95, 106
  study objectives, 123-124
  technology transfer, 57-58, 62-63
Institutional review boards, 78
Insurance, see Health insurance
Internet resources, 226-232
Iowa Consortium for Substance Abuse
      Research and Evaluation, 95-98,
      107

J

Jails, see Prisons and jails
Joint Commission on Accreditation of
      Healthcare Organizations, 20,
      100

K

Kentucky, 22
Knowledge development, see headings
      beginning "Research"
Knowledge dissemination/transfer, see
      Information dissemination;
      Technology transfer

L

LAAM, 49, 149, 151, 166, 201, 209, 212
Language, see Foreign language speakers
Law, see Crime and criminal justice system;
      Informed consent; Regulatory
      issues
Legislation
  federal
      ADAMHA Reorganization Act of
          1992, 95-96
      Harrison Act, 199
      Mental Health Parity Act, vi
      Narcotic Addict Rehabilitation Act,
          22
      women's services, 36
  state
      driving while under the influence, 19,
          239

Length of treatment, *see* Duration of
treatment
Levo-alpha-acetylmethadol/levomethadyl
acetate, *see* LAAM
Licensing and certification, professional, 8,
44, 115, 165, 175
Local factors, *see* Community-based drug
treatment organizations;
Community-level factors, other
Local government, 17, 42, 43, 114

M

Managed care organizations, general, 2, 3,
7, 11, 12, 17, 18, 24, 27, 29, 63,
64, 65-66, 90, 95, 101, 186, 235-
236, 248
see also Community-based drug
treatment organizations; Health
maintenance organizations
Management information systems, 8, 100,
101, 111, 113, 115, 127
Alcohol and Drug Services Survey, 188-
189
TEDIS, 232
training in, 77
see also Databases
Managers, *see* Administrators and managers
Marijuana, 22, 193, 194, 206, 239
Marital status and therapy, 153, 168, 169
Massachusetts, 22
Mass media, 10, 240, 248
Mathematica study, *vi*
Medicaid, 42, 94, 96, 176, 197
Medical education, 12-13, 47-48, 62-63,
210-211, 213
continuing medical education, 8, 12, 15,
48, 62-64
Medical interventions, 24, 31, 56, 94-94,
112, 173
acupuncture, 37-38, 150, 175, 195, 244
Alcohol and Drug Services Survey, 188
Medicaid, 42, 94, 96, 176, 197
Medicare, 94, 197
NIH heroin addiction treatment
guidelines, 204, 206
primary care, 35, 36, 101
women, 34, 154
see also Biopsychological factors;
Detoxification methods and
centers; Hospitals; Saliva testing;
Urine testing

Medicare, 94, 197
Men, 85, 192
Mental Health Parity Act, *vi*
Mental Health Services Administration, *see*
Center for Substance Abuse
Treatment
Mental illness, other than alcohol/drug
abuse, 16-17, 25, 38-39, 68, 84,
203, 238, 249-250
adolescents, 239
outcome monitoring, 154-155, 157, 160,
170, 171, 172, 173, 175, 176
suicide, 168, 239
see also Biopsychological factors;
Psychiatric treatment
Mentors, 45, 48, 111, 244
Methadone, 22, 30-31, 32-33, 34, 35, 47,
49-50, 58, 62, 80, 149
Alcohol and Drug Services Survey, 188,
192
LAAM, 49, 149, 151, 166
NIH treatment guidelines, 201-214
passim
nonmethadone treatments *vs*, 37, 208,
209
outcome monitoring, 151, 154, 155,
158, 164-166, 170-172
withdrawal from, 166, 204, 208
Methamphetamines, 194, 229-230
Methodology, *see* Research methodology
Minority groups, 7, 47, 91, 101, 114, 139,
142, 152, 153, 194, 214, 237,
238
adolescents, 239
see also specific groups
Mississippi, 30, 141
"Money with strings," *see* Incentives,
financial
Motivation, *see* Attitudes; Behavioral
interventions; Contingency
management
Multi-problem addicts, 16-17, 25, 34, 38-
39, 46, 168-174, 212, 239, 250
Multiple substance abusers, 27, 38, 158,
174, 209
Multiple treatment modalities, 17, 30, 31,
34-35, 103, 168-174, 175
Myths of addiction, *see* Stigma

N

Naltrexone, 28, 33, 80, 166-168, 201, 207-208
  alcohol abuse treatment, 33, 167
Narcotic Addict Rehabilitation Act, 22
Narcotics Anonymous, 140, 162-164, 175
National Acupuncture Detoxification Association, 37
National Advisory Council on Alcohol Abuse and Alcoholism, 95
National AIDS Demonstration Research, 105
National Alliance for the Mentally Ill, 47
National Alliance of Methadone Advocates, 47
National Association of Alcohol and Drug Abuse Counselors, 20
National Association of State Alcohol and Drug Abuse Directors, 65
National Cancer Institute
  see also Community Clinical Oncology Program
National Committee on Quality Assurance
  see also Health Plan Employer Data and Information Set
National Institute of Mental Health, 94
National Institute on Alcohol Abuse and Alcoholism, 7, 9, 10, 13-15, 74, 94, 95, 100, 102, 104, 108, 116, 117
  Project MATCH, 155, 159, 162, 170, 173
National Institute on Drug Abuse, v, vii, 7, 74, 94, 114, 124
  AIDS, 105, 142
  acupuncture, 37-38
  definitional issues, 23
  grant review, 106
  information development/dissemination, 9, 10, 12-15, 28, 48-49, 58, 116-118, 119-120, 136
  methamphetamine abuse, 229-230
  NIH heroin addiction treatment guidelines, 213
  prevention demonstrations, 102-103, 108
  service delivery approaches, 34, 116
  technology transfer, 12-13, 48-49, 58, 119-120, 136
  understudied approaches, 37
  Web site, 58

National Institutes of Health, v, 15, 101, 106, 107
  heroin treatment guidelines, 198-225
  methadone maintenance, 32-33
Native Americans, 3, 20, 73-74, 98-99, 194
Navajo Nation, 20, 96, 98-99, 108
New Hampshire, 30
New Jersey, 22
New Mexico, 20, 131
New York, 22
NIDA, see National Institute on Drug Abuse
Non-residential treatment, see Outpatient treatment
Non-traditional interventions, 87, 244
  acupuncture, 37-38, 150, 175, 195, 244
  relaxation therapy, 175
North Dakota, 30
Not-for-profit organizations, 74, 137, 237
  abusers, recovering, 22
  Alcohol and Drugs Services Study, 188, 189, 191, 196, 197
  foundations, 18-19, 46, 141
  HMOs, 140
  market forces and, 59
  Treatment Episode Data Set, 232

O

Office for Treatment Improvement, 94
Office of National Drug Control Policy, 22, 94, 213
  methadone maintenance, 32
Ohio, 31
Opiates, 22, 32-33, 49-50, 194
  biopsychological factors, 200-201, 203-204, 212
  dependence defined, 204
  outcome monitoring, 153, 154, 155, 158
  relapse and relapse prevention, 200, 202, 205, 208, 212
  treatment guidelines, 61, 198-225
  withdrawal from, 151, 166, 207-208, 244
  see Buprenorphine; Heroin; LAAM; Methadone; Naltrexone
Organizational factors, general, 4-5, 9, 40-42, 56, 94, 116, 237
  ADAMHA reorganization, 94-95
  Alcohol and Drug Services Survey, 188-190

change models, 59-60, 66-69, 82-86, 87
cultural, *vii*, 5, 27-29, 60, 85-86, 108,
   112, 136
funding, 196-197
institutional review boards, 78
learning, 6, 76, 79, 111-112, 113
see also Administrators and managers;
      For-profit organizations;
      Infrastructure; Not-for-profit
      organizations
Orlaam™, *see* LAAM
Outcome monitoring, 10-12, 14, 17, 25, 39,
      41, 49, 61-64, 93, 95, 96, 99-
      100, 118
   alcohol abusers, 153-160 *passim*, 167,
      168, 169
   cocaine users, 153, 155, 159, 160-161,
      163, 164, 167-168, 171
   consumer participation, 11
   crime and criminal justice system, 152,
      160, 165, 171, 176, 209
   definitional issues, 149, 174-175, 176
   employment variables, 157-158, 160,
      165, 169, 171, 172, 173
   family factors, 158-159, 160, 167, 168,
      173, 175, 176
   goals, controversy, 38
   heroin abusers, 153, 158
   homeless persons, 103-104
   hospitals, 150, 159-161, 169
   inpatient treatments, 149, 150-155
      passim, 158, 159-163, 170, 172
   relapse, 154, 157, 158, 159, 163, 164,
      170, 171, 172, 195
   residential treatment, 150, 155, 159-
      160, 172
   self-reporting, 152, 160
   social factors, 158-159, 160, 172
   socioeconomic status, 142-143, 152,
      203, 239, 243
   top-down incentives, 65
   variables, 35, 152-176
   see also Evidence-based treatments
Outpatient treatment, 22, 37, 49, 137, 138,
      149, 243
   Alcohol and Drug Services Survey, 188,
      192, 193
   outcome monitoring, 150, 159-161, 171,
      172
   see also Counseling and counselors

Outreach, 7, 42, 87, 242-243
   adolescents, 87, 239-240
   Community Reinforcement Approach,
      169-170, 240-242
   cost factors, 239-240, 243
   crime and criminal justice system, 239,
      243
   HIV-infected persons, 105, 114

                              P

Parents, 8, 65, 153, 203
   see also Children; Families
Patient Outcome Research Teams, 63-64
Peer support, 22, 24, 27, 41, 44, 45, 75,
      138, 164, 243, 244
   Alcoholics Anonymous, 24, 27-29, 85,
      138, 140, 160, 162-164, 169, 175
   Narcotics Anonymous, 140, 162-164,
      175
   Synanon, 22
   see also Group therapy
Performance Partnership Grants, 65
Pharmacotherapy, *see* Drugs to treat
      abusers
Physicians, 48, 62, 101, 210
   see also Medical education
Physicians in Residence program, 48
Policy and policymakers, general, *vi*, 1-8
      passim, 14, 18, 29, 40, 49-51, 56,
      90-91, 96, 97, 113, 114-115,
      127, 247-248
   historical perspectives, 21-23
   knowledge development/dissemination,
      7-8, 9-11, 19, 31-32, 113
   report at hand, panelists, 126
   war on drugs, 22
   see also Funding; Legislation
Political and ideological factors, *vi*, 16, 19-
      20, 51-52, 94
   see also Cultural factors; Religious
      factors
Practice-based research networks, 6, 12, 57,
      69, 79, 119
   see also Community Clinical Oncology
      Program
Practice guidelines, 61-64, 75, 248
   heroin addiction treatment, NIH
      guidelines, 198-225
   see Clinical protocols

Pregnancy, 36, 49, 65, 153, 195, 207, 239
Preventive interventions, 87, 91, 95, 96, 97, 102-104, 108, 249
 academic research, 102-103
 school-based, 73-74, 97, 102-103, 240
 see also Followup treatment;
   Identification of abusers;
   Outreach
Prisons and jails, 43, 137
 cocaine abusers, 249
 cost-effectiveness, 49
 historical perspectives, 22, 25
 opiate offense incarceration, 200
Professional education, 2, 4, 6, 12-13, 15, 69-70, 76, 97, 107, 119-120
 counselors, 84
 guidelines, 62-63, 210-211
 Internet sites, 228
 licensing/certification, 8, 44, 115, 165, 175
 practice-based research networks, 6, 12, 57, 69, 79, 119
 see also Academic programs and research; Medical education
Program of Assertive Community Treatment, 67-68
Project MATCH, 155, 159, 162, 170, 173
Psychiatric treatment, 16, 25, 61, 150, 152, 154, 170, 172, 203
Psychological factors, *see* Biopsychological factors
Public education, 4, 6, 14, 113, 118
 school-based preventive interventions, 73-74, 97, 102-103, 240
 see also Mass media
Puerto Ricans, 139

Q

Quality control, 39, 76, 93, 99
 see also Evaluation methodology;
   Standards

R

Racial factors, *see* Minority groups; White persons
Referral, 100, 170-174
 Alcohol and Drug Services Survey, 191
 clinical protocols, 6, 96, 100, 161
 self-referral, 191, 192

Regulatory issues, 6, 19, 21, 24, 90-91, 113, 138, 141, 211-212
 state barriers, 40
 see also Legislation; Standards
Relapse and relapse prevention, 16, 30, 33, 34, 58, 100, 236
 opiates, NIH statement, 200, 202, 205, 208, 212
 outcome monitoring, 154, 157, 158, 159, 163, 164, 170, 171, 172, 195
Relaxation therapy, 175
Religious factors, 24, 85-86, 138, 140, 244
Research, general, *vii*, 2, 4-11, 14, 56, 111-114, 116
 academic/CBO collaboration, 12-13, 76, 79, 87, 96, 98-99, 102-103, 140, 141, 144
 agenda building, 21
 clinical settings, researchers in, 6, 12, 57, 69, 79, 89-110, 119
 cost of practice linkages, 4, 76-77, 111-112
 cultural factors, *vii*, 24, 77, 96
 direct CBO contributions to, 73-88
 Internet sites, 228
 misuse of, 6, 90, 113
 models, 111-114, 127, 247
  CBOs as researchers, 5-6, 58-70, 83, 85, 123-124, 131
  researchers as such, 5-6, 95-105, 123-124
 NIH heroin addiction treatment guidelines, 212-214
 practice-based research networks, 6, 12, 57, 69, 79, 119
 small projects, 7, 76, 84, 114, 148
 social factors, *vii*, 92-93, 94, 158-159
 training strategies, 12-13, 15
 understudied approaches, 35-40
 underutilized, 32-34, 116-117, 135-136, 147-176
 see also Academic programs and research; Data collection; Information dissemination; Outcome monitoring; Technology transfer; Theory
Research methodology, 80-82, 90, 91-92, 94, 95
 Alcohol and Drug Services Study, 187-188
 applied social science, 91-92

clinical trials, 32, 37, 38, 62, 68, 79, 86,
    90, 100-101, 106, 148, 152, 174
cost factors, 81, 101
detoxification, literature review, 148-
    176
evidence-based treatments, 10-11, 14,
    17, 56, 59-60, 63-64, 118
homeless persons, 103-104
longitudinal studies, 249
NIH heroin addiction treatment
    guidelines, 199
quasi-experimental, 86, 249
report at hand, v-vii, 20-21, 123-134
    participants, 128-130, 132-134
see also Evaluation methodology
Research recommendations, 1, 18, 123-124,
    247-250
    CSAT role, 10, 13-15, 18, 74, 94, 100,
        117-118, 120
    implementation of research, vii, 4-7,
        111-114, 148
    NIDA role, 9, 10, 12-15, 28, 48-49, 58,
        116-118, 119-120, 136
    small research projects, 7, 76, 84, 114,
        148
    technology transfer, 12-13, 48-49, 58,
        119-120, 136
    treatment facilities placement, 38
Residential treatment, 27-28, 80, 86, 137,
    138, 141
    Alcohol and Drug Services Survey, 188,
        189, 192, 193
    outcome monitoring, 150, 155, 159-160,
        172
    see also Detoxification methods and
        centers; Halfway houses;
        Hospitals
Revia™, see Naltrexone
Runaways, 239
Rural areas, 7, 20, 99, 250

                                S

Saliva testing, 204
SAMHSA, see Substance Abuse and Mental
    Health Services Administration
Scorecards, 11, 61-63, 118
Screening, see Identification of abusers
Self-help, see Peer support
Self-reporting, 152, 160

Severity of addiction, 154, 168, 170, 173-
    174, 206, 236, 249
    Addiction Severity Index, 103, 155-156,
        172
    duration of abuse, 153
Smoking, 148, 195
Social factors, general, 20, 80, 87, 97, 139,
    142-143
    community defined, 136-137
    outcome monitoring, 158-159, 160, 172
    research, vii, 92-93, 94, 158-159
    see also Community-level factors;
        Cultural factors; Socioeconomic
        status
Social support and services, 20, 31, 34, 86,
    97, 116-117, 137, 140, 141
    Alcohol and Drug Services Survey, 187-
        197
    Medicaid, 42, 94, 96, 176, 197
    Medicare, 94, 197
    welfare, 2, 7, 191, 192, 249
    see also Children; Families; Group
        therapy; Parents; Stakeholders
Socioeconomic status, 142-143, 152, 203,
    239, 243
    see also Homeless persons
South Dakota, 30
Special Action Office for Drug Abuse
    Prevention, 22
Stakeholders, general, 3, 9, 19, 20, 57, 70,
    93, 100, 116, 151
Standards, 10, 75, 100
    clinical, 6, 12, 96, 100, 161, 233-234
    consumer participation, 8, 12, 119
    data collection, 104
    funding and, 141
    level of care, 100
    practice guidelines, 61-64, 75, 198-225,
        248
    professional, 44, 62-63, 115
        licensing/certification, 8, 44, 115,
            165, 175
State government, vii, 2, 8, 14, 114, 115,
    118
    AIDS, 105
    administrators, 31, 35
    consumer participation, 12
    professional licensing/certification, 8, 44,
        115, 165, 175
    service delivery monitoring, 9, 116
    see also Block grants

State-level actions, 22-23, 95-86
  service delivery approaches, 35
  see also District of Columbia; State
    government; *specific states*
Statistics, 93
  access to treatment, 16
  addiction and dependency, national
    figures, 1, 16, 200, 205-206
  Alcohol and Drug Services Survey, 187-
    188
  cancer treatment, 68
  counselor training, 44
  naltrexone treatment, 33
  outpatient treatment, 37
  see also Databases; Data collection;
    Management information systems
STEP ONE, 89-90
Stigma, 9, 11, 16, 17, 25, 32, 46-48, 49-50,
    116, 153, 205, 210, 213
Structural factors, *see* Infrastructure;
    Organizational factors
Substance Abuse Prevention and Treatment
    Block Grant, 7, 114
Substance Abuse and Mental Health
    Services Administration, *v, vi*, 17-
    18, 68, 94-95, 106, 138, 187,
    232
Suicide, 168, 239
Synanon, 22

T

Technical assistance, 31, 42, 49, 58, 77,
    104, 250
Technology transfer, 4, 9, 18, 21, 48-49,
    116, 117, 123-124
  bidirectional, general, 2, 3, 18, 23, 36,
    58-59, 66-68, 121, 123, 135-137,
    144, 186-197
  CSAT role, 58, 59-60, 115, 120, 136
  definitional issues, 57-58
  lag time, 19, 29, 31, 250
  models, 57-59, 60-62, 77
  NIDA role, 12-13, 48-49, 58, 119-120,
    136
  trust-building and, *xv*, 3, 5, 56, 57, 66-
    70, 74, 98, 112
  see also Medical education
Telephone contacts, 248
Television, 10
Texas, 20, 22, 77

Theory, 79, 81, 87, 90, 91-93
  counseling, 80
  etiology of drug addiction, 1, 16, 31,
    150, 202-204
Therapeutic community, *see* Synanon
Time factors
  community defined, 137
  duration of abuse, 153; *see also* Severity
    of addiction
  duration of treatment, 35, 147, 149,
    150, 151, 154, 161-162, 166,
    181, 207, 209, 248
  research/implementation lag, 19, 29, 31,
    250
  state implementation of federal
    requirements, 19
Tobacco, 148
Training, *see* Education and training
Transportation services, 49, 195, 247
Treatment Assistance Publication Series, 58-
    59
Treatment Episode Data Set, 232
Treatment Improvement Exchange, 59
Trust building, *xv*, 3, 5, 56, 57, 66-70, 74,
    98, 112
Tuberculosis, 25, 65, 195

U

University-based programs, *see* Academic
    programs and research
University of Rhode Island Change
    Assessment, 157
Urban areas, 7, 160
Urine testing, 33, 49, 151, 160, 164, 166,
    187, 204

V

Vermont, 30
Videotapes, 58

W

Washington, D.C., *see* District of Columbia
Washington State, 20
Welfare programs, 2, 7, 249
  Alcohol and Drug Services Survey, 191,
    192
  Medicaid, 42, 94, 96, 176, 197

West Virginia, 30
WESVAR, 188
White persons, 192, 193, 194
Withdrawal, 149, 155, 202, 203, 204
    alcohol, 49
    methadone, withdrawal from, 166, 204,
        208
    opiates, 151, 166, 207-208, 244

see also Detoxification methods and
        centers; Drugs to treat abusers
Women, 34, 36, 140, 153-154, 194, 237,
        238
    see also Pregnancy
Wraparound services, 20, 34